6/14

MINDFULNESS AND PSYCHOTHERAPY

Mindfulness and Psychotherapy

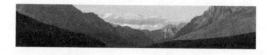

SECOND EDITION

Edited by
CHRISTOPHER K. GERMER
RONALD D. SIEGEL
PAUL R. FULTON

THE GUILFORD PRESS
New York   London

© 2013 The Guilford Press
A Division of Guilford Publications, Inc.
72 Spring Street, New York, NY 10012
www.guilford.com

Printed in the United States of America

This book is printed on acid-free paper.

Last digit is print number: 9 8 7 6 5 4 3 2 1

The authors have checked with sources believed to be reliable in their
efforts to provide information that is complete and generally in accord
with the standards of practice that are accepted at the time of publication.
However, in view of the possibility of human error or changes in
behavioral, mental health, or medical sciences, neither the authors, nor
the editors and publisher, nor any other party who has been involved in
the preparation or publication of this work warrants that the information
contained herein is in every respect accurate or complete, and they are not
responsible for any errors or omissions or the results obtained from the use
of such information. Readers are encouraged to confirm the information
contained in this book with other sources.

Library of Congress Cataloging-in-Publication Data

Mindfulness and psychotherapy, second edition / [edited by] Christopher K. Germer,
Ronald D. Siegel, Paul R. Fulton. — Second edition.
     pages cm
  Includes bibliographical references and index.
  ISBN 978-1-4625-1137-2 (hardback : acid-free paper)
  1. Meditation—Therapeutic use. 2. Meditation—Buddhism. 3. Psychotherapy.
I. Germer, Christopher K., editor of compilation. II. Siegel, Ronald D., editor of
compilation. III. Fulton, Paul R., editor of compilation.
  RC489.M43M56 2013
  616.89′14—dc23

                                                                2013004104

45.00

Clinical case illustrations either have been disguised or are composites
of different individuals.

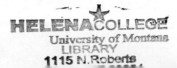

About the Editors

Christopher K. Germer, PhD, a clinical psychologist in private practice specializing in mindfulness- and compassion-oriented psychotherapy, is Clinical Instructor in Psychology at the Harvard Medical School/Cambridge Health Alliance, and a founding faculty member of the Institute for Meditation and Psychotherapy (IMP). He has been integrating the principles and practices of meditation into psychotherapy since 1978. Dr. Germer is a co-developer of the Mindful Self-Compassion training program, author of *The Mindful Path to Self-Compassion*, and coeditor of *Wisdom and Compassion in Psychotherapy*. He conducts workshops and lectures internationally on mindfulness and self-compassion.

Ronald D. Siegel, PsyD, is Assistant Clinical Professor of Psychology at Harvard Medical School/Cambridge Health Alliance, where he has taught for over 30 years. He is a long-time student of mindfulness meditation and serves on the board of directors and faculty of IMP. Dr. Siegel teaches internationally about mindfulness and psychotherapy and mind–body treatment, while maintaining a private clinical practice in Lincoln, Massachusetts. His books include *The Mindfulness Solution*, *Wisdom and Compassion in Psychotherapy*, *Back Sense*, and *Sitting Together: Essential Skills for Mindfulness-Based Psychotherapy*.

Paul R. Fulton, EdD, has a private practice in psychotherapy in Newton, Massachusetts, and is Clinical Instructor in Psychology at the Harvard Medical School/Cambridge Health Alliance. He was formerly the president of IMP and is currently director of the Certificate Program in Mindfulness and Psychotherapy. Dr. Fulton received lay ordination as a Zen Buddhist in 1972, has been a student of psychology and meditation for over 44 years, and is on the board of directors of the Barre Center for Buddhist Studies. He teaches mindfulness to clinicians internationally and has authored a number of book chapters and articles.

Contributors

Judson A. Brewer, MD, PhD, is an addiction psychiatrist at the Yale University School of Medicine and West Haven Veterans Hospital. He has been practicing insight meditation since 1996, studying with Ginny Morgan and Joseph Goldstein, among other teachers. Dr. Brewer has been studying and delivering mindfulness training to clinical populations since 2006, with an emphasis on individuals with addictions. His research focuses on testing the efficacy of mindfulness training for clinical populations with addictions and determining the underlying neurobiological mechanisms of mindfulness, using modalities such as neuroimaging. Dr. Brewer is currently Assistant Professor at Yale and Medical Director of the Yale Therapeutic Neuroscience Clinic.

John Briere, PhD, is Associate Professor of Psychiatry and Psychology, Director of the Psychological Trauma Program, and Center Director of the Adolescent Trauma Training Center (National Child Traumatic Stress Network) at the University of Southern California. A past president of the International Society for Traumatic Stress Studies (ISTSS), he is a recipient of the Award for Outstanding Contributions to the Science of Trauma Psychology from the American Psychological Association and the Robert S. Laufer Memorial Award for Scientific Achievement from ISTSS. Dr. Briere is author or coauthor of over 100 articles and chapters, 10 books, and 8 trauma-related psychological tests. He teaches on the topics of trauma, therapy, and mindfulness practices internationally.

Paul R. Fulton, EdD (see "About the Editors").

Christopher K. Germer, PhD (see "About the Editors").

Trudy A. Goodman, PhD, is executive director, founder, and guiding teacher of InsightLA, a nonprofit organization for mindfulness education and meditation training since 2002. She is one of the first mindfulness-based stress reduction trainers, with its creator, Dr. Jon Kabat-Zinn. Dr. Goodman is also guiding teacher and cofounder of the Institute for Meditation and Psychotherapy (IMP) in Cambridge, Massachusetts. She created family mindfulness programs with Susan Kaiser Greenland and has worked with children all her life. Dr. Goodman teaches at retreats and workshops nationwide. She is a contributing author to *Clinical Handbook of Mindfulness* and *Wisdom and Compassion in Psychotherapy.*

Gregory Kramer, PhD, is a meditation teacher, author, and cofounder and guiding teacher of the Metta Foundation. Since 1974, he has studied with esteemed monastics, including Anagarika Dhammadina, Ven. Balangoda Ananda Maitreya Mahanayaka Thera, Achan Sobin Namto, and Ven. Punnaji Mahathera. Dr. Kramer is author of *Insight Dialogue: The Interpersonal Path to Freedom*; *Meditating Together, Speaking from Silence: The Practice of Insight Dialogue*; *Seeding the Heart: Practicing Lovingkindness with Children*; and *Dharma Contemplation: Meditating Together with Wisdom Texts.* He pioneered online meditation and contemplation practices and cofounded Harvest with Heart, a hunger project in the Northeast United States, and Spiritual City Forum, an interfaith dialogue program in Portland, Oregon.

Sara W. Lazar, PhD, is a scientist in the Psychiatry Department at Massachusetts General Hospital and Instructor in Psychology at Harvard Medical School. The focus of her research is the neurobiology of meditation. Dr. Lazar uses magnetic resonance imaging to investigate the neural correlates of beneficial changes associated with meditation practice, both in healthy individuals and clinical populations. She has been practicing yoga and mindfulness meditation since 1994 and serves as Science Advisor to IMP.

Stephanie P. Morgan, PsyD, MSW, is a clinical psychologist and social worker. She has been a student of meditation in the vipassana and Zen traditions for the past 35 years. Dr. Morgan was Instructor in Psychology at Harvard Medical School from 1990 to 1994, where she trained psychology interns in mindfulness and self-care skills. She is currently on the faculty of IMP and in private practice in Manchester, Massachusetts.

Susan T. Morgan, MSN, RN, CS, is a clinical nurse specialist in private practice in Cambridge, Massachusetts. She was Coordinator of the Yale Adult Pervasive Developmental Disorders Research Clinic for 5 years. Following this position, she was a clinician at the Harvard University Health Services and introduced mindfulness meditation to college students in the context of psychotherapy. Ms. Morgan has been practicing Buddhist meditation for 20 years and is currently completing a 4-year silent meditation retreat. Since 2000, she has co-led retreats for psychotherapists with an emphasis on loving-kindness and body awareness.

William D. Morgan, PsyD, is a clinical psychologist in private practice in Cambridge and Quincy, Massachusetts. He is a board member of IMP and has participated in many years of intensive retreats in the Theravadin, Zen, and Tibetan schools of Buddhism during his 40 years of meditation practice. Dr. Morgan has led mindfulness retreats for mental health professionals for the past 15 years.

Andrew Olendzki, PhD, is Senior Scholar at the Barre Center for Buddhist Studies, an institution dedicated to the integration of academic understanding and meditative insight. He has taught at several New England colleges (including

Harvard, Brandeis, Smith, Amherst, and Lesley) and was the executive director of the Insight Meditation Society. Dr. Olendzki is author of *Unlimiting Mind: The Radically Experiential Psychology of Buddhism* and a frequent contributor to *Tricycle* magazine.

Susan M. Orsillo, PhD, is Professor of Psychology at Suffolk University in Boston. Her current research focuses on the role of emotional response styles, most notably experiential avoidance, in potentially maintaining psychological difficulties. In collaboration with her doctoral students in clinical psychology, Dr. Orsillo has developed and tested a number of prevention and treatment programs that integrate acceptance and mindfulness with evidence-based behavioral approaches. With Dr. Lizabeth Roemer, she has been studying the efficacy of an acceptance-based behavioral therapy for generalized anxiety disorder and comorbid conditions, mechanisms and processes of change, and applicability to clients from diverse backgrounds, with support from grants from the National Institute of Mental Health.

Thomas Pedulla, LICSW, is a clinical social worker and psychotherapist in private practice in Arlington, Massachusetts, where he works with individuals and leads mindfulness-based cognitive therapy groups. Before a deepening interest in mindfulness meditation led him to change careers, he worked for over two decades as an advertising copywriter and creative director. A faculty and board member at IMP, Mr. Pedulla has also served on the board at the Cambridge Insight Meditation Center. He has been a practitioner of meditation in the vipassana tradition for over 25 years. He is coauthor of *Sitting Together: Essential Skills for Mindfulness-Based Psychotherapy.*

Susan M. Pollak, MTS, EdD, is President of IMP and a psychologist in private practice in Cambridge, Massachusetts. She is Clinical Instructor in Psychology at the Cambridge Health Alliance/Harvard Medical School, where she has been teaching a course on meditation and psychotherapy since 1994. Dr. Pollak is coauthor of *Sitting Together: Essential Skills for Mindfulness-Based Psychotherapy,* coeditor of *The Cultural Transition,* and a contributing author to *Mapping the Moral Domain* and *Evocative Objects.*

Lizabeth Roemer, PhD, is Professor of Psychology at the University of Massachusetts–Boston. Along with her clinical psychology doctoral students, her research examines the role of mindfulness, acceptance, and valued action in a range of clinical presentations, including anxiety disorders, posttraumatic functioning, and responses to racist experiences. With Dr. Susan Orsillo, she has been studying the efficacy of an acceptance-based behavioral therapy for generalized anxiety disorder and comorbid conditions, mechanisms and processes of change, and applicability to clients from diverse backgrounds, with support from grants from the National Institute of Mental Health.

Ronald D. Siegel, PsyD (see "About the Editors").

Charles W. Styron, PsyD, is a clinical psychologist in private practice in Watertown and Walpole, Massachusetts, as well as a consulting psychologist for

Caritas Norwood Hospital in Norwood, Massachusetts. He specializes in individual adult psychotherapy and neuropsychological testing. Dr. Styron has been a practitioner and teacher in the Shambhala and Tibetan Vajrayana Buddhist traditions for 34 years, and a faculty and board member of IMP since its inception. He was formerly an architect.

Janet L. Surrey, PhD, is a clinical psychologist and Founding Scholar of the Jean Baker Miller Training Institute at the Stone Center, Wellesley College. She was on the faculty of Harvard Medical School for 25 years and is currently on the faculty and board of IMP. She is a graduate of the Spirit Rock Meditation Center Community Dharma Leader Program and is currently in the Teacher Training Program of the Metta Foundation. Dr. Surrey has been consulting and teaching relational–cultural theory nationally and internationally for over 20 years, and has been working to synthesize Buddhist and relational psychology. Her publications include *Women's Growth In Connection*; *Women's Growth In Diversity*; *Mothering against the Odds: Diverse Voices of Contemporary Mothers*; *We Have to Talk: Healing Dialogues between Women and Men*; and *Bill W. and Dr. Bob: The Story of the Founding of Alcoholics Anonymous*.

Preface

*T*his book is not about anything special. It is about a simple form of awareness—mindfulness—that is available to anyone at any moment. As you start to read this Preface, for example, your attention may be absorbed in the words you're reading or you may be wondering whether this book will be worth your trouble. Do you know where your attention is? Has it already wandered from this page? It's natural for the mind to wander, but are you aware when it does so, and what you're thinking about? And what's the quality of your awareness—relaxed, curious, and alert, or perhaps a little distracted and anxious? Mindfulness is simply about being aware of where your mind is from one moment to the next, with gentle acceptance. This kind of openhearted attention can have a deeply transformative effect on our daily lives. We can learn to enjoy very ordinary things—such as the flavor of an apple—or to tolerate great hardship—such as the death of a loved one—just by learning to be mindful.

This is also a book *by* clinicians *for* clinicians. The first edition, published in 2005, was the fruit of over 20 years of monthly meetings by a small group of psychotherapists who found themselves drawn to the twin practices of mindfulness meditation and psychotherapy. As curiosity about mindfulness grew in the psychotherapy community and other clinicians asked to participate in our discussions, we expanded the discourse into the public arena. Our first conference was held in 1994, and 2 years later we formed the Institute for Meditation and Psychotherapy (IMP). IMP now sponsors a wide range of continuing education programs locally, nationally, and online.

Much has happened in our field since the first edition of this book. The number of articles on mindfulness in the literature has expanded exponentially, along with brain-imaging techniques that can measure the effects of mindfulness on the brain even after days or weeks of meditation. Randomized controlled clinical trials of mindfulness-based interventions and meta-analyses of those studies now clearly demonstrate the effectiveness of mindfulness for a wide range of psychological disorders and patient populations. Mindfulness seems to have become a model of therapy in its own right—alongside cognitive-behavioral, psychodynamic, humanistic, and systems approaches—and is recognized as a mechanism of action in psychotherapy in general.

All this rapid growth means that our small band of therapists has had the pleasure of particpating in exciting conversations with clinicians, scientists, scholars, and meditation teachers from throughout the world, made all the more accessible by the expansion of the Internet. The current edition of this book is an effort to distill the enormous volume of new theory and research to what is most interesting and essential for the practicing clinician. Chapters by leading experts on trauma, addiction, and neuroscience have been added to the book, and almost all of the earlier chapters have been updated, resulting in a book of mostly new text.

Although the authors of this book have grown older over the past three decades, the direct experience of mindfulness has not. Mindfulness is a renewable source of energy and delight. It can be easily experienced by anyone, but cannot be easily described. Mindful awareness is mostly experiential and nonverbal (i.e., sensory, somatic, intuitive, emotional), and it requires some practice to develop. Like any acquired skill, the experience of mindfulness becomes steadier with increased practice.

The question that arises most readily in the minds of clinicians is how to *integrate* mindfulness into our daily practice of psychotherapy. This question soon leads to many others at the interface of mindfulness and psychotherapy, including:

- What really is mindfulness?
- Is mindfulness a new therapy, or a common factor in all therapy?
- What does sitting in meditation have to do with relating to another human being in psychotherapy?
- What can a mindfulness approach offer to patients suffering from conditions such as anxiety, depression, trauma, substance abuse, or chronic pain?
- Can we teach mindfulness to children? If so, how?
- How and when should mindfulness be introduced into psychotherapy?
- What can mindfulness meditation accomplish that therapy cannot, and vice versa?

- What is the role of ethical conduct in cultivating mindfulness?
- How does mindfulness relate to wisdom and compassion?
- What can neuroscience contribute to our understanding of mindfulness?
- What is the relationship of therapeutic mindfulness to its ancient roots?
- Can Buddhist psychology contribute to the field of positive psychology?

This book will surely raise more questions than it answers. We hope it will contribute to the robust conversation currently happening within our profession.

Some readers may be wondering about the link between mindfulness and Buddhist psychology or philosophy. Mindfulness is at the heart of Buddhist psychology. Most of the authors of this volume consider themselves students of Buddhist psychology and meditation, rather than Buddhists per se. As the saying goes, "It's better to be a Buddha than a Buddhist." Similarly, when mindfulness skills are taught in therapy, clients do not need to take up a new religion or exotic lifestyle to benefit from them. As the theory and practice of mindfulness become increasingly rooted in science, concern about this issue seems to be diminishing.

A challenge of this book has been to maintain a consistent voice as we present a broad range of perspectives from 18 different authors. Our optimistic goal was to stitch together an attractive patchwork quilt.

Part of stitching this book together was to arrive at a consistent use of the words *client* or *patient*. Our profession has not settled that discussion yet, nor have we. However, after some exploration, we decided to use the word *patient* more often in the text. Etymologically, *patient* means "one who bears suffering," whereas *client* means "one who puts himself under the protection of a patron." Since doctor means "teacher," it can be said that we are doctoring patients, or "teaching people who bear suffering." This meaning is parallel to the original use of mindfulness 2,500 years ago—it is a teaching that alleviates suffering.

Mindfulness is an opportunity to be fully alive and awake to our own lives. Most therapists do not forget what a privilege it is to participate so deeply in the lives of our fellow human beings. We love, laugh, and cry together, yearn and fear together, succeed and fail together, and, on good days, heal together. As the years go by, the fleeting nature of each precious encounter becomes more apparent. We want to make the most of each moment of therapy. It is in this spirit that we offer this book to our colleagues.

Acknowledgments

Numerous people have contributed to the development of this book. Each of the authors had the privilege of learning over many years from teachers and colleagues in the clinical world as well as the world of meditation. While the particular contributions found in these pages are our own, they are based on the insights of others who came before. We would like to thank, in particular, some of the individuals that have influenced one or more of us as psychotherapists and/or meditation students: Dan Brown, Richard Chasin, Pema Chödrön, His Holiness the Dalai Lama, Jay Efran, Jack Engler, Robert Fox, Joseph Goldstein, Thich Nhat Hanh, Les Havens, Judith Jordan, Jon Kabat-Zinn, Anna Klegon, Jack Kornfield, Robert Levine, Narayan Liebenson-Grady, Joanna Macy, Jean Baker Miller, Norby Mintz, Sakyong Mipham, Ginny Morgan, Ram Das, Larry Rosenberg, Paul Russell, Sharon Salzberg, Seung Sahn, Irene Stiver, Larry Strasburger, Maurine Stuart, Shunryu Suzuki, Vimala Thaker, Chögyam Trungpa, and Rama Jyoti Vernon.

Many others offered direct and indirect support for our work: Kristy Arbon for her administrative care; Jerry Bass, Doriana Chialant, Rob Guerette, Ed Hauben, Jerry Murphy, Nancy Riemer, and Mark Sorensen for their wise guidance; Chris Willard for his contribution to the chapter on mindfulness and children; and David Black for the remarkable resource the *Mindfulness Research Monthly*. Thanks also to the National Institute of Mental Health (Grant No. MH074589) for funding the work described in Chapter 9.

We are especially grateful to Senior Editor Jim Nageotte at The Guilford Press, who patiently shepherded this book from idea to actuality and whose insights and innumerable suggestions contributed greatly to the final manuscript; to Senior Assistant Editor Jane Keislar, who kept us all on the same page; to our endlessly patient Senior Production Editor, Laura Patchkofsky; to Paul Gordon, who never fails to create a beautiful book cover; and to the many unseen hands at The Guilford Press who work in concert with one another to make publishing a book as seamless as possible for harried authors.

In all our efforts, we are reminded of our late friend and colleague Phil Aranow, whose prescience and steadfast vision led to the establishment of the Institute for Meditation and Psychotherapy, and whose memory guides us still.

We are also very grateful to our patients, who have trusted us with their minds and hearts, and who have taught us most of what we know about clinical work.

Finally, we cannot say enough to thank our families and friends for their love, support, and sacrifice during the process of bringing this second edition to fruition.

Contents

Part I

The Meaning of Mindfulness

As interest in mindfulness grows among clinicians and researchers, the term has taken on ever-expanding meanings. To understand how mindfulness practices can inform psychotherapy, and how psychotherapy can enrich mindfulness practice, it's helpful to have a clear understanding of what mindfulness is, and how mindfulness practice relates to traditional forms of psychotherapy.

To lay this groundwork, Chapter 1 provides a primer on mindfulness and psychotherapy—what mindfulness is, its possible roles in psychotherapy, the various skills involved in mindfulness practice, the history of mindfulness in both scientific and Buddhist psychology, and mindfulness as a new model of psychotherapy. Building on this base, Chapter 2 examines parallels and differences between Buddhist psychology and foundational Western psychotherapeutic approaches, exploring what each tradition might offer the other.

1

Mindfulness

What Is It? What Does It Matter?

Christopher K. Germer

> To live is so startling, it leaves but little room for
> other occupations. . . .
>   —EMILY DICKINSON (1872)

*P*sychotherapists are in the business of alleviating emotional suffering. Suffering arrives in innumerable guises: as stress, anxiety, depression, behavior problems, interpersonal conflict, confusion, despair. It is the common denominator of all clinical diagnoses and is endemic to the human condition. Some of our suffering is existential, in the form of sickness, old age, and dying. Some suffering has a more personal flavor. The cause of our individual difficulties may include past conditioning, present circumstances, genetic predisposition, or any number of interacting factors. *Mindfulness*, a deceptively simple way of relating to experience, has long been used to lessen the sting of life's difficulties, especially those that are self-imposed. In this volume we illustrate the potential of mindfulness for enhancing psychotherapy.

People are clear about one thing when they enter therapy—*they want to feel better*. They often have a number of ideas about how to accomplish this goal, although therapy doesn't necessarily proceed as expected.

3

For example, a young woman with panic disorder—let's call her Lynn—might phone a therapist, hoping to escape the emotional turmoil of her condition. Lynn may be seeking freedom *from* her anxiety, but as therapy progresses, Lynn actually discovers freedom *in* her anxiety. How does this occur? A strong therapeutic alliance may provide Lynn with courage and safety to begin to explore her panic more closely. Through self-monitoring, Lynn becomes aware of the sensations of anxiety in her body and the thoughts associated with them. She learns how to cope with panic by talking herself through it. When Lynn feels ready, she directly experiences the sensations of anxiety that trigger a panic attack and tests herself in a mall or on an airplane. This whole process requires that Lynn first turn *toward* the anxiety. A compassionate "bait and switch" has occurred.

Therapists who work in a more relational or psychodynamic model may observe a similar process. As connection deepens between the patient and the therapist, the conversation becomes more spontaneous and authentic, and the patient acquires the freedom to explore what is really troubling him or her in a more open, curious way. With the support of the relationship, the patient is gently exposed to what is going on inside. The patient discovers that he or she need not avoid experience to feel better.

We know that many seemingly dissimilar forms of psychotherapy work (Seligman, 1995; Wampold, 2012). Is there a common curative factor across various modalities that can be identified and refined, perhaps even *trained*? Mindfulness is proving itself to be such an ingredient.

A SPECIAL RELATIONSHIP TO SUFFERING

Successful therapy changes the patient's *relationship* to his or her suffering. Obviously, if we are less upset by events in our lives, our suffering will decrease. But how can we be less disturbed by *unpleasant* experiences? Life includes pain. Don't the body and mind instinctively resist or avoid painful experiences? Mindfulness is a skill that allows us to be less reactive to what is happening in the moment. It is a way of relating to *all* experience—positive, negative, and neutral—such that our overall suffering diminishes and our sense of well-being increases.

To be mindful is to wake up, to recognize what is happening in the present moment with a friendly attitude. Unfortunately, we're rarely mindful. We are usually caught up in distracting thoughts or in opinions about what is happening in the moment. This is mind*less*ness. Examples of mindlessness include the following (adapted from the *Mindful Attention Awareness Scale* [Brown & Ryan, 2003]):

- Rushing through activities without being attentive to them.
- Breaking or spilling things because of carelessness, inattention, or thinking of something else.
- Failing to notice subtle feelings of physical tension or discomfort.
- Forgetting a person's name almost as soon as we've heard it.
- Finding ourselves preoccupied with the future or the past.
- Snacking without being aware of eating.

Mind*ful*ness, in contrast, focuses our attention on the task at hand. When we're mindful, our attention is not entangled in the past or future, and we are not rejecting or clinging to what is occurring at the moment. We are present in an openhearted way. This kind of attention generates energy, clearheadedness, and joy. Fortunately, it is a skill that can be cultivated by anyone.

When Gertrude Stein (1922/1993, p. 187) wrote "A rose is a rose is a rose is a rose," she was bringing the reader back again and again to the simple rose. She was suggesting, perhaps, what a rose is *not*. It is not a romantic relationship that ended tragically 4 years ago; it is not an imperative to trim the hedges over the weekend—it is just a rose. Perceiving with this kind of "bare attention" is commonly associated with mindfulness.

Most people in psychotherapy are preoccupied with past or future events. For example, people who are depressed often feel regret, sadness, or guilt about the past, and people who are anxious fear the future. Suffering seems to increase as we stray from the present moment. As our attention gets absorbed in mental activity and we begin to ruminate, unaware that we're ruminating, our daily lives can become sorrowful indeed. Some of our patients feel as if they are stuck in a movie theatre, watching the same upsetting movie over and over, unable to leave. Mindfulness can help us to step out of our conditioning and see things anew—to see a rose as it is.

DEFINITIONS OF MINDFULNESS

The term *mindfulness* is an English translation of the Pali word *sati*. Pali was the language of Buddhist psychology 2,500 years ago, and mindfulness is the core teaching of this tradition. *Sati* connotes *awareness, attention*, and *remembering*.

What is awareness? Brown and Ryan (2003) define awareness and attention under the umbrella of consciousness:

> *Consciousness* encompasses both awareness and attention. *Awareness* is the background "radar" of consciousness, continually monitoring the inner and outer environment. One may be aware of stimuli without them being at the center of attention. *Attention* is a process of focusing conscious awareness, providing heightened sensitivity to a limited range of experience (Westen, 1999). In actuality, awareness and attention are intertwined, such that attention continually pulls "figures" out of the "ground" of awareness, holding them focally for varying lengths of time. (p. 822)

You are using both awareness and attention as you read these words. A tea kettle whistling in the background might command your attention if it gets loud enough, particularly if you would like a cup of tea. Similarly, we may drive a familiar route on "autopilot," vaguely aware of the road, but respond immediately if a child runs in front of us. Mindfulness is the opposite of functioning on autopilot, the opposite of daydreaming; it is paying attention to what is salient in the present moment.

Mindfulness also involves *remembering*, but not dwelling in memories. It involves remembering to reorient our attention and awareness to current experience in a wholehearted, receptive manner. This reorientation requires the *intention* to disentangle our attention from our reverie and fully experience the present moment.

The word *mindfulness* can be used to describe a theoretical *construct* (the idea of mindfulness), *practices* for cultivating mindfulness (such as meditation), or psychological *processes* (mechanisms of action in the mind and brain). A basic definition of mindfulness is "moment-by-moment awareness." Other definitions include "keeping one's consciousness alive to the present reality" (Hanh, 1976, p. 11); "the clear and single-minded awareness of what actually happens to us and in us at the successive moments of perception" (Nyanaponika, 1972, p. 5); and "the awareness that emerges through paying attention, on purpose, in the present moment, and non-judgmentally to the unfolding of experience moment by moment" (Kabat-Zinn, 2003, p. 145). Ultimately, mindfulness cannot be fully captured with words because it's a subtle, nonverbal experience (Gunaratana, 2002). It's the difference between *feeling* a sound in your body and *describing* what you might be hearing.

Therapeutic Mindfulness

A precise definition of mindfulness may further elude us because modern definitions diverge from their multidimensional Buddhist roots

(Grossman, 2011; Olendzki, 2011), and different traditions within Buddhist psychology don't necesssarily agree on the meaning of mindfulness (Williams & Kabat-Zinn, 2011). Practical approaches to defining mindfulness in clinical settings include discovering commonalities found in various training programs (Carmody, 2009) or investigating what seems to be useful to patients in mindfulness-oriented treatment. In a consensus opinion among experts, Bishop and colleagues (2004) proposed a two-component model of mindfulness: "The first component involves the self-regulation of attention so that it is maintained on immediate experience, thereby allowing for increased recognition of mental events in the present moment. The second component involves adopting a particular orientation towards one's experience that is characterized by curiosity, openness, and acceptance" (p. 232).

Although attention regulation has received the most consideration in the psychological literature over the past decade, the *quality* of mindful awareness is particularly important in clinical settings, characterized by nonjudgment, acceptance, loving-kindness, and compassion. Jon Kabat-Zinn (2005), the leading pioneer of mindfulness in health care, has defined mindfulness as "open-hearted, moment-to-moment, nonjudgmental awareness" (p. 24). We need a compassionate response to our own pain when we're dealing with intense and unremitting emotions (Feldman & Kuyken, 2011; Germer, 2009). If the therapist or the patient turns away from uncomfortable experience with anxiety or disgust, our ability to work with that experience significantly diminishes.

From the mindfulness perspective, *acceptance* refers to the ability to allow our experience to be just as it is *in the present moment*—accepting both pleasurable and painful experiences as they arise. Acceptance is not about endorsing bad behavior. Rather, moment-to-moment acceptance is a prerequisite for behavior change. "Change is the brother of acceptance, but it is the younger brother" (Christensen & Jacobson, 2000, p. 11). Mindfulness-oriented clinicians also see *self*-acceptance as central to the therapy process (Brach, 2003; Linehan, 1993a). In the words of Carl Rogers, "The curious paradox of life is that when I accept myself just as I am, then I can change" (Rogers, 1961, p. 17).

The short definition of mindfulness we use in this volume is *awareness* of *present experience* with *acceptance*. These three components can be found in most discussions of mindfulness in both the psychotherapy and Buddhist literature. The components are thoroughly comingled in a moment of mindfulness, but in ordinary life the presence of one element of mindfulness doesn't necessarily imply the others. For example, our awareness may be absorbed in the past rather than the present, such as in blind rage about a perceived injustice. We may also have awareness without acceptance, such as in the experience of shame. Likewise, acceptance can exist without awareness, as in premature forgiveness; and present-centeredness without awareness may arise in a moment of intoxication. Therapists can use these three elements as a measure of mindfulness in themselves and in their patients. Are we aware of what is arising in and around us, in this very moment, with an attitude of warmhearted acceptance?

MINDFULNESS AND LEVELS OF PRACTICE

Mindfulness must be experienced to be known. People may practice mindfulness with varying degrees of intensity. At one end of a continuum of practice is everyday mindfulness. Even in our often pressured and distracted daily lives, it's possible to have mindful moments. We can momentarily disengage from our activities by taking a long, conscious breath, gathering our attention, and then asking ourselves,

> "What am I sensing in my body right now?"
> "What am I feeling?"
> "What am I thinking?"
> "What is vivid and alive in my awareness?"

We don't even need to be calm to have some mindful awareness, such as when we discover, "I'm really angry right now." This is mindfulness in daily life—and how it commonly occurs in psychotherapy as well.

At the other end of the continuum we find monastics and laypeople who spend a considerable amount of time in meditation. When we have the opportunity to sit for sustained periods with closed eyes, in a silent place, sharpening concentration on one thing (e.g., the breath), the mind becomes like a microscope that can detect minute mental activity. The following instruction is an example of intensive meditation practice:

> Should an itching sensation be felt in any part of the body, keep the mind on that part and make a mental note *itching*. . . . Should the itching continue and become too strong and you intend to rub the itching part, be sure to make a mental note *intending*. Slowly lift the hand, simultaneously noting the action of *lifting*, and *touching* when the hand touches the part that itches. Rub slowly in complete awareness of *rubbing*. When the itching sensation has disappeared and you intend to discontinue the rubbing, be mindful of making the usual mental note of *intending*. Slowly withdraw the hand, concurrently making a mental note of the action, *withdrawing*.

When the hand rests in its usual place touching the leg, *touching*. (Mahasi, 1971, pp. 5–6)

This level of precise and subtle awareness, in which we can even detect "intending," clearly requires an unusual level of dedication on the part of the practitioner. Remarkably, the instruction above is considered a "basic" instruction. Mahasi Sayadaw writes that, at more advanced stages, "Some meditators perceive distinctly three phases: noticing an object, its ceasing, and the passing away of the consciousness that cognizes that ceasing—all in quick succession" (1971, p. 15).

Moments of mindfulness have certain common aspects regardless of where they lie on the practice continuum. In everyday life, the actual moment of awakening, of mindfulness, is roughly the same for the experienced meditator and the novice. Mindful moments are:

- *Nonconceptual.* Mindfulness is embodied, intuitive awareness, disentangled from thought processes.
- *Nonverbal.* The experience of mindfulness cannot be captured in words because awareness occurs before words arise in the mind.
- *Present-centered.* Mindfulness is always in the present moment. Absorption in thoughts temporarily removes us from the present moment.
- *Nonjudgmental.* Awareness cannot occur freely if we don't like what we are experiencing.
- *Participatory.* Mindfulness is not detached witnessing. It is experiencing the mind and body in an intimate, yet unencumbered, manner.
- *Liberating.* Every moment of mindful awareness provides a bit of freedom from conditioned suffering, a little space around our discomfort.

These qualities occur simultaneously in each moment of mindfulness. Mindfulness *practice* is a conscious attempt to return to the present moment with warmhearted awareness, again and again, with all the qualities listed above. Mindfulness itself is not unusual; *continuity* of mindfulness is rare indeed.

WISDOM AND COMPASSION

Mindfulness is not a goal in itself—the aim of fostering it is freedom from suffering. As mindfulness deepens, wisdom and compassion are likely to arise, and these qualities naturally lead to psychological freedom (Germer & Siegel, 2012). For example, mindfulness practice frees us from repetitive thinking, which, in turn, allows us to see how fluid and ever-changing our lives actually are, including our sense of self. This insight liberates us from the constant need to promote ourselves in society and defend ourselves from petty insults. That is considered *wisdom* in Buddhist psychology—insight into impermanence and the illusion of a fixed "self," and understanding how we create misery for ourselves by fighting present-moment reality.

The Greek philosopher Heraclitus wrote, "Applicants for wisdom do what I have done: inquire within" (Hillman, 2003, p. xiii). The Buddha said, "Come and see" (Pali: *ehipassiko*). The close association between contemplative insight and wisdom is why mindfulness meditation is also know as *insight meditation*—the practice of looking within to see things as they are, beneath our conditioned perceptions and reactions, to liberate the heart and mind.

Wisdom and compassion are "two wings of a bird" (Dalai Lama, 2003, p. 56; Germer & Siegel, 2012). *Compassion* refers to the ability to open to suffering (in ourselves and others) along with the wish to alleviate it. It emerges naturally out of wisdom—the deep awareness and acceptance of things as they really are. Compassion can also be directly cultivated through deliberate practices. As therapists, if we feel compassionately toward a patient but have no wisdom, we are liable to become overwhelmed with emotion, unable to see a path out of suffering, and conclude that the treatment is hopeless. Conversely, if we are wise—if we grasp the complex nature of a patient's situation and can see our way through but are out of touch with the patient's despair—our therapeutic suggestions will fall on deaf ears. Therapists need both wisdom and compassion, and can use mindfulness practices to develop them.

PSYCHOTHERAPISTS AND MINDFULNESS

Mindfulness has gone mainstream in the United States (Ryan, 2012). In a 2007 survey, 9.4% of Americans said they practiced meditation in the past year, up from 7.6% only 5 years earlier (National Center for Complementary and Alternative Medicine, 2007). This is not surprising, given that science is highly influential in modern society and the science community has shown vigorous interest in meditation. In clinical circles, meditation has become one of the most researched psychotherapeutic methods (Walsh & Shapiro, 2006). Clinicians are drawn to mindfulness from a variety of directions: personal, clinical, and scientific.

A Brief History of Mindfulness in Psychotherapy

The formal introduction of Eastern thought to Western philosophy and psychology can be traced to the late 1700s when British scholars began to translate Indian spiritual texts such as the *Bhagavad Gita*. These teachings, along with Buddhist writing, took root in America through the writings of "transcendentalists" such as Henry David Thoreau, who wrote in *Walden* (1854/2012): "I sat in my sunny doorway from sunrise til noon, rapt in reverie. . . . I realized what the Orientals mean by contemplation" (p. 61). In the early 1900s, William James remarked to his class at Harvard College, "This [Buddhist psychology] is the psychology everybody will be studying twenty-five years from now" (Epstein, 1995, pp. 1–2). James's prediction has largely come true, although it was off by a number of years.

The field of psychoanalysis has also flirted with Buddhist psychology for a long time. Freud exchanged letters with a friend in 1930 in which he admitted that Eastern philosophy was alien to him and perhaps "beyond the limits of [his] nature" (cited in Epstein, 1995, p. 2). That did not stop Freud from writing in *Civilization and Its Discontents* (1961a) that the "oceanic feeling" in meditation was an essentially regressive experience. Franz Alexander (1931) added a paper entitled "Buddhist Training as an Artificial Catatonia." Other psychodynamic theorists were more complimentary, notably Carl Jung, who wrote a commentary on the *Tibetan Book of the Dead* in 1927 and had a lifelong curiosity about Eastern psychology.

World War II opened the minds of many Westerners to Asian psychologies, notably Zen Buddhism. Shoma Morita, in Japan, developed a Zen-based residential therapy for anxiety that encouraged patients to experience their fears without trying to change or stop them, very akin to modern, mindfulness-oriented psychotherapy (Morita, 1928/1998). Following the war, D. T. Suzuki dialogued with Erich Fromm and Karen Horney (Fromm, Suzuki, & DeMartino, 1960; Horney, 1945) and inspired visionaries and artists such as Alan Watts, John Cage, and the beat writers Jack Kerouac and Alan Ginsberg. (See McCown, Reibel, & Micozzi, 2011, and Fields, 1992, for more extensive historical reviews of Buddhist psychology in the West.)

The seed of mindfulness was planted in the minds of many therapists who were drawn as young adults in the 1960s and 1970s to Eastern philosophy and meditation as a path to emotional freedom. Fritz Perls (2012) studied Zen in Japan in 1962 and, though disappointed by his experience, remarked, "The experienced phenomenon is the ultimate Gestalt!" In the late 1960s, young people flocked to classes on

Trancendental Meditation (TM; Mahesh Yogi, 1968/2001; Rosenthal, 2012) as ideas of enlightenment followed the Beatles and other famous pilgrims back from India. Former Harvard psychologist Ram Dass's book *Be Here Now* (1971), a mixture of Hindu and Buddhist ideas, sold over a million copies. Yoga, which is essentially mindfulness in movement (Boccio, 2004; Hartranft, 2003), also traveled west at the time. Gradually, clinicians began connecting their personal meditation practice with their clinical work.

Studies on meditation flourished; for example, cardiologist Herbert Benson (1975) became well known for his use of meditation to treat heart disease. Clinical psychology kept pace with research on meditation as an adjunct to psychotherapy or as psychotherapy itself (Smith, 1975). In 1977, the American Psychiatric Association called for a formal examination of the clinical effectiveness of meditation. The majority of the journal articles at the time studied concentration meditation, such as TM and Benson's *relaxation response*. During the 1990s, however, the preponderance of studies switched to mindfulness meditation (Smith, 2004). Jon Kabat-Zinn opened the Center for Mindfulness in 1979, at the University of Massachusetts Medical School, and taught mindfulness-based stress reduction (MBSR) to treat chronic conditions for which physicians could offer no further help. By 2012, there were over 700 MBSR programs offered worldwide (Center for Mindfulness, 2012) and MBSR had become the main mindfulness training program used in psychological research.

Whereas only 365 peer-reviewed articles on mindfulness appeared in the psychological literature (PsycINFO) in 2005 when the first edition of this book was published, by 2013 there were over 2,200 articles and over 60 mindfulness treatment and research centers in the United States alone (see Figure 1.1).

We now have mindfulness-based structured interventions for treating a broad range of mental and physical disorders, randomized controlled trials supporting these interventions, and reviews and meta-analyses of those studies. Furthermore, sophisticated neurobiological research is demonstrating the power of mind training to change the structure and function of the brain (see Chapter 15). (See *www.mindfulexperience.org* for a comprehensive, regularly updated mindfulness research database.)

We seem to be witnessing the emergence of a new, unified model of psychotherapy based on the construct of mindfulness. Mindfulness is both *transtheoretical* (it appeals to a wide range of therapists, e.g., behavioral, psychodynamic, humanistic, family systems) and *transdiagnostic*

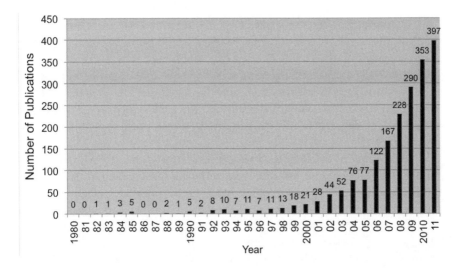

FIGURE 1.1. Number of mindfulness publications by year: 1980–2011. Figure provided by David S. Black, PhD, Institute for Prevention Research, Keck School of Medicine, University of Southern California, and reprinted by permission of the author (*www.mindfulexperience.org*).

(it appears to alleviate diverse mental and physical disorders). Mindfulness is reconnecting practitioners to their scientific colleagues as empirically supported, mindfulness-based treatment programs and neurobiological research are illuminating how mindfulness alleviates suffering. Therapists are exploring meditation both for personal well-being as well as for cultivating beneficial therapeutic qualities (see Chapters 3 and 5), and patients are seeking therapists who meditate and have a compatible approach to emotional healing. In short, mindfulness appears to be drawing clinical theory, research, and practice closer together and helping to integrate the private and professional lives of therapists.

A Word about Buddhism

Mindfulness lies at the heart of Buddhist psychology. Psychotherapists are likely to find early Buddhist psychology compatible with their interests because it shares the goal of alleviating suffering and the value of empirical inquiry. Whereas Western science explores phenomena through objective, third-person observation, Buddhist psychology is a systematic, first-person approach relatively devoid of a priori assumptions (Wallace, 2007; see also Chapter 2).

It cannot be overemphasized that Buddhist psychology is not a religion in the familiar, theistic sense, although Buddhists in some Eastern cultures worship the Buddha's teachings and image. The historical Buddha (563–483 B.C.E.) is understood to have been a human being, not a god, and his life's work was dedicated to alleviating psychological suffering. According to Buddhist tradition, when he discovered a path to freedom, he decided (reluctantly at first) to teach others what he had learned.

According to legend, when people met the Buddha after his realization/enlightenment, he did not seem quite like other men. When they asked him who he was, he replied that he was "Buddha," which simply meant, *a person who is awake*. He reportedly taught for a total of 45 years and had many students, rich and poor. He spoke in simple language using stories and ideas from popular Indian culture. In his first sermon on the Four Noble Truths, he put forth these foundational ideas:

1. The human condition involves suffering.
2. The conflict between how things are and how we desire them to be causes this suffering.
3. Suffering can be reduced or even eliminated by changing our attitude toward unpleasant experience.
4. There are eight general strategies (the Eightfold Path) to bring suffering to an end (see Chapter 2 and the Appendix).

The Buddha died at age 80, probably from contaminated food eaten at the home of a poor follower.

The Buddha is said to have discovered how to end suffering without any props or religious rituals. Cultures have venerated his image, but the Buddha enjoined his students not to worship him. Students were asked to discover the truth of his teachings *through their own experience*. Belief in notions such as karma or rebirth are unnecessary to derive full benefit from Buddhist psychology (Batchelor, 1997), which is primarily a practical way to know the mind, shape the mind, and free the mind (Nyanaponika, 1965; Olendzki, 2010). Mindfulness is the core practice of Buddhist psychology, and the body of Buddhist psychology—including the Buddha's original teachings and later writings of the *Abhidharma*—can be considered the theoretical basis for mindfulness practice (Bodhi, 2000; Nyanaponika, 1949/1998). Reading early Buddhist texts will convince the clinician that the Buddha was essentially a psychologist.

Chapter 14 and the Appendix of this book provide a more comprehensive historical and conceptual background to mindfulness practice.

states of mind, such as distraction or the arising of pride; and (4) *mental objects*, which include qualities that foster well-being, such as energy and tranquility, or qualities that inhibit wellness, such as anger and sloth. Although the distinction between thoughts and emotions apparently did not exist in the East at the time of the Buddha, mindfulness of emotions is certainly very important in modern psychotherapy.

Three Types of Mindfulness Meditation

Three kinds of meditation are typically taught under the umbrella of *mindfulness meditation* in the West (Salzberg, 2011; see also Chapter 7): (1) focused attention (concentration), (2) open monitoring (mindfulness per se), and (3) loving-kindness and compassion. The first two types have been emphasized in the theory and practice of mindfulness in psychotherapy (Carmody et al., 2011) and in early Buddhist texts. However, the practice of loving-kindness and compassion has generated considerable interest in the last few years (Hofman, Grossman, & Hinton, 2011). Neurological evidence suggests that the mental skills cultivated by these three meditation types represent overlapping, yet distinct, brain processes (Brewer, Mallik, et al., 2011; Desbordes et al., 2012; Dickenson, Berkman, Arch, & Lieberman, 2013; Lee et al., 2012; Leung et al., 2013; Lutz, Slagter, Dunne, & Davidson, 2008; Tang & Posner, 2013), and preexisting brain function might even determine a preference for one practice over another (Mascaro, Rilling, Negi, & Raison, 2013). A common element in all mindfulness meditation techniques is the centrality of openhearted, moment-to-moment awareness.

Focused Attention

Focused attention, or concentration meditation, can be compared to a laser light beam that illuminates any object toward which it is directed. Examples of internal objects of meditation include the sensation of breathing, selected words or phrases, or a single location on the body. Objects of external focus might be an image, a sound, a candle flame, or even a dot on the wall. Concentration is generally easier when the object is pleasant. The instruction for this type of meditation is, "When you notice that your mind has wandered, gently bring it back to [the object of attention]."

Concentration meditation helps cultivate a calm, unruffled mind. (The Pali word for focused attention, *samatha*, connotes both tranquility and concentration.) Our attention becomes steady and relaxed when

MINDFULNESS PRACTICE

Mindfulness occurs naturally in everyday life, but requires practice to be maintained. We all periodically wake up to our present experience, only to slip quickly back into ordinary discursive thinking. Even when we feel particularly attentive while doing therapy, for example, we are only *intermittently* mindful. Our minds become easily absorbed in associations to what our patients are saying or doing. We may then have a moment of awakening from our reverie, reorient ourselves to the patient, and resume our exploration of what the patient is communicating. Soon, however, we again slip away in distracted thinking. Sometimes the content of our distraction is a meaningful clue to what is occurring in the therapy room. Sometimes it is not. Continuity of mindfulness requires a strong intention and persistence.

Formal and Informal Practice

Mindfulness can be learned through training that is either formal or informal. *Formal mindfulness practice* refers to meditation, and is an opportunity to experience mindfulness at its deepest levels. It's like going to the mental gym. Sustained, disciplined introspection allows the practitioner to train attention, systematically observe the mind's contents, and learn how the mind works.

Informal mindfulness practice refers to the application of mindfulness skills in everyday life. Any mental event can be an object of awareness—we can direct attention to our breathing, listen to ambient sounds in the environment, label our emotions, or notice body sensations while brushing our teeth. Two common exercises for cultivating mindfulness in daily life are mindful walking and mindful eating. In walking meditation, we attend to the sequential, moment-to-moment, kinesthetic sense of walking. From the outside, it looks like a slow-motion movie. On the inside, we are silently noting "lifting . . . stepping . . . placing. . . . " In eating meditation, we eat slowly and silently, noticing the sight of the food on the plate, the sensations of the food in the mouth, the muscle movements of chewing, the flavors of the food, and the process of swallowing. This can make an ordinary meal exceptionally interesting, and is used in mindfulness-based strategies to manage compulsive eating (Kristeller & Wolever, 2011).

There are four foundations of mindfulness in traditional Buddhist practice: (1) the *body*, including breathing and posture; (2) *feeling tone*, such as the pleasant, unpleasant, or neutral quality of sensations; (3)

the mind is drawn to a single object, again and again, and away from the many concerns (real and imagined) that occupy us throughout the day. In psychotherapy, focused attention is a way of anchoring the mind when a person is buffeted with strong emotions. We might direct the patient's attention to feeling the sensation of his or her feet touching the floor, or air entering and leaving the lungs. Here is a simple concentration practice.

Breath Meditation

Find a quiet place and sit in a posture that is both upright and relaxed. Take a few slow, easy breaths to settle your body and mind. Then let your eyelids gently close, fully or partially.

- Explore your body with your awareness and try to discover where you can feel your breathing most easily. Some people feel it around the nostrils, perhaps as a cool breeze on the upper lip. Others notice the chest rising and falling most easily, and still others feel the breath in the abdomen as the belly expands and contracts.
- Just feel the physical sensations of breathing in and breathing out.
- When you notice that your mind has wandered, just feel the breath again.
- There is no need to control the breath. Let your body *breathe you*—as it does naturally.
- Don't worry how often your mind wanders. Each time you notice that your attention has gone elsewhere, simply return to the breath as you might redirect a toddler or puppy gone astray.
- When you wish to end your meditation, gently open your eyes.

Open Monitoring

Open monitoring meditation can be compared to a searchlight (vs. a laser beam in concentration meditation) that illuminates a wider range of objects as they arise in consciousness, one at a time. Being receptive to *whatever* sound in the environment is most evident at a given moment is an example of open monitoring, whereas deliberately listening to the sound of a bell is focused attention.

We can use open monitoring to notice our intentions, sensations, emotions, thoughts, and/or behaviors. A common use of open monitoring in clinical practice is to develop interoceptive awareness of body sensations (Farb, Segal, & Anderson, 2012; Michalak, Burg, & Heidenreich, 2012). Other therapeutic practices label emotions (e.g., *sadness*, *shame, fear*) and core beliefs (e.g., "I'm unlovable," "I'm defective"), which can help us get a little perspective on our distressing feelings and thoughts. In formal meditation, the transition from focused attention to open monitoring begins when we invite ourselves to "note what took our attention away" when the mind wanders from our chosen object of awareness (e.g., the breath), rather than simply returning to the object. *Noting* can involve a moment of recognition ("aha!") or naming our experience as *thinking, judging,* or *worrying.* The instruction for full open monitoring (also referred to as *choiceless awareness*) is to "notice whatever predominates in your field of awareness, moment to moment."

Open monitoring develops the capacity for relaxed awareness in which conscious attention moves naturally among the changing elements of experience. Over time, it helps us develop insight into our personal conditioning and how the mind functions. Whereas concentration calms the mind by focusing on a single object, open monitoring cultivates equanimity in the midst of random and unexpected life events.

Technically speaking, *mindfulness* refers to the skill of open monitoring. The Pali word for open monitoring is *vipassana*, which means *seeing clearly.* The unique feature of vipassana meditation, insight meditation, or mindfulness meditation is open monitoring. However, *mindfulness* is now used more broadly in mainstream Western culture to describe all three meditation skills being described here: (1) focused attention, (2) open monitoring, and (3) loving-kindness and compassion. The following exercise is an open monitoring practice that helps to regulate difficult emotions.

Mindfulness of Emotion in the Body

Start by finding a comfortable position, close your eyes fully or partially, and take three relaxing breaths.

- Locate your breathing where you can feel it most easily. Feel how the breath moves in the body, and when your attention wanders, gently return to feeling the movement of the breath.
- After a few minutes, start to notice *physical sensations* of stress that you're holding in your body, perhaps in your neck, jaw, belly, or forehead.
- Also notice if you're holding any *difficult emotions*, such as worry about the future or uneasiness about the past. Understand that every human body bears stress and worry throughout the day.
- See if you can *name* the emotion in your body. Perhaps a feeling of sadness, anger, fear, loneliness, or shame? Repeat the label a

few times to yourself in a soft, kind voice, and then return to the breath.

- Now choose a *single location in your body* where stress may be expressing itself most strongly, perhaps as an ache in the heart region or tension in the stomach. In your mind, incline gently toward that spot as you might toward a newborn child.
- Continue to breathe naturally, allowing the sensation to be there, just as it is. Feel your breathing in the midst of your other body sensations.
- Allow the gentle, rhythmic motion of the breath to soften and soothe your body. If you wish, place your hand over your heart as you continue to breathe.
- When you're ready, gently open your eyes.

Loving-kindness and Compassion

Loving-kindness and compassion describe the *quality* of mindful awareness—the attitude or emotion—rather than the direction of awareness. Think of the difference between the light in an operating room versus candlelight at dinner. Loving-kindness warms up the experience of meditation, bringing in the qualities of tenderness, soothing, comfort, ease, care, and connection. These qualities are particularly important when we're dealing with difficult emotions that constrict our awareness and activate our defenses. An example of a loving-kindness (Pali: *metta*) meditation is the slow repetiton of phrases such as "May I be safe" or "May I be happy and free from suffering." The purpose of a loving-kindness meditation is to plant seeds of goodwill toward ourselves and others, over and over, which eventually sprout into positive thoughts, emotions, and behaviors. In the broadest sense, any meditation that evokes a sense of happiness and warmth can be considered loving-kindness meditation.

Loving-kindness is a "state of mind which aspires that all sentient beings may enjoy happiness," whereas compassion (Pali: *karuna*) is "the wish that all sentient beings may be free from suffering" (Dalai Lama, 2003, p. 67). Compassion occurs when loving-kindness meets suffering. Both loving-kindness and compassion are positive emotions that improve our health and well-being (Fredrickson, 2012; Fredrickson, Cohn, Coffey, Pek, & Finkel, 2008; Klimecki, Leiberg, Lamm, & Singer, 2012). They shift our awareness from *worried* attention to *loving* attention and open our field of perception, helping us become more mindful.

In psychotherapy, compassion often takes the form of *self*-compassion. For example, a compassion meditation that includes oneself is the practice of inhaling warmth and tenderness for ourselves with each inbreath, and exhaling the same for others with the outbreath (see Chapter 4). This meditation can be practiced by clinicians during difficult moments in therapy, or by our patients in their daily lives. It is a modification of the Tibetan Buddhist *tonglen* meditation in which we breathe in the suffering of others and breathe out compassion for others (Chödrön, 2001).

To enhance self-compassion in traditional loving-kindness meditation (using phrases as the primary focus of attention), the words could change a little, such as "May I be kind to myself" or "May I accept myself as I am," to reflect the presence of suffering, or we can simply place a hand over the heart and feel the warmth and gentle touch (Neff & Germer, in press).

Loving-kindness Meditation[1]

This exercise is designed to bring warmth and goodwill into your life. Sit in a comfortable position, close your eyes fully or partially, and allow your mind and body to settle with a few deep breaths.

- Put your hands over your heart to remind yourself that you are bringing not only attention, but *loving* attention, to your experience. For a few minutes, feel the warmth of your hands and their gentle pressure over your heart. Allow yourself to be soothed by the rhythmic movement of your breath beneath your hands.
- Now bring to mind a person or other living being who naturally makes you smile. This could be a child, your grandmother, your cat or dog—whoever brings happiness to your heart. Feel what it's like to be in that being's presence. Allow yourself to enjoy the good company.
- Next, recognize how vulnerable this loved one is—just like you, subject to many difficulties in life. Also, this being wishes to be happy and free from suffering, just like you and every other living being. Repeat softly and gently, allowing the significance of your words to resonate in your heart.

    May you be safe.
    May you be peaceful.
    May you be healthy.
    May you live with ease.
- Should you notice that your mind has wandered, return to the image of your loved one. Savor any warm feelings that may arise. Go slowly.

---

[1]This loving-kindness meditation is adapted from the mindful self-compassion training program codeveloped by Kristin Neff and the author.

- Now visualize your own body in your mind's eye and feel the sensations of your body, just as they are. Notice any discomfort or uneasiness that may be there. Offer kindness to yourself.
    May I be safe.
    May I be peaceful.
    May I be healthy.
    May I live with ease.
- If you wish to use different phrases that speak more authentically to you, please do so. You can ask yourself, "What do I need to hear right now?" Use language that inclines the heart tenderly toward yourself, as if you were relating to a beloved child or a dear friend.
- If and when emotional resistance arises, let it linger in the background and return to the phases, or refocus on your loved one or your breath.
- Whenever you are ready, gently open your eyes.

Practicing the Three Skills

Beginning meditators often have misconceptions about what mindfulness meditation is and does. Mindfulness meditation is not a relaxation exercise; sometimes its effect is quite the opposite, as when the object of awareness is disturbing. It's not a test of your concentration; the nature of the mind is to wander (see *default mode network* in the later section, "Mechanisms of Action"). Mindfulness is not a way to avoid difficulties in life; on the contrary, it brings us closer to our difficulties before we can "decenter" from them. And it does not bypass our personality problems; rather, it is a slow, gentle process of coming to grips with who we are. Finally, mindfulness meditation is not about achieving a different state of mind; it's about settling into our current experience in a relaxed, alert, and openhearted way.

Mindfulness practice may use any of the senses: seeing, hearing, listening, smelling, and touching. The mind itself is also considered a sense organ in Buddhist psychology because thoughts and images can be objects of conscious awareness, similar to the other senses. However, due to the seductive and evanescent nature of thoughts, it's much easier to start mindfulness practice by focusing on bodily sensations, later expanding to noticing emotions in the body or naming emotions, and eventually noticing repetitive thoughts, such as familiar attitudes or core beliefs about oneself.

Typically, mindfulness meditation begins with returning awareness to an object of attention, such as the breath, again and again. When the mind settles down, after minutes or days, we can direct our awareness—ply the searchlight—to include other experiences, such as other body sensations, emotions, or thoughts and images. If the mind loses its stability by becoming entangled in regret or worry, we can take refuge in a sensory object any time, perhaps by feeling the rhythmic motion of breathing. Finally, if we find that we're struggling with the process, we can offer ourselves a little compassion with a hand on the heart or kind words. The seasoned mindfulness practitioner may move flexibly from one technique to another, even within a 30-minute meditation, endeavoring to maintain warmhearted, moment-to-moment awareness. The three skills of mindfulness meditation help us to abide peacefully in the midst of all arising experience—pleasant, unpleasant, and neutral.

Many people wonder, "Which is the best practice for me?" Since mindfulness meditation is highly personal, the answer may be found by asking, "What do my mind and heart need at this moment to be more aware, present, and accepting?"

Mindfulness-Oriented Psychotherapy

There are three key ways, along a continuum from implicit to explicit application, to integrate mindfulness into therapeutic work. A clinician may (1) practice mindfulness, formally or informally, to cultivate therapeutic presence; (2) use a theoretical frame of reference informed by insights derived from mindfulness practice, the psychological literature on mindfulness, or Buddhist psychology (mindfulness-*informed* psychotherapy); or (3) explicitly teach patients how to practice mindfulness (mindfulness-*based* psychotherapy). Collectively, we refer to this range of approaches as *mindfulness-oriented* psychotherapy. (See the companion handbook to this volume, *Sitting Together: Essential Skills for Mindfulness-Based Psychotherapy* [Pollak, Pedulla, & Siegel, in press], for detailed guidelines on how to integrate personal practice, clinical theory, and meditation exercises into your clinical practice.)

Practicing Therapist

Aspiring clinicans often ask, "How do I become a mindfulness-oriented psychotherapist?" The simplest answer is, "Get the best clinical training you can find . . . and meditate." The psychological benefits of mindfulness meditation are now well established (Hill & Updegraff, 2012; Hofmann, Sawyer, Witt, & Oh, 2010; Hölzel, Lazar, et al., 2011; Keng, Smoski, & Robins, 2011), including benefits specifically for counselors and health care professionals (Irving, Dobkin, & Park, 2009; Krasner et al., 2009; Shapiro, Brown, & Biegel, 2007). Favorable effects include decreased stress and anxiety and enhanced counseling skills such as empathy and compassion (Buser, Buser, Peterson, & Serydarian, 2012; Christopher et al., 2011; Davis & Hayes, 2011). However, research on the impact of therapist mindfulness on patient outcomes remains inconclusive (Excuriex & Labbe, 2011; Ryan, Safran, Doran, & Moran, 2012; see also Chapter 3), perhaps because self-report mindfulness scales are used instead of examining how often a therapist actually meditates. Theoretically, practicing meditation should improve our clinical outcomes because meditation appears to activate brain pathways associated with therapeutic qualities such as body regulation, empathic attunement, balanced emotions, and response flexibility (D. Siegel, 2009a, 2010a).

Mindfulness practice seems related to *therapeutic presence*. Presence is a *way of being* in the consultation room (Brach, 2012a, 2012b; Bruce, Manber, Shapiro, & Constantino, 2010; Childs, 2007; Cigolla & Brown, 2011; Collum & Gehart, 2010; Geller & Greenberg, 2012). It is defined as "an *availability and openness* to all aspects of the client's experience, *openness to one's own experience* in being with the client, and the *capacity to respond* to the client from this experience" (Bugental, cited in Geller & Greenberg, 2002, p. 72). This process can lead a patient to "feeling felt" (Siegel, 2009a, p. 155). Carl Rogers (1961) considered therapeutic presence to subsume empathy, unconditional positive regard, and genuineness. Chapters 3–5 consider these important subjects in greater depth.

Mindfulness-Informed Psychotherapy

Therapists who practice mindfulness-*informed* psychotherapy have a theoretical frame of reference that is influenced by insights from the practice and study of mindfulness, but they don't necessarily teach mindfulness exercises to patients. Their work usually includes a relational/psychodynamic understanding that values the therapeutic *relationship* as a central vehicle of transformation. Mindful awareness is taught to patients through language, facial expressions, voice tones, and other often subtle microcommunications. Therapists may pay particular attention to ways in which their patients resist mental or emotional experience and how their patients could bring more mindfulness and acceptance to their lives.

Mindfulness-informed psychotherapy borrows ideas from both Western and Buddhist psychology, as well as from the personal experience of practitioners. A number of books integrate mindfulness concepts into relational psychotherapy: see Epstein (2008), Hick and Bien

(2010), Magid (2002), Molino (1998), Safran (2003), Stern (2004), Unno (2006), Wallin (2007), Welwood (2000), and Wilson and Dufrene (2011). Of course, given the potential of human connections to heal emotional wounds (Cozolino, 2010; Karlson, 2011; D. Siegel, 2010a), the therapy relationship can be considered a key component of all forms of mindfulness-oriented psychotherapy.

Mindfulness-Based Psychotherapy

Mindfulness-*based* therapists teach their patients mindfulness exercises that can be practiced between sessions. It makes sense for patients to practice mindfulness between sessions because the benefits of mindfulness appear to be *dose-dependent* (Lazar et al., 2005; Pace et al., 2009; Rubia, 2009), and 1 hour per week of therapeutic mind training may not suffice for some troubled individuals. Daily formal and informal meditation practice could increase that number to 6 or 7 hours per week. Mindfulness-based clinicians often include techniques drawn from the cognitive-behavioral tradition, and mindfulness-based treatment protocols have been developed for a wide range of psychological conditions (see the section "Mindfulness Model of Therapy" below). The proliferation of structured treatments is encouraging clinicians to experiment with mindfulness exercises in therapy even if they utilize only a few elements of a given protocol.

There are now hundreds of excellent professional and self-help books that teach skills applicable to mindfulness, acceptance, and compassion-based therapy, including these: Brach (2012b, 2013), Didonna (2009), Forsyth and Eifert (2008), Germer (2009), Hanson and Mendius (2009), Harris and Hayes (2009), Hayes and Smith (2005), Kabat-Zinn (1990, 2005, 2011), Kabat-Zinn and Kabat-Zinn (1998), Koerner and Linehan (2011), Linehan (1993b), McCown and colleagues (2011), Neff (2011), Orsillo and Roemer (2011), Pollak and colleagues (in press), Salzberg (2011), Segal, Williams, and Teasdale (2012), R. Siegel (2010), Stahl and Goldstein (2010), Willard (2010), and Williams, Teasdale, Segal, and Kabat-Zinn (2007).

THE MINDFULNESS MODEL OF PSYCHOTHERAPY

When therapists are asked, "What is your theoretical orientation?", they typically respond by mentioning cognitive-behavioral, psychodynamic/psychoanalytic, humanistic/existential, or systems-oriented psychotherapy. Increasingly, however, the answer seems to be *mindfulness*. Therapists who have not felt entirely at home with existing theories of psychotherapy often remark, after discovering mindfulness-oriented therapy, "Oh, that's what I do already—I just didn't know it!" So is it useful to think of mindfulness (including acceptance and compassion) as a new model of therapy?

Theories or models of therapy are an attempt to cluster together different therapies based on common characteristics. A psychotherapeutic model generally includes the following elements (Gurman & Messer, 2011; Wampold, 2012): (1) a worldview, (2) an understanding of pathology and health, (3) an approach to the practice of therapy, (4) an understanding of the therapeutic relationship, (5) identifiable mechanisms of action, (6) a range of treatment applications, (7) ethical considerations, and (8) research support.

An argument can be made that mindfulness is not a model of therapy at all, but merely a curative process that underlies all therapies. For example, don't systematic desensitization of a snake phobia, emotion regulation in DBT, and free association in psychoanalysis share the common process of *awareness* of *present experience* with *acceptance*? Additionally, perhaps mindfulness should be left alone—allowed to be an elusive, preconceptual construct that inspires direct, personal inquiry. Why try to systematize it, creating a straw figure that we subsequently need to dismantle to keep mindfulness alive in the therapy room? Perhaps mindfulness is really a "model of no-model" (P. R. Fulton, personal communication, January 12, 2013)? With these cautions in mind, we invite our readers to explore a *middle way*. Can mindfulness as a model of therapy advance our understanding, even as we hold our constructions lightly and return regularly to the moment-to-moment, felt sense of being in the therapy room?

Worldview

All psychological theories and therapies are embedded in metatheories or worldviews. Each of us has a world view, an inclination to perceive the world in a particular way (Johnson, Germer, Efran, & Overton, 1988). The metatheoretical frame of reference for mindfulness is *contextualism* (Hayes, 2002a; Pepper, 1942).

Worldviews explain the nature of reality (ontology), describe how we know reality (epistemology), account for causality, and contain a concept of personality. The contextual worldview makes the following assumptions:

- *Nature of reality*. Activity and change are fundamental conditions of life. The world is an interconnected web of activity.
- *How we know reality*. All knowledge of reality is constructed, created by each individual within a particular context. There is no absolute reality that we can know.
- *Causality*. Change is continuous and events are multidetermined. Apparent causality depends on its context.
- *Personality*. The personality is best described as single moments of awareness continuously cobbled together to form a functional, coherent whole.

Buddhist Psychology and Contextualism

The assumptions of Buddhist psychology closely correspond to the contextual worldview. We need only to turn to the three characteristics of existence in Buddhist psychology: (1) suffering (*dhukka* in Pali), (2) impermanence (*anicca*), and (3) no-self (*anatta*). *Suffering* refers to the dissatisfaction we inevitably feel when things are not as we wish them to be. Our likes and dislikes are co-constructed with the environment, but we can become substantially happier by changing our *relationship* to experience. The Buddhist notion of *impermanence* is precisely the ontology of contextualism—everything is constantly changing, including who we think we are. Finally, the condition of *no-self* (no fixed, separate self) is also the contextual view of personhood. The *self* is "an orchestra without a conductor" (Singer, 2005) consisting of many parts spontaneously co-arising and disappearing. (More will be said about these characteristics of existence in the following chapters.) Another key concept in Buddhist philosophy is *dependent co-origination*, which is a fancy expression for a multidetermined universe—causality in contextualism. The most accurate causal description of any event would be the *universe of interacting causes* at a particular point in time.

Pathology and Health

Buddhist psychology assumes that the way we construct our private realities is mostly delusional; we unconsciously elaborate on current events based on our past experience and current desires, leading to errors and unnecessary suffering. The antidote—mindful attention—allows us to understand our conditioning and to see things more clearly. What we see, however, is not some absolute truth; rather, we see *through* the delusion of our conceptualizations. Noticing this tendency toward delusionary thoughts and beliefs, we learn to hold our constructions more lightly.

This new, softer approach to our own conceptions extends to our view of symptoms. Complaints, problems, or symptoms are not stable entities that are to be diagnosed and then excised. What creates and sustains symptoms is *resistance*, that is, our instinctive, often preverbal tendency to ward off discomfort by tensing our muscles, thinking too much, drinking too much, or engaging defenses to reestablish our equilibrium. This kind of *experiential avoidance* (Hayes, Strosahl, & Wilson, 1999) may help in the short run, but it keeps us frozen in place and amplifies our difficulties in the long run. Consider the dictum, "What we resist, persists." A good example is "trying to fall asleep"—sustained efforts to fight sleeplessness are likely to result in chronic insomnia (see Chapter 10). Our level of emotional suffering can be measured by the gap between our expectations and reality (what *is*).

In contrast, consider this dictum: "What we can *feel*, we can heal." Psychological health in the mindfulness paradigm is the capacity to be with moment-to-moment experience in a spacious, deeply accepting way, even when it's difficult. This state of mind is accompanied by healthy psychological qualities such as psychological flexibility, resilience, authenticity, patience, connection, kindness, compassion, and wisdom.

Practice of Therapy

All patients come to therapy with a resistant relationship toward their symptoms. The two main questions in the mind of a mindfulness-oriented psychotherapist are likely to be:

1. What pain is the patient resisting?
2. How can I help the patient find a more mindful, accepting, and compassionate relationship to his or her pain?

Therapy can take an infinite variety of forms, such as an authentic, compassionate dialogue; exposure therapy; cognitive restructuring; meditation; engaging in healthy activities; or prescribing medication. Regardless of the form, from a mindfulness perspective we're not seeking a life free of pain, but rather greater emotional freedom through a mindful, accepting, compassionate relationship to our inevitable difficulties.

It's a tall order to expect our patients to embrace their emotional distress overnight. Rather, we want to help them gradually be open to what's bothering them, moving from *curiosity* (turning toward discomfort), to *tolerance* (safely enduring discomfort), to *allowing* (letting discomfort come and go), to *friendship* (finding hidden value in our difficulties). This process reflects progressively relinquishing resistance.

The Therapeutic Relationship

Mindfulness-oriented psychotherapy is *idiographic*—that is, the structure and process depend on the unique qualities and capacities of the individual patient in his or her world. Just as the instructions for mindfulness meditation are to "notice what is most vivid and alive in your field of awareness," the mindfulness-oriented therapist is attuned to what is most alive for the patient, as well as what is simultaneously transpiring in the therapist's moment-to-moment experience and the ever-changing therapeutic alliance. Part II of this book explores the therapeutic relationship in greater depth.

Mechanisms of Action

How does mindfulness work? Various processes have been proposed from theoretical and neurological perspectives. For example, Hölzel, Lazar, and colleagues (2011) have identified six mechanisms of action—effects of formal mindfulness practice—for which we have neurological evidence:

1. *Attention regulation*—stability of awareness in spite of competing input
2. *Body awareness*—noticing subtle sensations, being conscious of one's emotions
3. *Emotion regulation*—decreased reactivity, not letting emotional reactions interfere with performance
4. *Reappraisal*—seeing difficulties as meaningful or benign, rather than as all bad
5. *Exposure*—global desensitization to whatever is present in the field of awareness
6. *Flexible sense of self*—disidentification with emotions and increasing adaptivity

Additional mechanisms with empirical support include *self-compassion* (Hölzel, Lazar, et al., 2011; Neff & Germer, 2013), *values clarification* (sense of purpose) and *flexibility* (cognitive, emotional, and behavioral adaptiveness) (Hayes et al., 1999; Shapiro, Carlson, Astin, & Freedman, 2006); *emotion differentiation* (awareness of emotional experiences) (Hill & Updegraff, 2012); and *metacognitive awareness* (Cocoran, Farb, Anderson, & Segal, 2010).

An important neurobiological effect of mindfulness meditation is that it deactivates the *default mode network* (DMN). Even when the brain is at rest, several regions along the midline of the brain remain active (Gusnard & Raichle, 200; Mason et al., 2007). The DMN is active whenever our minds wander—which, according to one study, happens 46.9% of our waking lives (Killingsworth & Gilbert, 2010) and very often in meditation as well. What is the mind doing? Mostly it seems to be taking excursions into the past and the future, trying to resolve problems both real and imagined. These excursions are good for survival purposes but less helpful for happiness, and activity in the DMN correlates with anxiety and depression (Broyd et al., 2009; Farb et al., 2010). The DMN is responsible for *narrative processing* (I–me–mine). In contrast, the moment-to-moment awareness of mindfulness activates different brain structures associated with *experiential processing* (Farb et al., 2007; see also Chapter 15). All three forms of mindfulness meditation described earlier—focused attention, open monitoring, and loving-kindness/compassion—help to deactivate the DMN (Brewer, Worhunsky, et al., 2011) or change its functional connectivity (Taylor et al., 2013).

Treatment Applicability

Mindfulness can be used to treat a wide range of disorders, from psychosis (Braehler et al., 2012; Langer, Cangas, Salcedo, & Fuentes, 2012) to stress management at the workplace (Davidson et al., 2003). And as a universal, healing capacity, mindfulness is making bedfellows of diverse approaches to mental health such as CBT, psychodynamic psychotherapy, humanistic/existential psychotherapy, behavioral medicine, and positive psychology.

Cognitive-Behavioral Therapy

CBT is the form of treatment that has been most extensively investigated empirically. We are currently in the "third wave" of CBT (Hayes, 2011). The first wave was behavior therapy, focusing on classical, Pavlovian conditioning and contingencies of reinforcement. The second was cognitive therapy aimed at altering dysfunctional thought patterns. The third wave is mindfulness, acceptance, and compassion-based psychotherapy, in which our *relationship* to our experience (intentions, sensations, emotions, feelings, behaviors) gradually shifts in the course of therapy.

The four pioneering, empirically supported, multicomponent, mindfulness-based treatment programs are mindfulness-based stress reduction (MBSR; Kabat-Zinn, 1990), mindfulness-based cognitive therapy (MBCT; Segal et al., 2012), dialectical behavior therapy (DBT; Linehan, 1993a), and acceptance and commitment therapy (ACT; Hayes et al., 1999). Many other mindfulness programs have grown out of these templates or were developed for specific populations, conditions, or skills training. These include mindfulness-based relapse prevention (Witkiewitz & Bowen, 2010); mindfulness-based eating awareness training (Kristeller & Wolever, 2011); MBCT for children (Semple, Lee, Rosa & Miller, 2010); MBSR for teens (Biegel, Brown, Shapiro, & Schubert, 2009); mindfulness and acceptance-based behavioral treatment of anxiety (Roemer, Orsillo, & Salters-Pedneault, 2008; see also Chapter 9); mindfulness-based relationship enhancement (Carson, Carson, Gill, & Baucom, 2004); mindful self-compassion training (Neff & Germer, 2013); and compassion-focused therapy (Gilbert, 2010a, 2010b).

Furthermore, the field of CBT has largely adopted the core concepts of mindfulness even in treatments where the word *mindfulness* isn't used, such as the "unified protocol for the transdiagnostic treatment of emotional disorders," by David Barlow and colleagues, which consists of four modules familiar to mindfulness-oriented therapists: (1) increasing emotional awareness, (2) facilitating flexibility in appraisals, (3) identifying and preventing behavioral avoidance, and (4) situational and interoceptive exposure to emotion cues (see Farchione et al., 2012).

Psychodynamic Psychotherapy

As mentioned earlier, psychodynamic theorists have recognized the value of Buddhist psychology at least since the time of Carl Jung (1927/2000). Psychoanalysis has historically shared common features with mindfulness practice—they are both introspective ventures, they assume that awareness and acceptance precede change, and they both recognize the importance of unconscious processes. The next chapter explores more fully the commonalities and differences between a traditional psychodynamic/psychoanalytic approach to treatment and the mindfulness perspective.

Humanistic/Existential Psychotherapy

Mindfulness practice was originally intended to address the suffering of existential conditions such as sickness, old age, and death—not clinical conditions since this category did not exist in the Buddha's time. Mindfulness has much in common with humanistic psychotherapy, which broadly encompasses existential, constructivist, and transpersonal approaches (Schneider & Leitner, 2002). The existential approach, like Buddhist psychology, "emphasizes the person's inherent capacities to become healthy and fully functioning. It concentrates on the present, on achieving consciousness of life as being partially under one's control, on accepting responsibility for decisions, and on learning to tolerate anxiety" (Shahrokh & Hales, 2003, p. 78).

For example, Gestalt therapy emphasizes phenomenological exploration (e.g., "I see that you crossed your legs") without interpretation or valuation, leading to the goal of simple awareness (Yontef, 1993). Hakomi was one of the first therapies to explicitly train mindfulness through body awareness of feelings, beliefs, and memories (Kurtz, 1990). The *focusing* work of Eugene Gendlin (1996), especially his idea of the preverbal, bodily *felt sense* of a psychological problem, is strikingly similar to interoceptive awareness training in mindfulness meditation. Sensorimotor psychotherapy (Ogden, Minton, & Pain, 2006) and emotion-focused therapy (Greenberg, 2010) also carefully direct a patient's attention to arising emotional experience. Constructivist psychotherapies, such as narrative therapy (Leiblich, McAdams, & Josselson, 2004), share the mindfulness-oriented notion that each person's reality is co-created by the individual in interaction with the environment. Transpersonal therapy and Buddhist psychology hold the common assumption that the person is indivisible from the wider universe, a theme that is explored in later chapters.

Behavioral Medicine

The health benefits of mindfulness seem to derive from a less reactive autonomic nervous system—in short, being less stressed. For example, meditation training significantly reduces cortisol in response to acute stress, compared to relaxation training (Tang et al., 2007). Mindfulness practice may also help patients maintain healthy habits: Asthma patients may be able to detect emotional states that can trigger attacks, diabetes patients might be more conscientious taking their insulin, and obese patients may be able "urge surf" when they feel hungry rather than acting upon the urge to eat (Bowen, Chawla, & Marlatt, 2011).

Mindfulness meditation has also been shown to improve immune function (Davidson et al., 2003) and both compassion meditation and mindfulness meditation have been shown to reduce stress-induced inflammation (Pace et al., 2009; Rosenkranz et al., 2013). Mindfulness training is even being integrated into biofeedback (Khazan, 2013).

Randomized controlled trails have demonstrated improvement through mindfulness training for a long list of ailments/conditions: irritable bowel syndrome (Zernicke et al., 2012), coping with diabetes (Gregg, Callaghan, Hayes, & Glenn-Lawson, 2007), coping with cancer (Hoffman et al., 2012), chronic pain (Wong et al., 2011), work stress (Wolever et al., 2012), chronic fatigue syndrome (Rimes & Winigrove, 2011), stress eating (Daubenmier et al., 2011), HIV quality of life (Duncan et al., 2012), smoking cessation (Brewer, Mallik, et al., 2011), hot flashes (Carmody et al., 2011), insomnia (Gross et al., 2011), effects of chronic medical disease (Bohlmeijer, Prenger, Taal, & Culjpers, 2010), and substance use disorders (Witkiewitz, Bowen, Douglas & Hsu, 2013). (See also Chapter 10.)

Spirituality

Spirituality has many meanings; we understand the word to refer to an appreciation of intangible, yet meaningful, aspects of our lives. The intangibles may be God, a life force, values (love, truth, peace), interpersonal connections, or perhaps a sense of transcendence.

Buddhist psychology offers an *immanent* approach to spirituality, suggesting that what we seek is happening right in front of our noses, in intimate contact with day-to-day experience. The thrust of spiritual aspiration within this immanent approach is to embrace each moment more wholeheartedly. In contrast, a *transcendent* approach is a "trickle-down" methodology in which repeated experiences of mystical union (e.g., closeness to God) gradually make our daily experience more complete. Although mystical states may occur during mindfulness meditation, they are still considered mental events and, hence, are not accorded special status. From the mindfulness perspective, freedom from suffering occurs when no mental events can snag our consciousness, even ecstatic ones. A balanced approach to spirituality probably entails both immanent and transcendent aspects—we live fully in our daily experience as we reach for what is beyond.

Positive Psychology

In Buddhist psychology, mental health is seen as complete freedom from suffering, generally referred to as *enlightenment*. From this perspective, we are all mentally ill!

Western psychology has made remarkable progress in understanding the biological, psychological, and social roots of a troubled mind, but it has generally neglected positive experiences such as those characterized by well-being, contentment, love, courage, spirituality, wisdom, altruism, civility, and tolerance (Seligman & Csikszentmihalyi, 2000). Buddhist psychology is a comprehensive mind training program that cultivates happiness, and mindfulness is at the core of the program. There is a curious paradox in the Buddhist approach to positive psychology: The more fully we can embrace *un*happiness, the deeper and more abiding our sense of well-being. (Positive psychology is discussed further in Chapter 16.)

Ethical Issues

Buddhist psychology does not distinguish between "good" and "bad" actions, which are often merely social conventions, but rather between "wholesome" and "unwholesome" actions. *Wholesome actions* are those that diminish suffering for oneself and others, whereas *unwholesome actions* increase suffering. Mindful attention allows us to carefully observe the consequences of our thoughts, words, and deeds. This harming–nonharming ethical distinction is entirely consistent with a secular psychotherapeutic agenda.

Within mindfulness, acceptance, and compassion-based psychotherapy, *values* have a high priority. ACT, for example, includes exercises for patients to discover their core values ("What do you want your life to stand for?") and to identify obstacles to achieving those goals ("Are you willing to openly experience what gets in your way?"). Our *intentions* often determine our emotions, thoughts, words, and actions, so they are also an important object of awareness in both mindfulness training (Monteiro, Nutall, & Musten, 2010) and psychotherapy (see Chapter 6).

Research Support

In her 2003 review of the empirical literature on mindfulness, Ruth Baer wrote that mindfulness-based treatments are "probably efficacious" and en route to becoming "well established." Since then, numerous reviews and meta-analyses of the outcome research clearly indicate that mindfulness, acceptance, and compassion-based treatments effectively promote mental and physical health (Chen et al., 2012; Chiesa, Calati & Serretti, 2011; Davis & Hayes, 2011; Fjorback, Arendt, Ornbol, Fink, & Walach, 2011; Greeeson, 2009; Grossman, Niemann, Schmidt, & Walach, 2004;

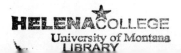

Hoffman et al., 2010, 2011; Keng et al., 2011; Piet & Hougaard, 2011; Rubia, 2009; Vøllestad, Nielsen, & Nielsen, 2012). However, although mindfulness research is quite advanced, there is still an urgent need for active control groups in outcome research and behavioral measures of mindfulness rather than reliance on self-report (Grossman, 2011; see also Chapter 15).

Exciting new areas of research are continuously emerging. Among them are topics closely associated with mindful awareness, such as the impact of compassion, wisdom, and ethical behavior on mental health. In the field of neurobiology, we might explore more precisely the links between specific, self-reported mind states and their neurological substrates, maybe even adding real-time functional MRI neurofeedback to augment the brain-changing effects of meditation. Can we learn to customize mind training techniques to alter dysfunctional brain patterns of individual patients? The impact of mindfulness practice on gene expression is another scientific frontier, perhaps even as stress prophylaxis for the next generation? We still need additional research on the short- and long-term effects of the meditating therapist on treatment outcome. Finally, it may be fruitful to investigate the outer reaches of mindfulness—to what extent can human beings actually regulate their attention, attitudes, and emotions, and how might these enhanced capacities impact the quality of our lives and society in general?

DOES MINDFULNESS MATTER TO THERAPISTS?

In light of the exponential increase in professional publications on mindfulness since the new millennium began, mindfulness clearly matters to clinical scientists and practitioners. Padmasambhava, an eighth-century Tibetan teacher, said that "when the iron bird flies, the dharma [Buddhist teachings] will come to the West" (cited in Henley, 1994, p. 51). We are currently witnessing an unprecedented convergence of the Eastern traditions of contemplative psychology with modern scientific psychology and psychotherapy.

Psychotherapists are on the vanguard of that important convergence. To have at our disposal psychological techniques drawn from a 2,500-year-old tradition that appear to change the brain, shape our behavior for the better, and offer intuitive insights about how to live life more fully, is an opportunity that is difficult to ignore. Only time will tell what we make of it.

The remainder of this book explores how the simple human capacity for mindfulness may enrich our understanding and effectiveness as psychotherapists. The next chapter considers commonalities and divergences between the Buddhist tradition of mindfulness and Western psychotherapy. Part II examines how mindfulness can be cultivated by the psychotherapist and its effect on the therapy relationship. Part III explores the application of mindfulness to particular psychological conditions and patient populations. Part IV discusses the ancient Buddhist teachings on mindfulness, summarizes what we've learned about mindfulness from neuroscience, and explores the future of mindfulness within positive psychology. Finally, the Appendix provides a glossary of Buddhist terms.

2

Buddhist and Western Psychology

Seeking Common Ground

Paul R. Fulton
Ronald D. Siegel

> Whether you can observe a thing or not depends
> on the theory which you use. It is the theory which
> decides what can be observed.
> —ALBERT EINSTEIN (1926, cited in Salam, 1990)

*M*indfulness has been practiced to alleviate human psychological suffering for over 2,500 years, primarily in the form of mindfulness meditation. Western psychotherapy is quite new by comparison, originating in a very different time and place.

Can we nonetheless expect to find parallels between an ancient Asian practice of mind training and modern Western systems of psychological treatment? Are the problems of ancient India and the modern West so different that comparing their systems of healing is misguided? Or, is there some universality to human psychology and suffering that both traditions address? How does each tradition understand suffering and its treatment? This chapter examines Buddhist psychology and Western psychotherapy side by side and considers how mindfulness itself may be seen as a common factor contributing to the efficacy of both Western psychotherapy and formal meditation practice.

Of course, there are many varieties of both psychotherapy and meditation, and it would be impossible to review all of these here. Instead, we go back to beginnings and explore core similarities and differences between mindfulness meditation in one of its earliest forms, practiced as part of *vipassana* or insight meditation, and the psychodynamic and behavioral traditions out of which most modern psychotherapy has developed. These two psychotherapeutic traditions are chosen with the open-eyed understanding that there are many more forms of treatment, and even the psychodynamic and behavioral traditions are themselves diverse.

ALLEVIATING PSYCHOLOGICAL SUFFERING

Like Western psychotherapy, mindfulness meditation developed in response to psychological suffering. And like psychotherapy, the domain of mindfulness practice includes thoughts, feelings, perception, intentions, and behavior. Given this focus, Buddhist psychology naturally shares with its Western counterpart a basic framework for understanding psychological disorders. Both systems (1) identify symptoms, (2) describe their etiology, (3) suggest a prognosis, and (4) prescribe treatment. This formulation is found in the Four Noble Truths, reported to be the Buddha's first formal teaching (see also the Appendix). Even in his own time, the Buddha likened mental suffering to illness, and his prescribed "treatment" as akin to medical care (Bhikkhu, 2012a).

Before looking at both traditions within this framework, let's consider a clinical example that we will use to illustrate subsequent points:

Richard was a young man of 23, living in New York. He was socially insecure in high school, didn't excel at sports, and was often intimidated by other guys. He had several girlfriends throughout high school and college, but still felt uncertain of his attractiveness.

During his last year at college Richard became involved with Jessica, an unusually attractive and sensual young woman. They began a torrid sexual relationship, complicated, however, by the background presence of her previous boyfriend, who had moved away to California.

Jessica invited Richard to live with her. This made him anxious, and he told her that he didn't feel ready. After many painful conversations, she announced that she, too, had decided to go to California.

Richard was devastated. His mind alternated between intense longing and wild jealousy, as he imagined Jessica passionately making love with her ex-boyfriend. He had trouble sleeping and couldn't concentrate at work. He started smoking marijuana daily in an effort to loosen his attachment to Jessica. Every time he saw a romantic couple or passed someone who looked at all like Jessica, he was overwhelmed with sadness and anger.

Richard found his weekly psychotherapy to be supportive, but he remained miserable. Desperate to do *something*, he signed up for a 2-week intensive mindfulness meditation retreat.

Few psychotherapy patients choose to try intensive retreat practice when in an emotional crisis. Nonetheless, Richard's experience will help us examine how psychotherapy and meditation traditions can address a typical psychological problem. By amplifying the effects of mindfulness, Richard's retreat experience offers a window into the workings of the practice.

Symptoms

The symptoms that are the focus of Western psychotherapy include both unpleasant subjective states such as anxiety and depression, and patterns of maladaptive behavior such as phobic avoidance and compulsions. The presence of symptoms is seen as an expression of an underlying disorder to be diagnosed and treated. Richard's difficulty concentrating, repetitive intrusive thoughts and feelings, sleep disruption, and dependence on illegal drugs are not atypical.

The "symptom" addressed by mindfulness meditation is simply the suffering that is inescapable to all who exist. No mental state, however pleasant, can be held indefinitely, nor can unpleasant experiences be avoided. However, we are so conditioned to avoid discomfort and seek pleasure that our lives are colored by a sense of "unsatisfactoriness," of something missing. Such suffering may or may not rise to the level of a clinical diagnosis. Rather, it arises from deep misunderstanding about the nature of our lives and our minds. In this sense, suffering is seen not as a symptom of an underlying disorder, but as a result of the nature of our relationship to the existential realities of life. Although clinicians are now using mindfulness meditation to treat a wide variety of psychiatric disorders, the practice was originally intended to address universal, clinical *and* nonclinical aspects of human suffering.

Interestingly, many of the "symptoms" that mindfulness meditation addresses do not become apparent to an individual until he or she begins mindfulness practice. For example, meditators notice that it is very difficult to sit and be fully present to the breath or other experience—they find that their minds are constantly leaping forward into fantasies of the future or reviewing memories of the past. They also notice an unsettling array of reactivity, anxieties, and other emotions that may not have been apparent before they attempted to be mindful. This is not unlike what patients entering psychodynamic psychotherapy experience, as they begin to feel that they are more neurotic than they had originally thought, defending against all sorts of thoughts and feelings, and enacting neurotic patterns based on past injuries.

There are parallels to this phenomenon in behavioral treatments as well. Self-monitoring or completing behavioral inventories can make clients suddenly aware of just how pervasive their symptoms are. Being asked to approach feared activities in the name of treatment can also amplify symptoms dramatically.

> Richard's gross symptoms—his depression and obsessive thoughts of his girlfriend—were initially quite obvious to him and others. When he started meditating intensively on retreat, however, he also noticed that he was frequently awash in intense fears whose object he couldn't identify. In addition, his mind began to fill with sexual and violent imagery, "alternating between porn and slasher films," as he put it. (We return to these movies shortly.)

Etiology

Modern mental health clinicians see the complex etiology of psychological disorders as involving biological, psychological, and sociological factors. Both psychodynamic and behavioral traditions have concluded that much human suffering is caused by distortions in thoughts, feelings, and behavior. Here they find some common ground with mindfulness meditation traditions, however much they differ on the causes of these distortions.

Psychodynamic psychotherapists generally presume that distortions in thought and feeling, born usually of childhood experience, have created psychological scars that warp our responses to present circumstances. The defenses we develop to selectively avoid some experiences prevent us from seeing current reality clearly and restrict our emotional range and behavior (McWilliams, 2011). For example, in his therapy, it was apparent that Richard was highly conflicted about intimacy and commitment. These difficulties arose from an inflated self-image ("Why should I *settle* on any one woman!") that compensated for his feelings of inadequacy ("I'm not really much of a man"). Both of these ideas had roots in his childhood relationships.

Whereas early behaviorists focused on problematic reinforcement contingencies (e.g., Skinner, 1974), later cognitive-behavioral clinicians (e.g., Beck, 1976; Ellis, 1962) came to see thoughts, feelings, and images as important links in the causal chain leading up to maladaptive behaviors. They developed techniques for noticing these mental events as they pass through consciousness, identifying "irrational" or unrealistic thoughts as a cause of suffering. For Richard, the most obvious cognitive distortions involved catastrophizing—thoughts such as "I'll never find another woman like Jessica" and "I'll never enjoy life again."

Mindfulness meditation shares the observation that holding a variety of distorted core beliefs leads to suffering, though it takes a more radical perspective that adhering to *any or all* fixed beliefs, regardless of how realistic they are, is a cause of distress. In Buddhist psychology, the most pernicious of these distorted beliefs are those related to who and what we are. In addition, Buddhism adds the idea of "grasping" or "clinging" as an underlying cause of all suffering.

At their roots, psychodynamic psychology, behavioral psychology, and Buddhist mindfulness all rest on the idea of conditioning. However, conditioning is addressed differently by each tradition. Psychodynamic psychology is interested in understanding an individual's unique conditioning and how it informs the present through the misapplication of early adaptive strategies, and how early experience shapes the sense the individual makes of him- or herself and the world. Behavioral psychology, like mindfulness practice, is less interested in the way an individual constructs meaning than in helping an individual to see the role conditioning—learned behavior and thoughts—plays in present day life, thereby empowering him or her to modify responses and achieve more satisfactory outcomes. Buddhist psychology, however, is less concerned with "my" conditioning than in understanding how *all* experience is conditioned from moment to moment. Healing arises as one learns about the nature of conditioning in all moments of experience.

What all three traditions share, then, is a recognition that suffering is not random, not a consequence of divine retribution for sin, not a test for entrance into a future paradise, nor a result of moral weakness, but a natural consequence of conditions. This recognition offers hope for relief, because suffering arises from causes that can be understood—and, often, modified. Human suffering is rendered as part of a lawful natural order.

Prognosis

The prognosis for treatment in psychodynamic and behavioral traditions of course varies with the disorder being treated, and the same can be said of mindfulness meditation. Although the apparent emphasis on suffering and impermanence in Buddhist psychology may seem gloomy, it is actually remarkably optimistic. Given the pervasiveness of "symptoms" of repeated striving, frequent disappointment, and difficulty being fully present that we observe during meditation practice, it can be hard at first to imagine that this method can actually alleviate suffering.

In fact, the prognosis, as described in the Buddhist literature, is radically optimistic. It states that although no one is immune from suffering, there is the potential for its complete alleviation, though this level of freedom is afforded only to fully enlightened beings. However, even in its more modest application, mindfulness offers a surprisingly good prognosis; if we can learn to embrace life as it is, we will suffer less. In the case of Richard, he realized at the beginning of his retreat how he was continually absorbed in his thoughts and fantasies. He saw the possibility of grounding himself in the immediate reality of moment-to-moment sensory experience—that he could take refuge in the present. This realization brought the first ray of hope he had felt since Jessica announced her departure.

Treatment

All three of the traditions we have been discussing involve a combination of introspection and prescribed behavioral changes in their efforts to alleviate suffering. A brief overview reveals several parallels.

Introspection

Psychodynamic psychotherapy, with its historical emphasis on free association, begins by exploring the contents of the mind. Patients are encouraged to say whatever comes into awareness, and this material is examined for patterns that reveal underlying thoughts and feelings. It is through gaining insight into these contents, correcting distortions based on early experience, and healing psychic wounds that reducing suffering becomes possible.

In traditional CBT, irrational thoughts are labeled, challenged, and replaced with more rational thoughts, leading to more adaptive, satisfying behavior. The origin of irrational thoughts is seen as less important than correcting them. This approach has broadened recently with the development of mindfulness and acceptance-based CBT treatments, which borrow from ancient mindfulness practice the idea that learning to *accept* painful experiences, rather than seeking to be rid of them, can be transformative (Hayes, Follette, & Linehan, 2011).

Mindfulness meditation involves repeatedly observing the mind, moment by moment. It is less concerned with the content of a particular thought, memory, or idea than whether it is held more firmly than it deserves, whether it is mistaken as something more *real* than a mere thought. Mindfulness differs from the introspection practiced in psychodynamic therapy by the nature of the objects chosen for attention and by the sort of attention brought to them. Repeatedly *being with* and accepting moment-to-moment experience in mindfulness practice eventually leads to *insight* into the workings of the mind, which, as we will see, brings relief from suffering. It also allows the mindfulness practitioner to increasingly and wholeheartedly embrace the full range of human experience.

Behavior Change

In recent years many psychoanalysts have recognized the limits of insight, and even "working through," to effect change, and have come to value deliberate efforts at modifying behavior. In behaviorally oriented treatment, deliberate, practiced action obviously assumes a central role.

The mindfulness meditation tradition also includes prescriptions for behavior change. At first glance, these appear to depart radically from Western psychotherapeutic traditions in their emphasis on morality. Both psychoanalysis and behaviorism differentiate themselves from Western religions and other cultural institutions in their relative neutrality around moral issues. By remaining nonjudgmental, therapists seek to allow patients to explore their true feelings, whether or not the feelings are ethical or socially acceptable. In most settings, therapists take a similarly nonjudgmental stance toward their patients' behavior, despite being legally mandated to report certain conduct to outside agencies.

"Treatment" in the Buddhist tradition is described in a group of principles known as the Eightfold Path (see the Appendix). Three of these eight principles—Right Effort, Right Mindfulness, and Right Concentration—describe mental practices, and another three refer explicitly to moral conduct: Right Speech, Right Action, and Right Livelihood. Although these ethical guidelines include many of the prohibitions found in Western religions, they are presented somewhat differently in the Buddhist tradition. Practitioners are invited to watch their minds carefully to see the impact that following or not following these guidelines has on the quality of consciousness. This approach actually parallels what might occur in dynamic or cognitive-behavioral psychotherapy, wherein the patient is invited to observe the consequences of his or her behavior in order to make better-informed choices. The guidelines are thus recommended as a foundation for mindfulness meditation practice based on the observation that an individual engaged in unethical activities will find peace and tranquility elusive. Conducting oneself in a moral fashion is therefore seen as a practical—even therapeutic—matter. As one's understanding deepens, ethical conduct becomes a natural expression of one's insight (see Chapter 6).

INSIGHT AND THE DISCOVERY OF TRUTH

Increased awareness is presumed to lead to greater psychological and emotional freedom in both the psychodynamic and mindfulness traditions. Neither tradition deliberately seeks to cultivate a particular feeling state, but rather sees a greater sense of well-being as a consequence of the freedom won by replacing mental distortions with clear understanding. Insight is both the vehicle and the goal of both practices. Although each tradition speaks differently about what constitutes "truth," it is only by moving toward such truth—and not by the cultivation of comforting illusion—that freedom becomes possible.

In psychodynamic psychotherapy, *insight* refers to the recognition of what was formerly hidden, unconscious, distorted, or otherwise defended against. In the meditation tradition, *insight* is often described as the direct perception of the characteristics of existence: notably, the changing nature of all phenomena, the absence of an enduring essence in phenomena, and the suffering that arises from not seeing all this clearly. As we see how suffering arises from our mistaken clinging, we naturally let go, much as we reflexively let go of a burning object.

In both traditions, insight involves seeing how we've mistakenly come to believe that thoughts and perceptions are more real than they are—we loosen our identification with our thoughts and emotions. We come to see how what was once taken as "reality" is actually a mental construction, and how our adherence to that construction gives rise to suffering. Insight involves loosening our grip on rigid beliefs and fixed positions. Experientially, it feels like beliefs loosen their grip on us.

One way in which insight leads to diminished suffering is by the light it sheds on the nature of suffering itself. We begin to see the difference between the arising of raw experience and our responses to it. In ordinary, nonmindful awareness, our experience of events is an undifferentiated confounding of event and reaction. With close, mindful attention, we can distinguish the event from the quality of our relationship to it, and in the process, see how suffering arises in the reaction (broadly called *grasping*), but is not inherent in the raw experience itself, opening new avenues for freeing ourselves of unnecessarily painful mental reactions (see also Chapter 10).

Adherence to fixed, mistaken, and unhelpful thoughts is identified as a source of distress in CBT as well. Various CBT techniques seek to loosen a patient's identification with a distorted or rigid thought, or to replace a maladaptive idea with one that permits greater flexibility. Insight per se is less the focus of CBT, though it shares with insight meditation and psychodynamic therapy the purpose of loosening the grip of unreflectively held ideas.

Points of Departure: Insight, Thought, and Language

Despite theses similarities, the role and importance of thinking differ in CBT, psychodynamic therapy, and mindfulness meditation. In CBT, erroneous thinking is seen as a cause of distress, and correcting mistaken ideas is a mechanism of relief. That is, tightly held thoughts and ideas cause suffering to the degree to which they are unrealistic.

In psychodynamic psychotherapy, words are a necessary currency for the conduct of treatment; thoughts and feelings must be symbolically represented in language to be communicated. However, language is understood to be an imperfect and often disguised vehicle for communicating subtle subjective experience. The words we speak are assumed to mask underlying meanings that may be hidden from the speaker. It is not the expressed thought per se—accurate or inaccurate—that requires examination, but the underlying motivations, conflicts, and desires lying in disguised form behind the spoken word. Although treatment must rely on language, the therapist and patient learn to listen *beyond* the spoken word "with the third ear," to use Reik's (1949) expression, to the unspoken, the avoided, the accidental—to find the reality that lies imperfectly revealed and imperfectly disguised in thought.

As a method, mindfulness meditation is distinguished from these other traditions by its near total abandonment of thinking. The practice differs from reflection by the continuous effort to set aside thinking—or at least to avoid getting caught up in it—in favor of watching the arising and passing of all sensory, perceptual, and cognitive events. In this stance, thoughts are not granted any special status, and are observed in their arising and passing just as one might note an itch or passing sound.

Across its history, Buddhist psychology has been part of a vigorous and sophisticated philosophical tradition, trading in logic and argument. Despite this, it has generally regarded thinking, as a means of knowing or cultivating insight, as suspect—for it is shaped and confined by the structure, categories, and lexicon provided by language and culture.

In meditation practice, because words are regarded as relatively limited and primitive, our efforts to understand the world through intellect are therefore superficial. Indeed, discursive thought actually obscures direct seeing into the nature of things. For individuals new to meditation, the idea that active, alert attention can exist without thought is difficult to fathom. However, with experience, it becomes clear that the process of knowing becomes more penetrating, subtle, and direct as thought is set aside; in its absence, a clear awareness emerges.

Mindfulness practice involves direct attention unmediated by language. "Content," or the narrative story as is understood in therapy, is given little weight. In fact, when we are hijacked by discursive thinking about the past or future, we have left the domain of mindfulness practice.

This difference in method is essential to understand where psychotherapy and mindfulness meditation depart from one another. Mindfulness meditation is *not* intended to replace one meaning with another, to reframe experience through interpretation, or to rewrite a personal narrative. By operating at a more fundamental and refined level of attention, mindfulness meditation has a more primal and transformative power. It has a quality of deep certainty and insistence that is beyond refutation.

> Richard had been struggling in therapy to rewrite his personal narrative, and the process was going slowly. What began to give him hope was the direct, felt experience during his meditation retreat that *reality* was not the same as his thoughts. Yes, he was haunted by images of Jessica reunited with her old boyfriend, and by powerful, often painful emotions; but these existed against a backdrop of the more immediate reality of the present moment—sensations in his body, the taste of food, the color of the grass and sky. Along with this experience came the dawning realization that *all* of his concerns were actually just thoughts and fantasies.

GOALS

An important contribution of ethnopsychology to the mental health field over the past half-century has been the realization of how our understanding of psychological health and pathology is highly culture-bound (Barnouw, 1973; Kleinman, Kunstadter, Alexander, Russell, & James, 1978). All systems of psychological healing are embedded in a cultural context and are inevitably expressions of cultural beliefs and values. They all share the goal of helping to restore an individual to "normal" development, as normalcy is understood in that culture, or fuller participation in his or her society. It is thus not surprising, given their different origins, that there are significant differences between the goals of modern Western psychotherapy and those of the mindfulness meditation tradition.

The Western View of the Self

One salient quality of the Western concept of the person and the self is its emphasis on separateness. In contrast to non-Western cultures' conceptions of the person that emphasize embeddedness in the clan, in society, and in nature, we have tended to hold a view that is radical in its emphasis on separateness (Lee, 1959).

In Western psychological traditions, healthy development has meant becoming well individuated, not overly dependent on others, knowledgeable of one's own needs, appropriately respectful of one's own boundaries, with a clear and stable sense of identity and a sense of self marked by cohesion and esteem. Although this view has been critiqued by contemporary relational theorists (e.g., Gilligan, 1982; Miller & Stiver, 1997), it continues to form the backdrop for both psychodynamic and behavioral therapies.

It is no surprise, then, that patients in the West often enter psychotherapy complaining that they're missing one or more of these qualities. Naturally, psychotherapy seeks to restore individuals to fuller participation in the culturally normative conception of selfhood.

Treatment plans often express these cultural ideals by noting that treatment is intended to "improve self-esteem . . . identify her own needs in a relationship . . . establish a more cohesive sense of self . . . establish boundaries and learn to maintain them in relationships," and so on. Our emphasis on the autonomy of the individual (often against evidence from our own social sciences) has led to a large technical vocabulary to describe disorders of the self and the consequent impairments in relationships.

Although the psychology field speaks of behavior that is *adaptive* or *maladaptive*, rather than *healthy* or *sick*, it is still difficult to avoid our assumption that distress is a matter of health relative to an ideal of selfhood: "If I am suffering, there is something *wrong with me*."

> Richard's therapist discussed Richard's difficulties with self-esteem, and how his sense of self had become dependent upon the affections of his girlfriend. Richard felt that if only his sense of self were stronger, he wouldn't be so affected by Jessica's departure.

The Self in Buddhist Psychology

In its original context of Buddhist psychology, mindfulness was not a technique to help restore a sense of self as we ordinarily understand it. Its purpose was not to become someone, but to cultivate insight into "no-self" (Pali: *anatta*). The goals of psychotherapy and mindfulness meditation depart significantly on this point. Mindfulness meditation is intended for nothing short of total psychological, emotional, moral, and spiritual emancipation, commonly called *enlightenment*. This concept is elusive because it cannot be described in psychotherapeutic terms. Although mindfulness offers benefits conventionally recognized as psychotherapeutic, it also reaches to a "treatment goal" that lies outside of our culturally constituted conception of the healthy self—*it seeks to illuminate the insubstantiality of all phenomena, including the self.*

This notion of the insubstantiality of the self is one of the most challenging for Westerners who delve into mindfulness. However, the idea is not alien in contemporary science. All of the elements of our bodies and minds are in constant flux, and simple reflection demonstrates that the boundary between the human body and its environment is actually quite arbitrary. Every time I eat, breathe, or go to the bathroom, millions of molecules that were once the external environment become "me," and vice versa. Similarly, we may view an ant colony or beehive as a collection of individuals, but the communities are more meaningfully understood as complex organisms, much as our body can be seen as a collection of interdependent cells (Thomas, 1995).

Through mindfulness meditation we come to experience ourselves as constant flux, a field of movement, always changing, without reference to some essence to whom it is happening. Even our cherished self is seen as an event that arises when supporting conditions exist, and passes when they do not; it is more *state* than *trait*. As insight into the self-as-process grows, we begin to see the folly of accepting our naïve adherence to the idea that the "I" is fixed, enduring, or even truly "mine." This insight greatly reduces our concerns for self-protection or self-aggrandizement, and allows us to respond compassionately to others as we perceive our genuine interdependence with all of creation (see Chapters 5 and 14).

Ironically, in Buddhist psychology, the successful effort to establish a more stable sense of identity, self-esteem, security, and the like, is often seen as the condition of *pathology*, a delusion from which the path of mindfulness meditation begins. It is therefore not uncommon for modern writers to suggest that the goals of mindfulness meditation begin where the Western concept of self-development ends (Boorstein, 1994). In this analysis, Western psychotherapy brings a person so far along a path of development, and mindfulness meditation continues the process from that point. "Ordinary human unhappiness," Freud's description of the best expectable outcome of psychoanalysis (Freud & Breuer, 1895/1961), is described as the point of departure for a mindfulness meditation practice.

These differences are a fundamental point of departure between the two traditions. Because Western psychotherapy rests on the notion of a stable and cohesive self, it regards development and healing and as processes of *becoming*—becoming well, less flawed, individuated, becoming *someone*. By contrast, Buddhist practice is about stopping our incessant efforts to firm up our sense of permanence and to rest in the uncertainty that we observe. It is to enable us to put to rest this need to *become*.

Although this difference in the goals of Western and Buddhist psychological practice is profound, in some ways the gap is not so wide. This is because the *no-self* of Buddhist psychology does not involve eliminating adaptive ego functions; rather it describes an observing ego that is much more objective and much less identified with individual desires than we typically see in Western psychotherapy (Epstein, 1995).

Let's consider what "well-adjusted" individuals, each with a well-developed "sense of self," look like in our psychotherapy traditions. They are flexible and open to new experiences; resilient, richly feeling the ups and downs of life; and capable of close, loving relationships, and compassion toward others. They are able to see things from multiple perspectives; able to identify goals and pursue them, unhindered by internal conflict or a compulsion to exaggerate strengths or minimize weaknesses.

Enlightenment is traditionally understood as the permanent extinction of greed, hatred, and delusion. However, there is no "litmus test" by which we can positively identify an enlightened person. All of the qualities described above would be expected to develop from successful practice in the Buddhist tradition. Whereas intensive meditation practice may lead to profound transformation in ways invisible to an outside observer, in many ways an *enlightened* person might look a lot like the *healthy* individual described above. We see this overlap in Richard's mindfulness meditation experience:

> Because he was practicing intensely, Richard had moments in which his discursive thoughts quieted. He felt at peace, part of his natural surroundings, marveling at small events, such as a flower opening toward the sun, or the complex patterns of cracks in a stone wall. Personal fears and desires diminished in importance. Interspersed with sadness, sexual arousal, and violently jealous images, he felt moments of love and compassion toward Jessica. Richard was experiencing moments of *no-self* that produced effects a lot like those we would expect from the *healthy self* his psychotherapy was cultivating.

Instincts, "Root Causes," and Human Nature

As introspective practices, it is not surprising that both psychodynamic and mindfulness meditation traditions have observed that impulses in the human heart give rise to suffering. (Early on, behavioral psychology differentiated itself from psychodynamic schools by declaring that, since these impulses were inferred rather than directly observed, they were not a suitable object of study.)

Freud originally posited two biologically hardwired instinctual drives—erotic and aggressive—as the source of human motivation. Because these drives are enduring vestiges from our evolutionary past, a well-adjusted person can at best only accommodate to them in a socially permissible fashion. The cost of such accommodation is the need for psychological defenses, which enable some gratification of drives while (ideally) enabling us to get along with others. Human nature can never transcend the aggressive, ignorant, insatiable demands of the id.

Buddhist psychology describes three "root causes"—greed, hatred, and delusion—that give rise to suffering (see Chapter 14). The similarity of the first two of these root causes to Freud's instincts is evident: erotic drive = greed; aggressive drive = hatred. Both psychodynamic and mindfulness meditation traditions describe how these forces wreak havoc on mental life, and both suggest ways to understand and address their influence. Where they depart, however, is the ultimate status of these forces.

Where Freud saw the drives as immoveable, Buddhist psychology teaches that they can be uprooted once and for all. This goal is surely a stretch, but the idea that the instincts could be eradicated suggests a potential for human freedom absent in Western psychological traditions. In the mindfulness meditation tradition, the expressions of these forces in the life of a meditator are seen as hindrances to be recognized, worked with skillfully, and in the process of being fully known, overcome. Although the permanent extinction of these drives may be the province only of a fully enlightened being, as these forces are exposed to awareness through mindfulness, they gradually become weakened, and we grow incrementally in understanding and compassion.

Seeing our work as part of a path to complete psychological freedom can infuse it with a kind of hope and enthusiasm that working toward ordinary human unhappiness, or the adaptive life skills of behavior therapy, may not.

METHODS

Exposure

A noteworthy area of overlap among psychodynamic psychotherapy, behavior therapy, and insight meditation is their emphasis on *exposure*. In essence, all three traditions identify our propensity to avoid what is unpleasant as a cause of suffering, and work to counteract it.

Behaviorists articulate this perspective clearly in exposure and response prevention treatments for obsessive–compulsive disorder, phobias, and other anxiety disorders (Abramowitz, Deacon, & Whiteside, 2011; Barlow, 2004; Foa, Franklin, & Kozak, 1998). They describe how we develop conditioned fears of situations that have been unpleasant in the past, avoid them, and consequently miss the opportunity for the fears to be extinguished. For example, a boy who is bitten by a dog may develop a generalized fear of all dogs. If he subsequently avoids contact with dogs, he misses the corrective learning that dogs can be friendly, and he thereby gets stuck in persistent, unnecessary fear and avoidance.

Treatment for such fear and "experiential avoidance," to use the term of Hayes, Wilson, Gifford, Follette, and Strosahl (1996), involves bringing a person into contact with the feared stimulus and maintaining that contact until he or she learns through experience that it is actually harmless. In the case of the dog, we bring the child closer and closer to a nonaggressive dog, teaching him or her to tolerate the fear that arises, until finally the child can play with it.

In psychodynamic psychotherapy, exposure begins with discussion of thoughts, feelings, and memories that have been avoided because they are unpleasant or shameful—interoceptive exposure. In the trusting environment of the therapeutic relationship, patients learn that formerly forbidden memories or feelings are tolerable, and they come to accept them. In this way a patient becomes much freer, and he or she can relax the neurotic defenses associated with symptoms. As mentioned earlier, in current practice this exposure within the office is often followed by encouragement to face feared or challenging situations outside of the therapy hour.

Insight meditation functions similarly to psychodynamic psychotherapy in this arena. As one sits and follows the breath, inevitably thoughts, feelings, and images arise. The practitioner notices the persistent tendency to hold on to pleasant events and to reject unpleasant events—in short, to try to control experience. By following the instruction to neither pursue nor push away these experiences, meditators learn that they can tolerate unpleasant mental contents, that they need not fear them (Orsillo & Roemer, 2011; see also Chapter 9). The emphasis is on *knowing*, without any special need for expression, abreaction, or catharsis.

Through this practice, the meditator becomes comfortable with the contents of his or her mind. In this sense, mindfulness is like exposure therapy without discriminating among the objects and events to which one is being exposed.

On retreat Richard was visited by intense sadness and fear, erotic memories, and violent images involving the dismembering of Jessica and her ex-boyfriend. Sometimes his emotions were experienced as pain in the body—tightness in the throat, muscle tension elsewhere. Hours would pass with disturbing erotic and violent scenes playing like movies inside his head. Richard nonetheless tried to follow his instructions—he allowed the sensations and images to arise and neither pushed them away nor distracted himself.

Over time, things began to change. His aversion to these experiences relaxed. His grieving over Jessica's decision seemed to be accelerated by his unflinching exposure to the images and feelings. It was a cathartic experience, albeit a silent one. By the end of the 2 weeks Richard felt much more at peace.

The Interpersonal World

Most psychodynamic and behavioral psychotherapy is dyadic, occurring within a significant interpersonal relationship. Group and family treatments are also very interpersonal. Relationship issues are therefore very likely to come up and be addressed in psychotherapy.

In contrast, the traditionally solitary nature of meditation, and its focus on the present moment, may influence what material is *unlikely* to arise. The lore among meditators is replete with stories of individuals who fall into familiar neurotic interpersonal conflicts despite years of intensive meditation practice. Indeed, meditation practice can be misused as an escape from the turmoil of intimate relationships.

In classical psychodynamic psychotherapy, the analysis of transference is the principal tool of treatment. Although mindfulness meditation traditions enlist the relationship between a student and teacher as an essential element of practice, and may use the presence of other meditators for support, meditation is primarily solitary and makes no effort to understand transference and countertransference. Furthermore, Buddhist practice was first taught to monastics, and although it is now more available to lay practitioners, it has never placed primary emphasis on navigating the ordinary difficulties faced by laypeople in the worlds of work and love.

Structure and Support

Both meditation and psychotherapy advance by enabling the individual to examine his or her thoughts, feelings, and actions, without recourse to habitual avenues of escape and avoidance. Both traditions provide supports to facilitate this movement toward difficult experience.

Supports in Psychotherapy

The most essential support in psychotherapy is arguably the quality of the therapeutic relationship, particularly the therapist's stance of openness and acceptance (see Part II). In the face of genuine fearlessness on the part of the therapist, the patient may be emboldened to stand closer to painful or humiliating experiences and memories. So, too, do qualities of empathy, sustained interest, and genuine care, tempered by professional neutrality, establish an environment conducive to a therapeutic alliance. This is the "holding environment" described by D. W. Winnicott (1971).

The trust that is crucial to therapy is supported by the integrity of the therapist. Elements of this trust are codified in the therapist's absolute commitment to confidentiality and a clear statement of its limits (e.g., in the face of serious, imminent harm). Establishing and maintaining consistent appointment times (both starting and ending) also lend a sense of reliability. Genuine integrity is the basis of trust (see Chapter 6). Finally, the mutual trust in the efficacy of the therapy process and methods can enable patients to suspend some of their ordinary caution (Meyer et al., 2002).

Elements introduced by behavior therapy also lend support. The use of rating scales and inventories help to lend a sense of scientific legitimacy to the work. When "homework" is used in psychotherapy (and most therapists do so in some form; see Kazantzis & Dattilio, 2010; Scheel, Hanson, & Razzhavaikina, 2004), the patient can become more confident in his or her ability to continue the therapeutic work independently.

Supports in Meditation Practice

Mindfulness meditation is a well-developed practice, refined over centuries. As a result, many "bugs" have been worked out. Meditation practice can be arduous at times, but there are many sources of support for the individual's efforts, including elements of the structure of practice:

• *Traditional teachings as a map:* A student of meditation can turn to a long history of formal teachings for guidance. Though the focus of practice is one's own unique experience, these teachings describe where the practice is headed, what one may expect, and methods suited to different obstacles that may arise. These teachings provide a way to understand difficult or frightening experiences, so the student need not feel that he or she has "fallen off" the path. The map of these teachings provides a degree of predictability that is fortifying.

• *The community of like-minded people:* Historically, a community of monks and nuns has assured the continuity of instruction and practice. Today in the West, a community of like-minded individuals can similarly be enormously supportive. An individual is simply less likely to bolt from a difficult session of meditation if it is conducted in a room full of other silent meditators. Also, this practice can seem unusual or even exotic; being with others helps us to feel that the practice is legitimate and worthwhile. Through discussion with fellow meditators, one is also reassured to learn that the difficulties encountered are not unique; others endure physical pain, restlessness, doubt, and sleepiness.

• *Others' experience as models:* The example of countless others who have benefited over the course of centuries provides inspiration that can carry us through periods of difficulty. Having firsthand contact with an experienced teacher can be especially inspiring if that individual is wise and compassionate. An experienced teacher can also provide "customized" advice during difficult periods.

• *Success in practice as reinforcement:* As in the acquisition of any skill, having some success in mindfulness practice reinforces one's efforts. The task of paying sustained attention can seem impossible at first. However, the taste of even a little clarity is enormously rewarding and reinforcing. Once a student begins to experience insight, the practice becomes compelling. At a certain stage, mindfulness becomes fascinating, regardless of the contents of awareness.

• *Concentration* helps to contain the tumultuousness that can arise in mindfulness practice. Concentration grows naturally alongside mindfulness in meditation and is stabilizing, calming, and fortifying. With this growing stability, we become more adept at allowing attention to rest on difficult experiences without flinching. *Physical posture*—usually sitting upright with a straight spine—similarly supports practice efforts, helping us to remain alert, and feel "held" in facing whatever arises in our awareness (Suzuki, 1973).

• *Compassion and self-compassion:* One result of mindfulness meditation is enhanced feelings of interconnectedness. As we come to see that our desire for happiness and well-being, as well as our suffering, are shared by all others, compassion naturally arises for both ourselves and all living beings. This compassion helps us to be less judgmental of our meditation practice and to realize that the benefits of practice extend beyond ourselves.

EPISTEMOLOGY

Another important area of overlap between Western psychotherapeutic and mindfulness meditation traditions involves their methods of discovery. These methods are particularly worthy of attention in the current climate that emphasizes the search for empirically supported treatments.

We saw earlier that psychodynamic, behavioral, and mindfulness traditions all share an interest in seeing reality clearly, though they differ somewhat in their conclusions about that reality. Interestingly, although it predates the Western Renaissance by over two millennia, the Buddhist psychology from which mindfulness practice derives has a surprisingly modern attitude toward discovering "truth."

Insight meditation uses direct observation as the means for understanding the workings of the mind. Although maps and guidelines based on the observations of others are taught, the tradition strongly emphasizes that one should not accept any principle without first verifying it in one's own experience. While not based on the modern scientific experimental method, mindfulness meditation nonetheless is part of a highly empirical tradition.

Psychoanalysis, from which psychodynamic psychotherapy emerged, has historically seen itself as an empirical, scientific discipline. From Freud onward the enterprise has been interested in finding truth through observation. Freud believed that the method of psychoanalysis could yield scientific truth. However, modern critics have pointed out that many psychodynamic postulates cannot readily be tested experimentally, and more recent theorists have moved toward a more hermeneutic approach to arriving at meaning and "truth."

Of course, both psychodynamic traditions and Buddhist psychology have exhibited the human tendency to create orthodoxies, so that at times each has relied on received teachings in a way that inhibits discovery. Nevertheless, the direct apprehension of truth as revealed in experience is the most valued in the Buddhist tradition; no axioms or dogma, no matter how supported by accumulated data or promulgated by high authority, are to be accepted until tested in the laboratory of one's own experience. As the ninth-century Buddhist master Lin Chi reportedly put it, "If you meet the Buddha on the road, kill him"—answers are to be found within (Harris, 2006, p. 73).

Behavior therapy is a radically empirical tradition in a different sense, and has long tested its postulates experimentally. It differs from the other two traditions in an important regard: Rather than encouraging each practitioner or client to see if principles apply to his or her experience, the behavioral tradition looks to replicable peer-reviewed experiments to identify general principles that can be applied across individuals (though every treatment also becomes its own experiment).

Scientific methodology seeks to predict and control phenomena through observation, hypothesis generation, experimentation, and replication. It embodies an underlying belief consistent with the Western rational tradition that what is true is true independent of our apprehension of it; truth is objective.

The truth sought in Buddhist meditation is of a different sort. The purpose of systematic investigation in meditation is not to create a replicable model of reality that holds up to scientific scrutiny. Rather, it seeks understanding for a single purpose: to assist the individual practitioner to become free of suffering.

Despite these differences in approach, we're currently entering a new period in which principles of Buddhist psychology and effects of meditation practice are being examined by Western science. And the Dalai Lama (2005a) has repeatedly said, "If science proves some belief of Buddhism wrong, then Buddhism will have to change." It remains to be seen how these two great empirical traditions will continue to influence one another.

Psychotherapy and mindfulness are both concerned with finding relief from psychological suffering, making the effort to find common ground worthwhile. A respectful appraisal of each illuminates its respective strengths and limitations, helps to avoid reducing one to the other, and alerts us to the dangers of overlooking the integrity of each practice within its own tradition. Having tried to take such precautions, we can now turn to the ways mindfulness can expand and deepen the practice of psychotherapy.

Part II

The Therapy Relationship

*P*sychotherapy is, above all, a relational process. While mindfulness practices were refined for over two millennia by monks, nuns, and hermits, they are now proving themselves to be remarkably useful for developing our capacity for interpersonal relationships. It turns out that Buddhist psychology, from which many mindfulness practices derive, also contains valuable frameworks for structuring and deepening our connections with one another.

Chapter 3 explores mindfulness techniques as clinical training—how they enhance therapeutic presence, cultivate empathic attunement, and promote cognitive flexibility—all important factors in positive treatment outcome. Chapter 4 builds on this foundation, illustrating how mindfulness practices can be used to increase attention, how the seven factors of awakening in Buddhist psychology can help us to be more fully present in our work, and how practices designed to cultivate compassion can help prevent burnout and deepen our connection with patients. Chapter 5 then explores what may arguably be the West's greatest contribution to the evolution of mindfulness: practices designed explicitly to cultivate relational or interpersonal mindfulness in order to deepen our personal and professional relationships. Finally, Chapter 6 investigates how Buddhist ethical principles, which are traditionally considered the foundation of meditation practice, can help us to deepen our work as psychotherapists.

3

Mindfulness as Clinical Training

Paul R. Fulton

> The art of healing comes from nature, not from the
> physician. Therefore, the physician must start from
> nature, with an open mind.
> —PARACELSUS (1493–1541)

*T*here are many ways that mindfulness can be integrated into therapy, from the implicit influence of therapists' own mindful awareness of what happens in treatment to explicitly teaching mindfulness exercises to patients (see Chapter 1). This chapter addresses the implicit end of the spectrum—the influence of the therapist's own mindfulness practice—and argues for the value of mindfulness as training for clinicians irrespective of the theoretical approach or techniques used in treatment.

Mindfulness practice is increasingly being incorporated into clinical training (Aggs & Bambling, 2010; Christopher & Maris, 2010; Moore, 2008). Most research on the therapeutic application of mindfulness has focused on its use as a clinical intervention for specific disorders, but recent work is beginning to address the impact of mindfulness practice, especially MBSR training, on health care workers themselves (Bruce, Young, Turner, Vander Wal, & Linden, 2002; Cohen-Katz et al., 2005; Galantino, Baime, Maguire, Szapary, & Farrer, 2005; Irving et al., 2009; Martin-Asuero & Garcia-Banda, 2010; McCollum & Gehart, 2010; Shapiro, Astin, Bishop, & Cordova, 2005; Shapiro, Schwartz, & Bonner, 1998; Wang & Gao, 2010; Warneke, Quinn, Ogden, Towle, & Nelson,

2011). Not surprisingly, the research suggests that clinicians can reap the same beneficial effects of mindfulness training as has been previously reported for nonclinicians, such as reduced anxiety and depression (Shapiro et al., 1998), decreases in mood disturbance (Rosenzweig, Reibel, Greeson, Brainard, & Hojat, 2003), and increased empathy and self-compassion (Shapiro et al., 2005, 2007). Thus far, less research attention has been paid to the impact of the therapist's own level of mindful awareness and daily mindfulness practice on treatment outcome.

WHAT MATTERS IN PSYCHOTHERAPY?

To understand how therapists' own mindfulness might influence their patients, it may help first to consider what actually matters in treatment. One approach to identifying key factors in effective therapy is to develop and refine interventions whose efficacy can be established in randomized controlled trials (e.g., Clark, Fairburn, & Wessely, 2008; Siev, Huppert, & Chambless, 2009). By contrast, others have argued that effective treatment is due more to common factors such as the personal qualities of the clinician and the therapy relationship (Duncan & Miller, 2000), rather than particular techniques or approaches (Hatcher, 2010; Leichsenring, 2001; Luborsky et al., 2002; Rosenzweig, 1936; Stiles, 2009). Proponents of the common-factor approach often regard therapy as more art than science.

Although this debate is likely to go on for years, there is a *middle path* between these views, expressed in the conclusion of a large task force on effective treatment relationships (Norcross & Lambert, 2011, p. 1): "Like all complex human endeavors, many factors account for success and failure: the patient, the treatment method, the psychotherapist, the context, and the relationship between the therapist and the patient." Based on their review of research across these factors, the authors note, "the therapy relationship accounts for why clients improve (or fail to improve) as much as the particular treatment method" (p. 2). This chapter focuses specifically on the potential contribution of mindfulness to effective treatment relationships.

Mindfulness, Common Factors, and the Treatment Relationship

A number of meta-analyses has established a positive association between the treatment alliance and therapy outcome (Horvath, Del Re, Flückiger,

& Symonds, 2011; Tryon & Winograd, 2011; Wampold, 2001), even in structured CBT (Waddington, 2002) and pharmacological treatment (McKay, Imel, & Wampold, 2006). Importantly, it is the *patient's* assessment of the alliance that seems to be more predictive of positive outcomes than the therapist's view (Horvath et al., 2011; Orlinsky, Ronnestad, & Willutzki, 2004).

Meta-analyses have established the value of *empathy* in effective treatment relationships across theoretical orientation, symptom severity, and treatment format. Although empathy is an elusive factor to measure, "Overall, empathy accounts for as much and probably more outcome variance than does specific intervention" (Bohart, Elliott, Greenberg, & Watson, 2002, p. 96), even in protocol-based and pharmacological treatment (Wampold, Imel, & Miller, 2009). Some authors have gone so far as to claim that the relationship *is* the treatment (e.g., Duncan & Miller, 2000). Here, too, the patient's assessment of the therapist's empathy is more predictive of success than the therapists' own valuation (Elliot, Bohart, Watson, & Greenberg, 2011). It's not surprising that the qualities patients attribute to therapists in positive treatment alliances include empathy, warmth, understanding and acceptance, positive regard, collaboration, and consensus (Norcross & Wampold, 2011), and are short on behaviors such as blaming, ignoring, or rejecting (Lambert & Barley, 2001). Other meta-analyses of successful therapeutic relationships have focused on positive regard (Farber & Doolin, 2011), successful repair of ruptures in the therapeutic alliance (Safran, Muran, & Eubacks-Carter, 2011), and the genuineness of the therapist and the relationship (Kolden, Klein, Wang, & Austin, 2011).

Therapists differ along these dimensions; some are more effective than others (Huppert, Bufka, Barlow, Gorman, & Shear, 2001; Kim, Wampold, & Bolt, 2006), and these differences may outweigh the particular treatment method or theory embraced by the therapist (Lambert & Ogles, 2004; Luborsky et al., 1986; Wampold, 2001).

Given the importance of the therapy relationship, it stands to reason that methods for creating a strong alliance should be taught to clinicians to at least to the same extent as theory and technique. However, current graduate training programs generally emphasize models of treatment and technique over the less tangible qualities of the therapist, perhaps because it's simply easier to do so. Cultivating beneficial personal qualities in clinical trainees may be more complex and subtle than gaining knowledge of theory and specific treatment techniques (Crits-Christoph & Gibbons, 2003; Crits-Christoph, Gibbons, & Hearon, 2006; Lazarus, 1993; Norcross & Beutler, 1997). Instruction in therapy skills is essential, but the larger challenge is to find a way to help cultivate qualities associated with strong treatment relationships.

MINDFULNESS AS ADVANCED TRAINING

Mindfulness cultivates numerous qualities suited to establishing a strong therapeutic alliance. Factors that support the treatment relationship include the cultivation of attention (Lutz et al., 2009; Valentine & Sweet, 1999), compassion and empathy (Neff, 2003; Sweet & Johnson, 1990), therapeutic presence (Brown & Ryan, 2003; Geller & Greenberg, 2002; Thomson, 2000), self-attunement (Bruce et al., 2010), openness and acceptance (Bishop et al., 2004), dispassionate self-observation and self-insight (Chung, 1990), a broader perspective on suffering (Deikman, 2001), nonattachment (Tremlow, 2001), and a range of other factors (Henley, 1994; Siegel, 2009a).

To date, evidence establishing the link between a therapist's mindfulness and clinical outcomes is limited and equivocal, mostly resting on qualitative data and a small number of relatively brief trials. The most compelling study randomly assigned a group of day treatment therapists to practice Zen meditation for 9 weeks. At the end of this period, their clients showed greater improvement than those treated by nonmeditators on a number of dimensions, including symptom reduction, rate of change, and general well-being (Grepmair et al., 2007). Other research has shown either a positive impact of therapists' mindfulness on treatment outcome (Padilla, 2011), no impact (Stratton, 2006), or in some studies, negative correlations (Vinca & Hayes, 2007). For example, Stanley and colleagues (2006) found that therapists' mindfulness predicted *less* improvement in global functioning and symptom reduction. (These negative findings may be an artifact of the difficulty in measuring mindfulness: More mindful individuals tend to underestimate their level of mindfulness, whereas less mindful subjects frequently overestimate it [Davis & Hayes, 2011].)

Yet, it seems natural to infer that the influence of mindfulness on the therapist is consistent with the qualities underlying a successful treatment relationship. For example, if mindfulness cultivates empathy, and empathy is associated with an effective treatment relationship, it seems plausible that a therapist's mindfulness would positively influence outcomes. The growth of therapists' interest in mindfulness training suggests that this view may be gaining in popularity. As we wait for more nomothetic, larger-sample research, we can take a closer look at our own, qualitative therapy experience and that of mindfulness-oriented therapists in clinical practice. Some skills and qualities of mind that seem to be relevant to the treatment relationship and are enhanced by mindfulness practice are described below and in the three subsequent chapters.

Paying Attention

Every clinician knows the experience of a wandering mind during therapy. A colleague described attending a supervision group as a young trainee where a senior psychiatrist spoke in a confessional tone about his difficulty paying attention to his patients. The supervisor said that his mind wandered off regularly during each therapy session. The trainee, as a seasoned meditator, was shocked; she took for granted that therapists could pay close attention to their patients. "How could they do psychotherapy without paying attention?"

Inattention may be a response to what is—or is not—happening in the therapy hour. An emotionally disengaged patient can leave the therapist similarly distracted and bored. Or a therapist made anxious by the material offered by the patient may react by "tuning out," becoming restless, sleepy, or otherwise partially absent. The therapist's own inquiry, "What's happening with this patient that is making it hard for me to stay interested?", may or may not be sufficient to shake off the shroud of disinterest.

Some experienced therapists fall victim to inattention even more easily than eager novices, yet they can be adept at covering for lapses of attention by, for example, asking a probing question in a timely way. We can fake attention, believing that the patient is none the wiser, and therapy can continue in a lackluster way. By contrast, genuine interest and close attention are hard to fake. When we are alert and focused, our energy is quickened, and both parties are fully alert to the work at hand. A therapist's alertness may be enhanced by an emotionally engaged patient or the riveting account that he or she delivers, but we can't always rely on our patient to enliven our attention.

Mindfulness practice is an antidote to the wandering mind, and improved attention has been posited as an underlying mechanism of action in mindfulness meditation (Carmody, Baer, Lykins, & Olendzki, 2009; Hölzel, Lazar, et al., 2011; Lutz, Slagter, Dunne, & Davidson, 2008; Shapiro et al., 2006). Although it falls short of a permanent cure for daydreaming, mindfulness strengthens our capacity for attention (Jha, Krompinger, & Baime, 2007; van den Hurk, Giommi, Gielen,

Speckens, & Barendregt, 2010). Since we can be mindfully aware of any psychological event—including boredom or anxiety—every moment of therapy is an opportunity to practice mindfulness.

When bored, many of us seek excitement or stimulation. It's possible to create an entire lifestyle based on seeking thrills and novelty, such that ordinary life can feel aversively dull. Mindfulness meditation takes a different approach to generating interest. In training the mind to be attentive to the smallest details of experience, we become sensitive to simple events such as the taste of food, the sensations of walking, or the play of light on our office furniture. When we are alert, fascination is a natural response—even boredom flees in the face of interest.

Wholehearted attention from others is surprisingly uncommon, even worth *paying* for in psychotherapy. When we meet someone who is interested and utterly focused on our words, we feel that something special has occurred. We *know* we've been heard in an uncommon way. To pay genuine, wholehearted attention is a gift we can offer to anyone whom we encounter, whether children, partners, colleagues, or patients. In clinical encounters, such close attention vivifies the session. Fortunately, this level of attention can be learned, practiced, and deepened. Mindful attention, applied to the moment-to-moment therapeutic interaction, may enable us to *notice* when we have taken empathic leave from our patients, so that the breach can be repaired (Bruce et al., 2010). Such repairs are positively related to psychotherapy success (Safran et al., 2011).

There is a Japanese Zen expression, *ichigo ichie*, which translates roughly as "one opportunity, one encounter." It points to the fact that every moment is unique, unprecedented, and irreproducible. When we approach each moment with this understanding, it reminds us to pay attention to each new moment with fresh eyes.

Affect Tolerance, Emotional Regulation, and Fearlessness

When we practice mindfulness, strong emotions will be among the invited and uninvited guests. Intense feelings can be welcomed with the same attitude of acceptance and interest as any other mental event. Although strong emotions may be overpowering, when we set aside our fear and resistance, we discover that no emotion is ever permanent and that we can tolerate more than we suspected. *Tolerance* may be a poor word to use because it connotes a clenched-teeth, white-knuckle relationship to the emotion, as though we can muscle our way by sheer strength and willpower. *Mindful* tolerance is marked by a *softening into* and *embracing of* the experience, carrying the qualities of allowing and friendship (see Chapter 1). By becoming mindful of the fear of being overwhelmed, we may be less intimidated or possessed by it. Feelings are not so much endured as known.

Affect tolerance (also sometimes called *emotional regulation*) was first described in psychoanalytic terms by Elizabeth Zetzel (1970) and is currently considered a therapeutic mechanism in mindfulness meditation (Garland, Gaylord, & Fredrickson, 2011; Hölzel, Lazar, et al., 2011). Because of the importance of body sensations in the experience of emotion (that's why emotions are called *feelings*!), there is growing reason to believe that a new relationship to our bodily sensations—being more aware and accepting—can help us regulate emotion (Bechara & Naqvi, 2004).

Unsurprisingly, our own emotional awareness appears to be associated with our understanding of the emotional lives of *others* (Decety & Jackson, 2004). For example, Dan Siegel (2007) argues that our ability to become attuned to ourselves draws on the same neural circuitry that enables attunement to others; paying attention to ourselves appears neurologically related to empathic attunement to others. *Attunement* describes a relationship in which one person focuses on the internal world of another in such a way that the other "feels felt," understood, and connected (Bruce et al., 2010; Siegel, 1999). This process may rest on mirror neurons, which in lower primates have been found to fire in mimicry of observed movements of another (Carr, Iacoboni, Dubeau, Mazziotta, & Lenzi, 2003). That is, observing another's conduct seems to activate those neurons in the observer much as if the observer had conducted the activity him- or herself. Although this mechanism has not been yet demonstrated in human brains, it may provide a biological basis for understanding empathy and social conduct.

Bruce and colleagues (2010) suggest that mindfulness is a form of attunement to oneself. Furthermore, they speculate, "A psychotherapist's relationship to himself or herself has a direct bearing on his or her relationship to patients" (p. 87). That is, they hypothesize that therapists' own mindfulness enables attunement to their patients and, consequently, supports their patients' attunement to themselves.

Siegel (2007) suggests that mindfulness supports our ability to both be resonant with another's experience while simultaneously helping to reinforce the self-regulatory circuits that protect us from becoming overwhelmed. These are both crucial skills for a therapist—to be empathically connected, but to also maintain balance to avoid becoming flooded by another's pain.

Affect tolerance and emotional regulation are ordinarily considered skills to be cultivated by patients, though they are enormously important for therapists as well; if we cannot tolerate our own difficult emotions, we may find it difficult to sit with our patients' powerful affects. We are likely to distance ourselves from ourselves and then from our patients. This can all occur unconsciously.

> After several months of therapy, a middle-age man began to describe abuse he had suffered as a child, with great difficulty, in a tense and flat manner. The story he told was horrifying, and the therapist, a seasoned middle-age woman, was overwhelmed. She felt herself recoil and turn away from the graphic nature of what she was told. She frantically searched for a proper intervention or comforting statement, something to *do*. As a seasoned meditator, she noticed how she had shut down from the connection with the moment in an effort to manage her own horror. On noticing this, she turned her attention toward her own affective response, and then fully back to her patient, acknowledging to herself the intolerable helplessness she felt. When she finally spoke, she merely acknowledged to him that the memories of these events, too, must somehow be accommodated by simple virtue of the fact that they occurred. He later thanked her for her willingness not to abandon him, and to remain open in the face of such difficult emotions.

Mindfulness reveals that emotions, like all subjective phenomena, are transitory, which makes them less fearsome; as we come to know this directly, we are able to invite them in. This receptivity extends naturally to our patients, who are offered the opportunity to bring forward more of their own seemingly intolerable experience. Our receptivity in the face of difficult emotional content reassures patients that they need not censor themselves to protect themselves or the therapist. Emotions lose some of their threat. There is a Buddhist story that if a tablespoon of salt is added to a cup of water, it will be difficult to drink. But if that same tablespoon of salt is added to a clear pond, we can drink from it with no difficulty, though the salt is still present. Mindfulness practice transforms the mind into a larger pond. Difficult emotions remain, but their power to disturb is diffused in the openness of mind. We become much larger containers.

Practicing Acceptance

Mindfulness is acceptance in action; it is not a permanent state of mind but rather an *attitude* that is repeated each time we draw our attention back to our object of awareness. We return with full attention without regard for the pleasant or unpleasant qualities of the object. Everything is welcomed equally. In clinical terms, we might call this *mindful exposure*, setting aside strategies of behavioral or cognitive avoidance in order to find safety in the face of what is feared (Lovibond, Mitchell, Minard, Brady, & Menzies, 2009; see also Chapter 2).

In contrast, judgment and self-criticism are so deeply rooted in the human mind that we even criticize our own mindfulness practice. As any meditator knows, meditation can be difficult; in the beginning, it can seem impossible. It's all too common for us to compound our difficulty paying one-pointed attention with self-judgment about the process.

As mindfulness practice matures, the tendency toward self-criticism is mitigated by several developments. First, one begins to have moments, albeit temporary, of relatively steady, uninterrupted attention. This is one of the first rewards of consistent effort and it's self-reinforcing. A second shift occurs when thoughts arise but are taken simply as objects to be aware of, neither pursued nor rejected. When this happens, it is possible to *witness* self-judgment as just another thought, arising and passing. Judgment begins to lose its sting when seen in this impersonal light; we identify less with the message. By recognizing self-judgment and allowing it to pass, we avoid fueling a protracted litany of self-criticism. Turning again and again toward *all* that arises is the practice of self-acceptance. And like anything that is repeated, self-acceptance becomes stronger over time.

The practice of acceptance, nurtured in meditation, is likely to carry over into our work lives. Therapists have ample opportunities to watch the pendulum of judgment—self-congratulation and self-doubt—swing while practicing psychotherapy. Our judgments of others arise in direct proportion to judgments of ourselves, and conversely, when we're at peace with ourselves, we're less likely to find fault with others.

Clinicians are taught the importance of being accepting of their patients to cultivate a therapeutic alliance. However, judgment is pernicious; we can harbor many prejudices while flattering ourselves that we do not. Such unexamined views lower the headroom of patients' freedom as they subtly find their way into psychotherapy. An attuned patient may know well before the therapist that the therapist's ostensible acceptance is paper-thin. Mindfulness practice is a vehicle for the training of acceptance, both through exercising acceptance itself and by recognizing when it's absent. We can learn to extend the safety of genuine acceptance to our patients, sometimes providing them with their first truly safe relationship.

Empathy and Compassion

Despite the importance of empathy in the therapeutic relationship, research on empathy *training* is still lacking. In the psychotherapy literature, we find recommendations for teaching about communication styles and how to tailor therapists' relational stance to different patients' needs (Lambert & Barley, 2001). Even if these skills are teachable, however, they probably fall short of genuine empathy. Mindfulness practice can help. In Buddhist traditions, some forms of meditation are explicitly designed to cultivate compassion, which is essentially empathy with an attitude of loving-kindness and a wish to alleviate suffering.

Compassion for *ourselves* can arise as we open to our own suffering. The mere presence of suffering is not enough, however. Consider how some people become hardened by devastating loss or hardship. Mindfulness offers a way to change our relationship to suffering by letting go of our need to reject it. That makes mindfulness an act of kindness to oneself. Our own suffering becomes an opportunity for growth rather than merely a problem.

Compassion for *others* arises from the insight that no one is exempt from suffering and that everyone wishes to be free of it. In addition, moment-to moment awareness in meditation and everyday life begins to loosen our sense of a fixed, separate self. Compassion toward others is a natural expression of a growing understanding of how we are related to all things in ever-expanding circles of interdependence.

Equanimity and the Limits of Helpfulness

In the mindfulness tradition, *equanimity* has a number of meanings. It describes an attitude of nondiscriminating, open receptivity in which all experience is welcomed. It can also include the recognition that despite our best efforts and our most heartfelt wish for the welfare of others, there are real limits to what we can do to help. Therefore, even as our mindfulness practice begets empathy and compassion, our wish to be of assistance to others needs to be tempered by the sober recognition of our patients' ultimate responsibility for themselves.

During a visit to a residential treatment center, I spoke with an art therapist who described a very difficult patient who demanded help but rejected everything offered to her. The patient's hostile and belittling stance enlisted—and frustrated—the entire staff. The worse the patient behaved, the more committed the staff became to finding a solution to her difficulties.

Exhausted, angry, and sad, the art therapist ran out of ideas and patience. One day, looking at the patient across an activity room, she had the thought that there was nothing left to offer, and the patient was going to have to figure it out for herself. At that very moment, the patient looked at her, walked across the room, and for the first time ever, apologized for her disruptive behavior.

Although things may not always turn out this well, accepting limits to our helpfulness is a prerequisite to letting our patients assume greater responsibility for their own growth and well-being. Subscribing to the fantasy of therapy's unlimited reach can lead to disillusionment, anger, and unnecessarily prolonged treatment. Even as compassion motivates us to give our very best efforts to our patients, it needs to be balanced by the sober recognition of the absolute and genuine limits of our ability to change anybody other than ourselves. Holding this paradox of compassion and equanimity is familiar to therapists, and is well described by T. S. Eliot in *Ash Wednesday* (1930, p. 58):

> Teach us to care and not to care
> Teach us to sit still.

A therapist's confidence in the efficacy of his or her methods is associated with a positive treatment outcome (Frank, 1961; Wampold, 2001), perhaps because the placebo effect is strengthened (O'Regan, 1985). And yet this confidence factor can be overdone. Therapists and patients have been known to endlessly examine a problem to avoid the uncomfortable truth that some conditions of our lives cannot be changed. We need to distinguish what is fixable from what is not. In running toward an unrealistic cure, the opportunity to examine the broader reality of a problem can be lost. The greatest challenge of psychotherapy is to sit nobly and alert with a patient in the full flame of suffering. Those brave moments may be the most honest and transformative in therapy.

Gerald's life was excessively predictable and dull. By his own description, "the lights are on, but nobody's home." Gerald's treatment—one of many stints in psychotherapy—was nearly intolerable for his latest therapist, who persistently tried to discover an unsecured door or an unopened window into Gerald's inner life. The therapist felt genuinely helpless and despondent about the treatment. In desperation, the therapist observed aloud how they both seemed to feel helpless. Gerald brightened. Though Gerald had no real expectation that another round of therapy with another therapist would change anything, for the first time in many months he felt less alone in his helplessness.

The equanimity that is cultivated in mindfulness practice helps teach us humility and allows us to stop trying to fix things long enough to see what *is*. This stance can free both the therapist and the patient from the need to be "successful," giving the patient the freedom to inhabit his or her life as it is, or to change him- or herself from the firm foundation of radical acceptance.

Learning to See

One of the great, unheralded assets therapists possess is that they are not their patients. Whatever a therapist's struggles or blind spots may be, they are unlikely to be identical to those of the patient. This distance allows a degree of perspective. Perspective is further supported by training, which exposes the clinician to multiple points of view. A problem may often seem intractable because of the way the patient formulates it, but by skillfully reframing the problem, a therapist can open the patient to creative new opportunities.

Through the process of watching thoughts arise and pass away in mindfulness meditation, therapists can gain insight into the ways we construct our world and thereby cause much of our own suffering. This process of *insight* is not fundamentally different from the insight gained into personal conditioning through insight-oriented psychotherapy, but it further exposes the nature of attachment to mental constructions themselves (see Chapter 2). Reframing, from this perspective, is not merely replacing a patient's familiar self-understanding with another, but includes seeing how any stance or position is potentially entrapping.

By learning to see thoughts as events with no special reality, we come to appreciate our mind's incessant tendency to build imaginary scenarios that we inhabit as if they are real. As this capacity deepens, we simultaneously enhance our ability to see how others construct their worlds. This capacity is described by the Pali term *sampajañña*, often translated as "clear knowing" or "clear comprehension." Subjectively, it is experienced simply as seeing more clearly. For therapists, this clarity is manifested by becoming more astute observers of both our own and our patients' minds.

Letting Go and Starting Again

To be present, we need to let go. Attending to the present moment requires that we let go of what occupied our attention just a moment before. Therefore, as we practice *being with* a patient, we simultaneously learn to let go. This important paradox deserves further explanation.

The common idea about therapy is that understanding or insight about our past conditioning will naturally set our lives in a more positive direction. Experienced therapists, however, understand that insight may be necessary, but not always sufficient, for meaningful change. Enduring change requires the ongoing practice of alternative behaviors. Familiar habits and personal problems are rarely resolved suddenly; rather, we come to spend less time and attention perseverating on old ways of thinking, feeling, and behaving. We learn to let go, though subjectively it may feel as if patterns or preoccupations let *us* go.

One of the insights of mindfulness meditation is the *momentariness* of experience—that each moment arises anew from an infinite multiplicity of contributing factors. This means that in principle, each moment invites us to set aside unhelpful habits of thought and behavior and *start again*. This is letting go in action, and it's never too late.

Exposing Our Narcissistic Needs

One difficult aspect of mental functioning that is revealed by mindfulness practice is our incessant concern with self-esteem and self-image. This eternal dilemma befalls therapists as well. The desire to be an effective therapist is laudable, but it is easily confounded with the need to see ourselves in a positive light. Our professional self-esteem is perpetually renegotiated, often based on our assessment of our most recent therapy session. Therapy falters when our own narcissistic needs blur with needs of our patients.

While this tendency is not easily stopped, it can be seen and handled wisely by a mindful therapist. Mindfulness has the potential to take this examination to a more profound level, exposing the self as constructed and illusory. This gradual illumination occurs as we learn to let go of *all* constructions, including positive and negative *self* views (Goldin & Gross, 2010).

Buddhist meditation practice, especially on extended retreats, eventually yields the insight that there is no enduring, unchanging, or separate self (Olendzki, 2010; see also Chapter 12). This understanding is considered by Hölzel and colleagues (2011) to be a key way that mindfulness meditation improves lives. Even novice meditation practitioners can witness how their sense of self constantly changes, leading to recognition of the insubstantiality of their mental constructions. This process helps meditators of any degree of experience to disidentify with the contents of consciousness, a process sometimes called *decentering* (Carmody et al., 2009; Sauer & Baer, 2010).

Learning entails both seeing self as a construction as well as observing how that construction influences our daily life, including our clinical work. It is a kind of learning that helps us get out of our own way. For example, an analytically trained therapist may be convinced of the brilliance and correctness of an interpretation. Should the patient reject the interpretation, the therapist may insist on its accuracy out of an unconscious desire to avoid the loss of self-esteem associated with being wrong.

Overconfidence in our understanding can become an obstacle to new knowledge. As psychiatrist Thomas Szasz (2004) wrote: "Every act of conscious learning requires the willingness to suffer an injury to one's self-esteem. That is why young children, before they are aware of their own self-importance, learn so easily; and why older persons, especially if vain or important, cannot learn at all" (p. 40). Loosening our grip on being "the one who knows" opens us to genuine learning, and this openness can make us more creative and flexible as therapists.

Overcoming Infatuation with Theory

The Problem

Most professional training in psychotherapy focuses on theory, research, and clinical applications. Having this knowledge is an important hallmark of professionalism, and we naturally enjoy our mastery of it. Unfortunately, however, we may also confuse our models and theories for "truth," taking our theoretical constructions as something more real and deserving of our trust than they actually are.

Models of psychopathology and treatment are fundamental to being effective healers. For example, borderline personality disorder would be even more difficult to treat without the contributions of many skilled scientists and clinicians who illuminated the biopsychosocial etiology of the disorder and how it manifests in interpersonal relationships. Our diagnostic categories reduce staggering human variability in order to find underlying consistencies. Clinical categories may also be helpful to our patients, who need an explanation for their distress. For example, a man suffering from a delusion that he is being pursued by unseen enemies may not consider antipsychotic medication until he understands the nature of his illness. A woman who feels like a failure no matter how much success she achieves may be grateful to hear that she's suffering from clinical depression.

Our theoretical models of therapy also protect us from uncertainty and anxiety in our clinical work; even an inaccurate map is more reassuring than no map at all. Furthermore, as previously discussed, our confidence in the efficacy of our methods correlates with positive outcomes in therapy—because our patients need to feel that we know what we're doing, it helps if we do, too. However, unreflective attachment to our models and categories also poses risks. When we use a diagnostic label as a kind of shorthand, it can come to replace a more nuanced appraisal of the whole person. We may stop inquiring into the patient's world, convinced that we know enough. It becomes a cover for our ignorance, masquerading as knowledge and certainty. One example of this danger is "theory countertransference" (Miller, Duncan, & Hubble, 1997), in which a therapist unconsciously imposes his or her theoretical predispositions on the patient. The result is psychotherapy that conforms to and confirms the therapist's assumptions. As Abraham Maslow (1966) reportedly observed, if you only have a hammer, every problem looks like a nail.

When treatment stalls, we may try more of the same, or chalk the failure up to the patient's resistance.

> Adele presents for psychotherapy with distress about being bypassed for a promotion, ultimately leading to losing her job. She is angry and humiliated. Her therapist is convinced that her suffering is sign of an unresolved intrapsychic conflict that a "healthy" person would not experience, and that she needs more therapy to work this through.

In this example, her therapist could have suggested to Adele that her anger is justified and does not necessarily reflect unresolved personal problems; it's natural to be angry in such circumstances. Although there may be persistent maladaptive patterns in Adele's history, the therapist's formulation, embedded in a literature of disorders, inadvertently added to her burden. Adele's painful loss of a job became compounded by self-blame, wrapped in "objective" clinical terms, adding insult to injury.

Learning to Not Know

How can mindfulness meditation help us hold our models more lightly while doing therapy? One approach is to return our awareness again and again to our internal bodily experience in the consultation room, a shift in attention that inevitably helps us disentangle from our thoughts. By attending to *any* experience in the present moment, we also discover that we don't necessarily know what will happen next. We let go—albeit temporarily—of our wish to anticipate and control, taking refuge in "not knowing."

This attitude of not knowing is not alien to psychotherapy. Consider psychoanalyst W. R. Bion's (1967) classic admonition to rid oneself of preconceptions about a patient, cast off the bondage of memory and desire, and abandon even the wish to cure. Fortunately, there is some preliminary evidence that therapists indeed become more flexible and eclectic in orientation as their professional experience increases (Auerbach & Johnson, 1977; Schacht, 1991).

Mindfulness practice extends *not knowing* beyond an intellectual intention to "keep an open mind." Allowing thoughts to arise and pass helps us see clearly how we normally identify with our thoughts—we perceive the gap between the vast diversity of our experience and our narrow *ideas* about it. As one man said of his experience during an intensive mindfulness retreat, "It felt as though I had jumped out of an airplane without a parachute, which was terrifying until I realized there was no ground!"

Not knowing is valuable because it may enable therapy to progress unimpeded *and* because it is ultimately the truth of the matter: We actually know very little about our mysterious and complex lives. The following account by an elderly man illustrates the wisdom of not knowing:

> I have a friend, a woman I know already many years. One day she's mad at me—from nowhere it comes. I have insulted her, she tells me. How? I don't know. Why don't I know? Because I don't know her. She surprised me. That's good. That's how it should be. You cannot tell someone "I know you." People jump around. They're like a ball; rubbery, they bounce. The ball cannot be long in one place. Rubbery, it must jump. So what do you do to keep a person from jumping? The same as with a ball—make a little hole, and it goes flat. When you tell someone, "I know you," you put a little pin in. So what should you do? Leave them be. Don't try to make them stand still for your convenience. You don't ever know them. Let people surprise you. This, likewise, you could do concerning yourself.

To hold any fixed view, including a fixed view of our patients or ourselves, leads to suffering.

The invitation of mindfulness to *not know* should not be taken as license to give up clinical training and ongoing education. Rather, it is a process of trusting that an open and attuned mind (fortified by strong clinical training) will be far more responsive to the demands of being a therapist. Recognition of the limits of our knowledge restores our "beginner's mind"—which makes real learning possible, in and out of the therapy office.

The Possibility of Happiness

Mindfulness practice can make us happier (Davidson et al., 2003; Siegel, 2007). When our habitual, emotional reactions are held in mindful awareness and become less repetitive, a quiet joy begins to arise within us. Although I'm unaware of research that correlates the therapist's own happiness with treatment outcome, I suspect it helps. When referring a prospective patient to a colleague, I often take into consideration the therapist's general happiness and well-being. Therapists who have tasted calm joy implicitly teach their patients that happiness can emerge *in spite* of the conditions of our lives—that we can live more fully, right here, right now, in the midst of our inevitable challenges.

Mindfulness practice can develop many beneficial qualities of mind, only a few of which have been described here. These mental qualities invariably influence what we think, say, and do as therapists. In the next three chapters, we discuss ways that a clinician's own mindfulness practice, and related practices such as compassion training, can be enhanced while doing the work of psychotherapy.

4

Cultivating Attention and Compassion

William D. Morgan
Susan T. Morgan
Christopher K. Germer

Each of us literally chooses, by his way of attending to things, what sort of universe he shall appear to himself to inhabit.

—WILLIAM JAMES (1890)

*T*he last chapter identified a number of personal qualities and insights engendered in the therapist through mindfulness training that may positively affect treatment. This chapter addresses two of those: *attention* and *compassion*. In graduate training, aspiring therapists are not generally trained to enhance their capacity for attention and compassion. We assume that, as therapists, we have reasonable powers of attention, evidenced by years of schooling, and that we are good-hearted people whose natural compassion will continue to grow over the years and hopefully not succumb to compassion fatigue and burnout. These assumptions beg the question: "Can clinicians use specific techniques in and outside the consultation room to *enhance* their ability to pay attention to their patients and to deepen their compassion?"

ATTENTION

Sigmund Freud wrote that the analyst should have "evenly hovering attention" during the therapy hour, meaning that the analyst should "give equal notice to everything" and "withhold all conscious influences from his capacity to attend" (1912/1961b, pp. 111–112). This recommendation is remarkably similar to open monitoring in mindfulness practice. However, Freud did not offer any method to achieve this elusive goal beyond a personal analysis. The same receptive, nonpreferential state of mind surely supports other forms of therapy as well. It's hard to imagine anyone benefiting from therapy with a clinician who is preoccupied with a particular idea, self-absorbed, or shows little interest in the patient. We often ask therapists during workshops, "Given the choice, would you rather be 20% more attentive during your therapy hours, or would you rather have 20% more techniques at your disposal?" Most clinicians choose more attention.

Mindfulness as Attention Training

Although attention training may seem like a chore, there can be considerable delight and meaning in enhanced awareness. Meditation teachers Christina Feldman and Jack Kornfield (1991) note, "It is just simple attention that allows us to truly listen to the sound of the bird, to see deeply the glory of an autumn leaf, to touch the heart of another and be touched" (p. 83). Events that were previously too insignificant or mundane to merit our attention may become vivid and rich in detail. Consider the following clinical vignette:

> Josh and Karyn said that their marriage was never the same after the birth of their first child. Karyn believed that Josh just didn't appreciate how hard it was to be a mother, and Josh was convinced that Karyn was basically selfish—needing "personal time" whenever he returned home from a hard day in the office. Sitting in the same room with this couple, I (C. K. G.) could feel the chilliness that surrounded their relationship like a Boston winter. Even when Karyn noted that Josh was "improving" at responding to her needs, Josh slightly angled his head away from her and held his breath.
>
> Although I dreaded these therapy sessions, especially late in the afternoon, I resolved to remain curious to the soft feelings that might reside behind this couple's hard feelings. At one point when Josh turned his head away from Karyn, I asked Karyn if she noticed that. Actually, neither of them had noticed, and in their

brief moment of surprise and uncertainty, I asked Josh what his body language indicated. He declared that Karyn's use of the word *improving* was a "back-handed compliment." So I asked Josh what he *really* wants from Karyn. He said, "I guess I just want to be successful with Karyn—not to fail her all the time. I want to be a good husband." Karyn was amazed to hear this, believing all along that Josh didn't care what she thought or felt.

In this vignette, a seemingly insignificant body movement opened a robust, new conversation and reversed the couple's entrenched beliefs that began with arrival of their new baby.

There is now ample evidence that mindfulness meditation improves our ability to pay attention in a concentrated and sustained manner (Jha et al., 2007; Napoli, Krech, & Holley, 2005; Semple, 2010; Slagter et al., 2007; Tang & Posner, 2010; Valentine & Sweet, 1999). Neurological research also indicates that mindfulness meditation helps us engage less in self-referential thinking, especially when we're challenged by emotional distress (Farb et al., 2007, 2010), and meditation can help us recover more quickly from distractions (May et al., 2011; Moore & Malinowski, 2009; Reis, 2007).

As described in Chapter 1, we typically learn three skills under the umbrella of "mindfulness meditation": (1) *focused attention* or concentration, (2) *open monitoring* or mindfulness per se, and (3) *loving-kindness and compassion* (Salzberg, 2011). Experienced meditators blend these three practices to enhance their experience of mindfulness. Focused attention, such as returning awareness again and again to the breath or the soles of the feet, calms the mind. Open monitoring—noticing whatever arises in our field of perception—trains the mind to receive the vicissitudes of life with equanimity and insight. These two skills are the primary vehicles for clinicians to cultivate their capacity for sustained attention. The third skill, loving-kindness and compassion, provides comfort and soothing which, in turn, opens awareness. (Compassion is considered later in this chapter.)

Both focused attention and open monitoring can be practiced at home or while doing psychotherapy. When we're feeling distress during a therapy session, a simple strategy to calm ourselves is to take a conscious breath or to passively notice the body breathe itself. That's a focused attention practice. Our patients' emotional pain can also be a focal object during the therapy hour. When we feel lost or confused in a therapy session, it may help to ask the question, "Where is the patient's pain?" Maintaining this focus enabled the therapist above to explore the hidden meaning of Josh's reaction to Karyn's comment.

The meditation instruction for open monitoring is "pay attention to whatever is most salient and alive in your field of awareness." To do this in therapy, allow your gaze to soften—expand your visual field around your patient's face—and open yourself to notice whatever you're experiencing at the moment. What are you noticing in your patient or sensing in your own body? What emotions are present? What are you thinking? Open monitoring of *external* stimuli is what allowed the therapist in the vignette to recognize Josh's subtle head tilt. Monitoring of *internal* experience exposed the therapist to his discomfort in the therapy room, which, in turn, helped him refocus on the task of deepening this couple's understanding of one another.

Focused attention is like a headlight on a boat, illuminating only what is caught in the beam. Open monitoring allows us to also be aware of the barnacles stuck on the hull. In therapy, the barnacles are the sticky issues that hijack our attention and distract us from the therapeutic endeavor.

Mindfulness meditation also creates deep psychological changes that promote sustained attention. Originally known as *insight meditation*, mindfulness practice allows us observe how the mind works. Three key insights emerge over time:

1. Suffering arises in everyone's mind.
2. Our thoughts, feelings, and sensations are all transitory.
3. Our sense of self is also continuously in flux (see Chapter 14).

Each of these insights becomes a buffer between a stimulus and our usual reactivity. When we understand that suffering is universal—that *all* beings suffer—we're less likely to become overwhelmed by it. When we understand that our thoughts and feelings are all passing phenomena, we can more easily let go and refocus on the tasks at hand. And finally, when we don't spend our entire lives promoting and defending a particular sense of self (e.g., "I'm smart" "I'm pretty"), we're less ruminative and self-absorbed. Insights such as these are not mere intellectual concepts but psychological transformations that support our ability to pay attention in the therapy office.

Optimal Presence: The Seven Factors of Awakening

Mindfulness in the context of ancient Buddhist psychology is only one of seven interdependent qualities of mind (*factors of awakening*) that facilitate increased awareness. The privileged position of mindfulness is not an accident—the other six factors arise from mindfulness and together represent the full expression of mindfulness in our lives. A firm foundation in mindfulness provides a vantage point from which to recognize when the other six factors are active or not.

Unfortunately, our attention during an ordinary day is partial at best, often scattered, vague, or tepid, like a daydream while driving down a familiar highway. Attention becomes enhanced when we move into the passing lane of the highway, for example, or when we slice a tomato and the knife nears our fingers. "Crunch" moments in therapy also galvanize our attention. Some degree of attention to our present-moment experience is necessary to function in daily life, but our typical measure can hardly be characterized as full mindfulness.

How can we be optimally present in psychotherapy? What do moments that capture our attention, such as being with a patient who just lost her lifelong partner, contain that our less attentive moments lack? They include the seven factors of awakening: (1) mindfulness, (2) investigation, (3) energy, (4) joy, (5) tranquility, (6) concentration, and (7) equanimity (see the Appendix). The factors are like seven acrobats standing in a column on each other's shoulders. (The bottom acrobat is mindfulness.) Each must do his or her part, or else they will all fall. Optimal presence in therapy occurs when all the factors are active at the same time and in balance with one another.

Mindfulness

Mindfulness, the subject of this volume, can be defined as "knowing what you are experiencing *while* you're experiencing it" (G. Armstrong, lecture, January 9, 2008), or knowing *that* you are experiencing what you are experiencing—including preconceptual awareness of fluctuations in the field of awareness. The capacity for mindfulness creates a little space for reflection around our thoughts and feelings and allows us to make skillful, therapeutic choices.

Investigation

Investigation keeps our thoughts appropriately focused on the object at hand. Our attention is like a searchlight. For example, while sitting with a patient, investigation will keep the mind of the therapist actively engaged in trying to understand the patient better: "Where is the patient's pain?" "Why does the patient think this?" "What does he or she mean by that?" Investigation, or curiosity, enriches therapy by constantly probing for deeper layers of understanding.

Energy

Too much agitation or anxiety interferes with optimal presence, as does sluggishness or indifference. Neither of these states is conducive to effective therapeutic responses. This is illustrated by Hans Selye's (1956) well-known bell-shaped stress–response curve that depicts how performance increases up to a certain point of arousal, and thereafter drops as arousal continues to increase. Caffeine can sharpen attention up to a point, beyond which it creates agitation. To have optimal presence in therapy, we need calm energy; alert yet relaxed, neither restless nor drowsy. Balanced energy is the peak of the bell-shaped curve.

Joy

Joy is animated delight in what is happening in the moment, as though there is no place we would rather be. With joy, we see the present field of experience as an embarrassment of riches. In therapy, joy manifests as interest and warmth. Genuine interest cannot be faked; it is evident to both the patient and the therapist.

Tranquility

Tranquility is how we feel when there is little conflict or distress in the mind. It is serenity based not on the absence of thoughts and feelings, but on the acceptance of whatever is arising. There is alertness and joy in tranquility. Therapists require tranquility to act wisely and avoid the mistakes we make when our field of perception is narrowed by suffering.

Concentration

Concentration is the sustained quality of nondistraction, cultivated through the willing and repeated return of attention to a single object in the present moment, such as the inner state of the patient. Concentration provides the stability of mind to be mindful—to notice, for example, when we are angry, worried, or distracted, as well as to notice the presence or absence of the seven factors of awakening. In therapy, concentration also allows us to remain undistracted by concerns outside of the session.

Equanimity

Equanimity is the *even* in the "evenly hovering attention" that Freud recommended. It is the attentional rudder that keeps our awareness smooth and steady as the mind engages different elements of our experience. This is a subtle matter, as the mind is continuously steering toward that which is pleasant or interesting, and turning away from, or holding at arm's length, that which is less appealing. Equanimity encourages a posture of equal nearness to each moment within the therapeutic encounter.

When full presence is elusive, it can be helpful to do a brief inventory of these seven factors. If you discover a factor that needs strengthening, consider the available options. Ask yourself, "What do I need to be more attentive to my patient?" For example, nervous energy may mean that you need some physical exercise; loss of equanimity could indicate that you require clinical support or supervision; lack of interest suggests that the patient's motivation for being in therapy is not clear to you; and so forth. It can even help to keep a list of the factors of awakening nearby to remind yourself to be optimally present.

Cultivating Attention

William James (1890/2007) wrote, "The faculty of voluntarily bringing back a wandering attention, over and over again, is the very root of judgment, character, and will" (p. 424). Attention regulation is a key skill of an effective psychotherapist as well, knowing when the mind has wandered off, noting where it went, and returning it to the task at hand. The three types (or skills) of mindfulness meditation—focused attention, open monitoring, and loving-kindness/compassion—can be practiced either during formal practice periods or throughout the workday as an intermezzo between patients. In formal sitting practice, it is helpful to set aside a time and place where you're unlikely to be interrupted or distracted for however long you choose to practice. A gentle alarm clock will allow you to immerse yourself in the practice without vigilance to time. In the beginning, meditation periods should not be so long as to become tedious; 10 or 20 minutes are enough. When practicing in the office between patients, 3–5 minutes can suffice. Below are examples of mindfulness meditations that specifically train your capacity for focused attention (concentration) and open monitoring (mindfulness per se) (see also Chapter 1).

Concentration Meditation

- Find a comfortable posture. Close your eyes. Allow your body to be held, supported by the chair. Notice directly the sensation of your body in contact with the chair.

- Take two or three slow, deep breaths, relaxing with the exhalation. With each exhalation imagine the body becoming heavier and relaxing more fully.
- Allow the breath to find its natural, easy rhythm. Enjoy the relaxed simplicity of sitting and breathing.
- Where do you notice the flow of sensations of the breath most vividly—at the nose tip, the throat, the chest, or the diaphragm? Allow the attention to alight there easily, like a bird on a branch or a cork bobbing on the surface of the ocean.
- Whenever your attention wanders, and you notice that it has wandered, first reestablish the relaxed breath, then return your attention to the flowing sensations of breath where they are strongest.
- Allow yourself a few more breaths before slowly opening the eyes.

Mindfulness Meditation

- Find a comfortable posture. Close your eyes. Allow your body to be held, supported by the chair. Notice directly the sensation of your body in contact with the chair.
- Take two or three slow, deep breaths, relaxing with the exhalation. With each exhalation imagine the body becoming heavier and relaxing more fully.
- Allow the breath to find its natural, easy rhythm. Enjoy the relaxed simplicity of sitting and breathing.
- Keeping the mind open and spacious, allow whatever arises in your field of experience—visual images, sounds, physical sensations, feelings, thought formations—to come and go, to move freely.
- Try to maintain a receptive, nonpreferential stance to whatever is arising, as if you were gently flowing along in an ever-changing stream of experience.
- When you find yourself distracted, first return to the relaxed simplicity of sitting and breathing; then again open the field of awareness.
- Take a few more breaths before slowly opening the eyes.

You can experiment with these strategies for regulating attention. It's best not to think of meditation as a chore or a means to an end. Rather, let it be a psychologically rich endeavor—a rare chance to know what it's like to be fully alive in a human body, right here and right now. You will have pleasant, unpleasant, and neutral experiences in meditation. See if you can simply notice whatever arises in a loving way.

COMPASSION

Mind training within the tradition of Buddhist psychology has two main objectives: (1) the regulation of attention to cultivate wisdom and (2) the regulation of emotion to create a compassionate heart (Dalai Lama, 2005). At the time of this writing, mindfulness and acceptance-based treatments seem to emphasize the refinement of attention more than the transformation of emotions. Learning to relate to thoughts, feelings, and sensations with spacious awareness has been the key vehicle for regulating emotion in the emerging mindfulness therapy field.

However, there are additional techniques, such as loving-kindness (Pali: *metta*) and giving and taking (Tibetan: *tonglen*) meditations, that intentionally cultivate beneficial mind states as an antidote to difficult emotions such as anger and hatred. In addition to noticing all mental phenomena with open awareness, we can deliberately activate goodwill toward ourselves and others in the midst of these emotions. Some mindfulness practitioners might feel that these two approaches are at odds with one another, but it's important to remember that the purpose of mindfulness is to alleviate suffering, not choiceless awareness for its own sake. Different contemplative strategies, some more intentional than others, are useful depending on the conditions in our lives or our temperament. In Buddhist psychology, meditations that intentionally cultivate goodwill and positive emotions are drawn from the four *brahma viharas* (Pali), roughly translated as limitless qualities of heart—loving-kindness, compassion, empathic joy, and equanimity (see the Appendix). Here we focus particularly on compassion training because compassion deals with emotional suffering, the sine qua non of psychotherapy.

The Meaning of Compassion

The concept of compassion is a relatively new arrival to the field of psychotherapy, but it has been present all along under the umbrella of empathy. Interest in compassion seems to follow closely on the heels of mindfulness as our collective experience of mindfulness meditation deepens and grows (Germer & Siegel, 2012). For example, dedicated mindfulness meditators inevitably discover that suffering touches all human beings most of the time; that all our thoughts, feelings, and beliefs are transitory, like bubbles on a stream, and even our core sense of self is subject to change and is not separate from the rest of the world. These insights give way to an appreciation of our affinity with all beings, out of which compassion emerges.

Empathy

Empathy is classically understood as an "accurate understanding of the [patient's] world as seen from the inside. To sense the [patient's] private world as if it were your own, but without losing the 'as if' quality—this is empathy" (Rogers, 1961, p. 284). Self psychology pioneer Heinz Kohut stretched the definition and role of empathic understanding. He considered it an observational tool, a bond, a curative factor, and a necessity for psychological health (Lee & Martin, 1991). Empathy requires a particular sort of attention. Rollo May (1967) noted that empathy calls for "learning to relax, mentally and spiritually, as well as physically, learning to let one's self go into the other person with a willingness to be changed in the process" (p. 97). Empathy is considered a common factor in psychotherapy that "accounts for as much and probably more outcome variance than does specific intervention" (Bohart et al., 2002, p. 96; see also Norcross, 2001, and Chapter 3) with numerous implications for treatment (Elliot et al., 2011; Neumann et al., 2011).

Compassion

The word *compassion* derives from the Latin roots *pati* (to suffer) and *com* (with), and means to *suffer with* another person. Compassion is the shared experience of *suffering* in particular, rather than empathic resonance with all feeling states. Another important component of compassion is altruism, or the motivation to help others, which is often implied when we use the word *empathy* in psychotherapy. The Dalai Lama defines compassion as "the wish that all sentient beings may be free from suffering" (2003, p. 67). A shorthand definition of compassion is *the experience of suffering with the wish to alleviate it* (Siegel & Germer, 2012, p. 12). Compassion is different from pity, which implies an unequal standing between the giver and the receiver of kindness, and it's not the same as loving-kindness, which the Dalai Lama defines as a "state of mind which aspires that all sentient beings may enjoy happiness" (2003, p. 67). It may be said that when loving-kindness meets suffering (and remains loving!), it becomes compassion. Empathy is a prerequisite for compassion.

Self-Compassion

Compassion can also be directed toward oneself in response to one's own suffering (Germer, 2009; Neff, 2011). How do we typically react when we suffer, fail, or feel inadequate? We're likely to criticize ourselves for our shortcomings, isolate ourselves out of shame, and get stuck in our heads, asking "Why me?" We add insult to injury. An alternative response is self-compassion, consisting of (1) self-kindness, (2) a sense of common humanity ("I'm only human"), and (3) mindfulness (Neff, 2003). A growing body of research has shown that self-compassion is positively associated with emotional well-being and is consistently related to low levels of anxiety and depression (Neff, 2012; Neff, Kirkpatrick, & Rude, 2007).

Compassion is the attitude of mindfulness—goodwill in the face of suffering. When mindfulness is in full bloom in therapy, it feels like compassion. However, when we're overwhelmed with intense or disturbing emotions, we become self-critical ("I'm defective," "I'm unlovable") and our mindfulness becomes somewhat limited. This is the situation that many patients bring to therapy. They not only *feel* bad; they believe they *are* bad. They need to be rescued from shame, self-criticism, and self-doubt.

Mindfulness practices typically focus on moment-to-moment *experience*. However, sometimes we need to comfort and soothe the *experiencer* before we can attend mindfully to other elements of our lives. We need *self*-acceptance. Mindfulness says, in essence, "Feel the pain with spacious awareness and it will change." Self-compassion adds, "*Be kind to yourself* in the midst of the pain and it will change." Mindfulness asks, "What do you *know*?" and self-compassion asks, "What do you *need*?" Both approaches help to manage the spectrum of emotional challenges that we face with our patients.

Most efforts to integrate compassion training into psychotherapy focus on self-compassion. Research evidence suggests that self-compassion is an important underlying mechanism of change in psychotherapy (Baer, 2010; Barnard & Curry, 2011; Birne, Speca, & Carlson, 2010; Hofmann et al., 2011; Hollis-Walker & Colosimo, 2011; Kuyken et al., 2010; Patsiopoulos & Buchanan, 2011; Raque-Bogdan, Ericson, Jackson, Martin, & Bryan, 2011; Raes, 2010, 2011; Schanche, Stiles, McCollough, Swartberg, & Nielsen, 2011; Shapira & Mongrain, 2010; Van Dam, Sheppard, Forsyth, & Earleywine, 2011).

Paul Gilbert and his colleagues have developed a unique, empirically supported, compassion-oriented approach to psychotherapy called *compassion-focused therapy* (CFT; Gilbert, 2005, 2009a, 2009b, 2010a, 2010b, 2010c). This program emphasizes self-compassion, and has been applied to a wide range of disorders (Cree, 2010; Gilbert, 2010b; Gilbert & Proctor, 2006; Goss & Allen, 2010; Gumley, Braehler, Laithwaite, MacBeth, & Gilbert, 2010; Kolts, 2011; Lowens, 2010; Pauley

& McPhearson, 2010; Tirch, 2011). CFT recognizes that changing the *content* of our internal dialogue is often insufficient to change how we feel. Sometimes we need an entirely new approach—we need to "warm up the conversation" (P. Gilbert, personal communication, June 20, 2010). Compassion training may work by activating and transforming old attachment patterns, stored in the midbrain, which underlie much of our conscious, neocortical activity (Hart, 2010; Immordino-Yang, McColl, Damasio, & Damasio, 2009; Wilkinson, 2010).

Practicing compassion for *others* is also good for mental health (Cosley, McCoy, Saslow, & Epel, 2010; Crocker & Canevello, 2008; Dunn, Aknin, & Norton, 2008; Mongrain, Chin, & Shapira, 2010). Interestingly, however, giving support to others can increase our own self-compassion (Breines & Chen, 2012). However, *self*-compassion is generally considered the foundation for compassion toward others. As the Dalai Lama (2000/2010) said:

> For someone to develop genuine compassion towards others, first he or she must have a basis upon which to cultivate compassion, and that basis is the ability to connect to one's own feelings and to care for one's own welfare.... Caring for others requires caring for oneself.

This statement makes sense insofar as we cannot completely embrace another imperfect individual when we reject ourselves for similar imperfections.

The Power of Compassion

Compassion is a skill that can be learned, just like mindfulness. Richard Davidson and colleagues (Lutz, Greischar, Rawlings, Ricard, & Davidson, 2004) found that highly experienced compassion meditators (averaging 32,000 hours of meditation) showed gamma wave activity (signifying conscious awareness) that was 60 times stronger than controls. These changes were positively correlated with the number of hours of meditation practice. Functional magnetic resonance imaging (fMRI) demonstrated dramatic changes in the insula (social emotions and mind–body interaction), amygdala (response to suffering), and right temporal–parietal juncture (perspective taking) during compassion meditation (Lutz, Brefczynski-Lewis, et al., 2008). Shorter practice periods of only 2 weeks also revealed changes in the insula that, interestingly, are correlated with charitable giving (Davidson, 2012).

A number of structured, empirically supported programs have been established to deepen compassion, such as the compassion-cultivation training program (CCT; Jinpa et al., 2009), cognitive-based compassion training (CBCT; Dodson-Lavelle, 2011), and mindful self-compassion training (MSC; Neff & Germer, 2013). Mindfulness training programs such as MBSR have also been shown to increase self-compassion in conjunction with mindfulness (Birnie et al., 2010; Krüger, 2010; Shapiro et al., 2005, 2007).

Deliberate efforts to build the skills of compassion and empathy into clinical training are still relatively rare (Christopher, Chrisman, et al., 2011; Christopher & Maris, 2010; Greason & Cashwell, 2009; Richards, Campenni, & Muse-Burke, 2010; Shapiro et al., 2007) despite the established importance of empathy in psychotherapy (Norcross, 2001; Shapiro & Izett, 2007; see also Chapter 3). It stands to reason that any method that develops the therapist's capacity for empathy and compassion would contribute to a positive treatment relationship—and therefore to improved treatment outcomes.

Compassion Fatigue

Some clinicians are uneasy about compassion training, perhaps feeling they are already too compassionate and teetering on the edge of *compassion fatigue* (Figley, 2002). The literature on compassion fatigue recommends that the weary therapist distance him- or herself from the patient by maintaining clear professional boundaries, spending more time with friends, delegating responsibility to others, or getting supervision. These are important self-care strategies, but without mindful awareness and self-compassion, they may not empower the clinician to find emotional satisfaction while connecting with patients during stressful situations. Michael Kearney and colleagues (2009) note that "physicians with burnout who use self-care without self-awareness may feel as though they are drowning and barely able to come up for air, whereas self-care with self-awareness is like learning to breathe underwater" (p. 1160).

Clinicians may also wonder, "Can compassion—a mental state that embraces suffering—really be good for mental health?" This concern is likely to arise when we conflate the concepts of compassion and empathy. In fact, compassion fatigue should probably be renamed *empathy fatigue* (Klimecki & Singer, 2011; Ricard, 2010). Feeling the suffering of others as one's own suffering is indeed exhausting, but compassion has the added elements of tenderness, kinship, goodwill, and warmheartedness. The experience of compassion contains more loving-kindness than struggle. When we bring attention to it, compassion is like a mindful exhalation, a conscious letting go, with a corresponding sense of release.

Nonetheless, all clinicians are vulnerable to compassion fatigue, especially those who are highly motivated (Craig & Sprang, 2010; Sprang & Clark, 2007). Our brains are wired to feel the pain of others in our bodies as if it were our own (Decety & Cacioppo, 2011; Morrison, Lloyd, DiPellegrino, & Roberts, 2008). Compassion fatigue is a part of being human, not a sign of weakness. Below are two exercises that can help to alleviate vicarious suffering: one for self-compassion, the other for cultivating the equanimity that comes with wisdom. The first step toward overcoming compassion fatigue is to *recognize* when we're under stress. Perhaps you're worried about a patient? Is he or she "taking space in your head without paying rent"? If so, try one of the following exercises[1]:

Hand on Heart

- Put both hands over your heart.
- Feel the warmth of your hands. Enjoy the feeling of warmth.
- Notice the gentle pressure of your hands on your chest.
- Now feel your chest rising and falling beneath your hands as you breathe.
- Feel the rhythmic, soothing rhythm of your breath for a few minutes.

Equanimity Phrases

Repeat the following phrases slowly and quietly to yourself:

Everyone is on his or her own life journey.
I am not the cause of my patient's suffering, nor is it entirely within my power to alleviate it.
Though moments like this are difficult to bear, I may still try to help.

As we become more mindful of the onset of compassion fatigue, we may begin to notice how our breathing becomes shorter and shallower when we're under stress. Slowing and deepening the breath are other acts of self-compassion that can help to reestablish a more balanced flow of warmth in the session.

---

[1] The following four exercises were adapted from the mindful self-compassion training program codeveloped by Chris Germer and Kristin Neff.

Is Compassion Innate?

Compassion is a strength that has enabled people to survive and thrive. Charles Darwin himself considered "sympathy" to be the strongest of our instincts (Darwin, 1871/2010; Ekman, 2010). Cooperation between members of a tribe increases the chance that the offspring will reach reproductive age, improves group survival against external threat, and is a key factor in mate selection (Keltner, 2009; Keltner, Marsh, & Smith, 2010; Sussman & Cloninger, 2011). A significant portion of our brains, including the mirror neurons and much of the midbrain, are dedicated to social functioning (Cozolino, 2010; Hein & Singer, 2008; Kim et al., 2011; Siegel, 2007; Singer & Decety, 2011). The nervous system also has a built-in subsystem, based on oxytocin and the endorphins, that balances the threat and competition subsystems (Carter, 1998; Depue & Morrone-Strupinsky, 2005; Gilbert, 2009b). Therefore, when we cultivate compassion, we're merely strengthening caregiving tendencies that already exist (Bell, 2001).

Cultivating Compassion

Compassion can be brought into therapy by teaching specific practices to our patients (Germer, 2009; Gilbert, 2009b; Neff, 2011) or by the clinician embodying compassion and affectively resonating with a patient (D. Siegel, 2010a, 2010b). However, since we're all conditioned human beings with preferences and judgments, our compassion is a "relative potential" (Jordan, 1991), arising as a multitude of professional and personal variables are brought into delicate balance. Professional variables include clinical training and experience, the complexity of the patient population, the number of patients seen in a given day, and the work environment. Personal variables include the quality of primary relationships, current life stressors and one's ability to manage them, the quality of sleep, physical and mental health, and the stress of that day's demands. Our capacity for compassion fluctuates from day to day and moment to moment. The following exercises my help to strengthen the compassion habit, especially during therapy.

Loving-kindness Meditation

Traditionally, a loving-kindness (*metta*) meditation begins with directing loving-kindness toward *oneself*, based on the idea that all people are primarily interested in their own welfare, followed by focusing on a loved one, a friend, a neutral person, a challenging person, and then groups of people without differentiation. Nowadays, however, many people find it easier to generate warmth toward certain other living beings, such as a pet or a beloved grandparent, rather than themselves. Therefore, if you prefer, substitute any living being who naturally makes you smile as the object of this meditation.

Loving-kindness meditation uses phrases as well as images as meditation objects. Each person eventually discovers personalized phrases that work best for him or her. The words suggested in this exercise are designed to cultivate a compassionate response to suffering.

Loving-kindness with Self-Compassion Meditation

Set aside 20 minutes for the purpose of soothing yourself in the midst of difficult or stressful times. Sit in a comfortable position, reasonably upright and relaxed. Fully or partially close your eyes. Take a few deep breaths to settle into your body and into the present moment. Put your hand on your heart for a moment as a reminder to be kind to yourself.

- Form an image of yourself sitting down. Note your posture on the chair as if you were seeing yourself from the outside.
- Now bring your attention *inside* your body and feel the pulsation and vibration of your body. Locate your breathing where you can feel it most easily. Feel how your breath moves in your body, and when your attention wanders, gently feel the movement of your breath once again.
- After a few minutes, start to notice *areas of stress* that you're holding in your body, perhaps in your neck, jaw, belly, or forehead. Also notice if you're holding some *difficult emotions*, such as worry about the future or uneasiness about the past. Understand that every human body bears stress and worry throughout the day.
- Now offer yourself goodwill *because* of what you're holding in your body right now. Say the following phrases to yourself, softly and gently:

  May I be safe.
  May I be peaceful.
  May I be kind to myself.
  May I accept myself as I am.

- When you notice that your mind has wandered, return to the words or the experience of discomfort in your body or mind. Go slowly.
- If you are ever overwhelmed with emotion, you can always return to your breathing. You can also name the emotion, or find it in the body and soften that area. Then, when you're comfortable, return to the phrases.

- Finally, take a few breaths and just rest quietly in your own body, savoring the goodwill and compassion that flow naturally from your own heart. Know that you can return to the phrases anytime you wish.
- Gently open your eyes.

Phrases such as these can be used informally during therapy as well. When working with a difficult patient, feel free to include the patient in your phrases, such as "May you and I be . . ." or just focus on the patient, "May you be safe. . . ."

Difficult feelings will inevitably arise (Germer, 2009; Gilbert, McEwan, Matos, & Rivis, 2010). This is part of the transformative process and when that happens, allow the feelings to exist in the background. But if the meditation becomes too unpleasant, feel free to just focus on your breath, discover and allow the unpleasant emotion in your body, or perhaps stop meditating altogether and care for yourself behaviorally. The art of loving-kindness meditation is the gentle and gradual development of the mental habit of warmth and goodwill.

Giving and Taking Meditation

Giving and taking (*tonglen*) is a core practice in the Tibetan Buddhist tradition. Traditionally, it consists of breathing in the sufferings of others, quickly transforming those feelings inside, and then exhaling loving-kindness and compassion to a target person or persons. For beginners, the practice of inhaling the suffering of others can be challenging, so the following adaptation has been made.

Breathing Compassion In and Out

- Sit comfortably, close your eyes, and take a few relaxing breaths.
- Scan your body for stress, noting any physical sensations of tension. Also allow yourself to become aware of any stressful *emotions* that you may be holding in your field of awareness. If a challenging person comes to mind, let yourself be aware of the stress associated with that person. If you are experiencing the suffering of another person through empathy, let yourself be aware of that discomfort as well.
- Now, aware of the how your body carries stress, feel your body inhale and let yourself savor the nourishing sensation of breathing in. Let yourself be soothed by your inhalation.
- As you exhale, send out the same comfort and well-being to a person associated with your discomfort, or to the world in general.

- Continue breathing in and out, letting your body gradually find a natural, relaxed breathing rhythm.
- Try adding a kind word to each in-breath and each out-breath, such as *warmth*, *peace*, or *soothe*, or perhaps visualize yourself breathing golden light in and out. Experiment to see which approach evokes the feeling of compassion in you.
- Occasionally scan your inner landscape for any distress and respond by inhaling compassion for yourself and exhaling compassion for those who need it.
- Gently open your eyes.

You can also practice this meditation informally during therapy. When you experience distress during a session, turn your attention to your breath and gently draw compassion in and out with each breath.

The Greeting Exercise

This final exercise is another intermezzo we can practice on the hour, every hour. It reestablishes the intention to open to suffering with compassion and wisdom. Compassion practice is fundamentally about refining our intention to meet sorrow with kindness, and good feelings are an inevitable byproduct of good intentions.

Greeting Exercise

- Before you open the door for your next patient, take a moment to feel the rising and falling of your breath.
- Now visualize the person behind the door, a human being who is suffering, who was once a child, who has hopes and dreams just as you do, and who has tried to be happy and only partially succeeded, who feels vulnerable and afraid much of the time, and who is coming to you believing that you can relieve his or her suffering.
- Now open the door and say "hello."

Poet Naomi Shihab Nye (1995) wrote: "Before you can know kindness as the deepest thing, you must first know sorrow as the other deepest thing" (p. 42). But can we stay open to sorrow, our patients' and our own, long enough to transform it? The ability to regulate our attention using focused attention and open monitoring, and to cultivate goodwill with loving-kindness and compassion exercises, can go a long way toward that lofty goal.

5

Relational Mindfulness

Janet L. Surrey
Gregory Kramer

> Admirable friendship . . . is actually the whole of the
> holy life.
> —BUDDHA (*Upaddha Sutta*, cited in Bhikkhu, 2012b)

Relational mindfulness can be defined as the practice and cultivation of mindfulness in an engaged, person-to-person relational context. For the therapist, this means mindful awareness of his or her internal states, observing the moment-to-moment empathic connection with the patient, and continuous awareness of the changing relationship *between* both patient and therapist. This chapter explores therapy as a relational mindfulness practice and suggests the possibility of cultivating and enhancing relational awareness and competence through Insight Dialogue, a relational insight meditation practice developed by Gregory Kramer (2007). We also explore how relational meditation may deepen the practice of psychotherapy into a more fully engaged, liberating experience.[1]

---

[1] We recognize the ongoing work of the RIM (relational insight meditation) teaching team of the Metta Foundation Programs, especially team leader Sharon Beckman-Brindley, in conceptualizing and realizing the development of these practices for clinicians. The other team members are Phyllis Hicks, Mary Burns, Lori Ebert, and Fabio Giommi; the guiding teacher is Gregory Kramer. We acknowledge the relational emergence of the work cited in this chapter and our recognition that the body of work cannot be fully ascribed to any one or two individuals.

The importance of the therapeutic relationship has been recognized throughout the history of psychotherapy. Freud (1930/1961a) spoke of the transference relationship, and other early theorists emphasized the centrality of empathy in uncovering and releasing psychological suffering. Rogers (1961) wrote about accurate empathy, unconditional positive regard (or nonpossessive warmth), and therapist genuineness as critical factors in a healing relationship. Although scientific research has focused primarily on particular methodologies or interventions, there is now general agreement that relationship factors, regardless of the therapy approach, account for a significant portion of therapy outcome (see Chapter 4). Norcross (2011) brings an evidence-based approach to these relationship factors, spanning decades of research. He describes the most important relational elements as alliance building, empathy, unconditional positive regard and affirmation, and therapist congruence or genuineness. These are often presented as "personal characteristics" of therapists, not directly teachable, and many clinicians feel that they were not adequately trained in their cultivation. Buddhist depth psychology and meditation offer a new paradigm for training psychotherapists in relational development (including the factors of empathy, compassion, equanimity, resilience, and tranquility) and suggest new, untapped dimensions of transformation through relationship in clinical practice at every level of clinical experience.

Building on the previous two chapters, this chapter identifies and discusses key elements of therapeutic mindfulness. The connection between positive therapeutic outcome and therapist mindfulness has not yet been established scientifically (Davis & Hayes, 2011). One way to investigate this link is to identify factors known to be developed through mindfulness practice (affect regulation, acceptance, empathy, attention, etc.) and then investigate how these capacities might impact the therapy relationship. An even more direct path would be to study mindfulness *in vivo*—in the process of therapy itself. This chapter is a preliminary exploration of relational mindfulness in therapy. It is our hope that research investigating its effect and mechanisms of action will follow.

Mindfulness meditation, as it has been transmitted over centuries in monastic traditions, has been taught and practiced with an internal focus. However, mindfulness can also be practiced in engaged, mutually influencing interpersonal relationships (Kramer, Meleo-Meyer, & Turner, 2008). This approach may have particular relevance for clinical training because relational mindfulness practice has direct application to the relational component of psychotherapy. Learning to cultivate and sustain relational mindfulness during the multidimensional experience of therapy is potentially valuable for clinicians. It is one thing to cultivate equanimity and compassion for the suffering of all beings in private meditation; it's quite another to bear the rage and grief of a patient who may be experiencing you—the therapist—as the source of her or his suffering.

MIND, BRAIN, AND RELATIONSHIP

Psychotherapy is heir to religious, mystical, and shamanic traditions. The healing conversation, for example, has elements of both meditative contemplation and the confession booth. In the last century, Martin Buber (1970) wrote of true "meeting" or dialogue (the sacred "I–thou" relationship) as the place of healing and transformation. Currently, however, the practice of psychotherapy is located primarily within medicine and behavioral health, and is beginning to be understood in neurobiological terms. Banks (2010) writes:

> We now have data that shows that the brain re-regulates as a result of two people sitting in a room talking, responding to one another with facial signals, body posture responses, and empathy—that attuned "being with" the other person. This actually changes the way the brain works. And interestingly there is a change in both brains . . . revealing the mutuality of relationship. (p. 7)

Daniel Siegel (2007) has proposed a three-dimensional model of human experience that he calls the "triangle of reality." The three irreducible foundations of the triangle are *brain–body*, *mind*, and *relationship*. Each of these three elements influences the others. Siegel boldly added the relationship dimension, whereas many researchers are still working to understand how the brain and the mind impact each another, including in meditation (Davidson, 2009; Lazar et al., 2005)

Acknowledging the power of relationship grows out of an increasing appreciation of how relationship factors impact the developing brain and support mental and physical health factors such as resilience, immune functions, and stress reduction (Banks, 2010). In relational meditation, all three factors (brain, mind, and relationship) are engaged and offer us a unique opportunity to study their influence. This triangle of reality of three mutually influencing factors offers a greatly enlarged vision for our current theoretical and research models of healing factors.

Basic Relational Mindfulness Practice: "Breathing with"

- Sit facing a meditation partner on chairs or cushions, at a comfortable distance. (A bell can be rung at each step.)
- Close your eyes. Bring awareness to the internal experience of breathing—breathing in and breathing out in the presence of another person. (5 minutes)
- Open your eyes. Be aware of the other person in your visual field. Continue practicing mindfulness of your own breathing as you open your awareness to the other person. (1 minute)
- Extend your awareness to the breathing of the other. (3–5 minutes)
- Slowly expand the field of your awareness to *both* of you breathing. Notice any discomfort, pleasure, curiosity, or self-consciousness in this posture of seeing and being seen. Notice the flow—or shifts—in awareness between internal, external, or both. (5 minutes)
- Close your eyes and resume internal focus on your breathing. Notice any reactions or changes in mind–body states. (3 minutes)
- Open your eyes. Without words, find a way to express gratitude to your meditation partner for this time of practicing together. Allow a heartfelt wish for his or her happiness and well-being to arise, offering and then receiving these well-wishes. Rest in the flow. (3–5 minutes)
- Bell may be rung to signal the end of the meditation.

THE FLOW OF RELATIONSHIP

The essential practice of relational psychotherapy for the therapist is moment-to-moment attunement to self, other, and the relationship. These domains of experience co-arise and co-influence each other in an ongoing, ever-changing flow of experience. For the clinician committed to cultivating mindfulness while practicing therapy, absorption in these domains gradually increases and mindfulness becomes more continuous, pervading and illuminating therapeutic practice. Our aspiration becomes clear: how to be fully present in the relationship and to be a beneficial presence in the life of a particular patient as we explore the nature of his or her suffering together.

A heightened sense of therapeutic engagement can feel very special, even sacred. Segall (2003) writes:

> This kind of moment-to-moment attentiveness and compassionate non-egoistic focus is consistent with all forms of psychotherapy, but raising the commitment from one that is "only" professional to one that is also spiritual raises the seriousness of the therapeutic enterprise another notch. Being

fully present with the client in this way becomes part of the path of the therapist's own spiritual development. . . . Every therapeutic encounter becomes a sacred opportunity to make every word and moment count. (p. 169)

How can we incline ourselves toward such mutually uplifting experiences of therapeutic presence? I (J. L. S.) try to begin each session with the intention to anchor awareness in my breath and body (including contact points with the chair and the floor), and remind myself to sustain this form of embodied presence. Then I begin to enlarge my awareness to the physical experience of the patient in the room and to the flow of our relationship, the moment-to-moment, unfolding experience of connecting and disconnecting during the therapy hour. Again and again, I return to the felt experience of the patient, to the patient's experience of him- or herself and others in his or her life, to our relationship, and to the changing qualities of these co-emergent dimensions. Often I pause to interrupt timeworn habits from my role as a therapist (e.g., seeing something in a patient that I may have seen in past sessions and then assuming that this is what is happening right now) and anchor my awareness in the breath or sensations in my body. Over time, the field of relational mindfulness expands and becomes the larger "container" of all these internal, external, and relational experiences.

One of the Buddha's foundational mindfulness practices is to contemplate "internally, externally, and both internally and externally" (Nanamoli & Bodhi, 1995, p. 145). The scholar and Buddhist monk Analayo (2003) wrote:

> Contemplating internally serves as a basis for understanding similar phenomena in others during the second step of external contemplation. Indeed, to be aware of one's own feelings and reactions enables one to understand the feelings and reactions of others more easily. (p. 97)

Mindfulness, directed internally or externally, is known in Buddhist psychology as a *factor of awakening* (see Chapter 4), and this practice may lead our awareness beyond the duality of self- versus other-centeredness. Therapists can lose balance by practicing only other-centeredness, whereas solitary meditators can become overly focused on internal, self-oriented mindfulness. By practicing both, the distinction between internal and external becomes less significant, although the conventional difference between self and other remains. The willingness to experience fluid boundaries and to open to the flow and unfolding of relational experience characterizes clinical relational practice.

As interpersonal neurobiology has begun to demonstrate, the human brain, including the whole nervous system, is profoundly relational.

Self and *other* are mutually influencing and mutually regulating. For example, the presence of mirror neurons (Fadiga, Fogassi, Pavesi, & Rizzolatti, 1995), overlapping pathways of compassion and empathy in the brain (Decety, 2011; Decety & Meyer, 2008), and limbic resonance (Lewis, Amini, & Lannon, 2001) underlie our potential for mutuality. The release of fixed or rigid boundaries between self and other offers opportunities for deep, intersubjective knowing. This deconstruction of what are commonly thought to be stable, separate "selves" is the ground for working skillfully with change and growing in emotional freedom. The art of clinical practice is the capacity to see small changes in our patients, to sense new possibilities, and then to help actualize what is possible in patients' lives.

For example, my (J. L. S.) patient, Dave, always kept his eyes cast downward, especially when talking about suicidal thoughts. In one session, I observed his eyes scanning the office as he spoke. This fleeting perception of greater openness signaled to me that it was an opportunity to ask him more about his fears and hopes during his darkest moments. Relational mindfulness practice can deepen and make such experiential knowing more accessible, as well as guide therapeutic inquiry in a more aligned and penetrating direction.

The relational approach to psychotherapy (i.e., in which the relationship is the primary intervention) assumes that mutual influence is the ground of transformation. This subtle exchange, also known as *bidirectional exchange* (Jordan, Kaplan, Miller, Stiver, & Surrey, 1991) or *reciprocal causality* (Bandura, 1986), has also been described by Edward Tronick (2007) in his research on mother–baby interactions. He discovered that it was impossible to determine who initiated changes in facial microexpressions between mothers and their babies because they seemed to arise simultaneously. Miller and Stiver (1997) described such interreactivity in therapy as *relational movement,* an unseen realm of interbeing and interaction, or *movement-in-relationship*. Relationships are perpetually in motion, moving toward or away from deeper connection. The therapist mindfully guides the relationship toward deepening or sustaining mutual connection through recognizing and then addressing, repairing, and working to hold and heal disconnections.

THERAPY AS RELATIONAL PRACTICE

The aspiration of a psychotherapist practicing relational mindfulness is to promote the patient's self-discovery through unflinching compassionate presence. The patient's exploration can be guided or supported in many ways. The therapist can invite the patient to return to an unnoticed or fleeting experience ("Can we stay with what you just said for one more moment? It felt important"), to let go ("Can we let go of that thought for the moment and come back to the feeling in your body? I think there's a message here"), or to help the patient ground ("Something has triggered you, taken you away—let's come back to awareness of contact, body breathing, feet touching floor, awareness of being together, breathing together, right here and now").

I (J. L. S.) often experience how this sense of mutuality of awareness with a patient helps us both feel grounded and safe while enhancing intensity and clarity of insight. The shifts in perception that a process of mutual exchange offers—seeing through "my" eyes, seeing through "your" eyes, seeing what "we" see together—allow both patient and therapist to "see" beyond the limits of self-centered perception. As we release clinging and attachment to fixed views, new possibilities are awakened. Thich Nhat Hanh (2003) has described the co-arising of insight in community, compared to solitary meditation, as more clearly experienced, more memorable, more concentrated, and more sustainable in the process of awakening.

MINDFULNESS OF SELF-IN-RELATIONSHIP

From informal discussions with clinicians, we estimate that approximately 15% of the therapy hour is dedicated to background monitoring of self experience—the continuous awareness of internal, changing mind–body states (e.g., heartbeat increases when about to speak). The therapist may register, for example, countertransference reactions during which internally focused attention increases. We can attend to and work with this shift, often internally and silently (e.g., investigating, "What just triggered my anxiety and restless energy?"), while at the same time staying mindful of the patient and our relationship. The therapist can direct awareness internally to monitor empathic responses, to notice and release countertransference reactions, or simply to decide to postpone this internal work or to bring it into clinical supervision.

When working in a relational model, we try to remain open to our patients' perceptions of us, even if we would prefer not to be seen in a particular way. This openness is based on the insight that we are not the sole privileged "expert" on ourselves, that our self-image as a therapist may get in the way of knowing ourselves, and that information about our own blind spots can come from those with whom we are closely related, including our patients. The patient's own growth always remains the priority, however, as we attend to anything in ourselves that may be interfering or distracting from deep, mutual engagement.

Rogers (1980) and Norcross (2011) highlight therapist *genuineness* or *congruence* as an essential therapeutic factor. Although this quality is difficult to describe, it is supported by mindfulness of internal states. Norcross defines this factor as "the therapist's capacity to conscientiously communicate his or her experience with the client to the client" (p. 19). Rogers, Gendlin, Kiesler, and Truax (1967) write that "genuineness [in a therapist is] being [with] the feelings and attitudes which at the moment are flowing within him" (p. 100) and not hiding behind a professional role or denying feelings that are obvious in the encounter. *Congruence* is both a personal quality of the therapist as well an experienced quality of the relationship. It can be cultivated over time in clinical practice—mindfulness of deep listening and authentic speech—and may be one of the most important outcomes of an engaged relational meditation practice.

MINDFULNESS OF OTHER-IN-RELATIONSHIP

A relational therapist also practices moment-to-moment attentiveness to the actuality of the *patient*, how he or she is actually being and communicating verbally and nonverbally. In his book *Embracing the Beloved*, Stephen Levine (Levine & Levine, 1995) describes his meditative experience of moment-to-moment receptivity and open awareness in relationship to his partner Ondrea. He writes:

> Watching with merciful awareness the subtle emanations of another's body, their momentary awkwardness of movement, the slightly distended arch of their neck, the tilt of their head, the coloration of their skin, the tension around the mouth, the positioning of the hands and legs—in the changing of mind and body postures, the heart of each receives the process of the other. (p. 243)

He also describes a related practice of noting the qualities of one's own seeing:

> Noting when we bring a hard or soft gaze, noticing judgment, thinking, the level, depth, and sustaining of focus and how all this resonates with the conditions in the other . . . paying close attention moment to moment to the shifting qualities of "seeing" and "being seen." (p. 240)

Through descriptions of this changing moment-to-moment experience, Levine elegantly conveys how interrelated (or mutually co-arising) human beings actually are, and how deeply this can be known in close, ongoing relationships such as in therapy. Even qualities of how we see depend on sensing how the patient is feeling about being seen. These shifts and changes move faster than we can ever fixate on. In mindfulness practice, as we slow down and see more deeply into this process, we can make clearer choices and respond more effectively.

Empathic attunement in relationship, through relationship, has long been seen as central in therapy. Carl Rogers (1980) defined empathy as

> the therapist's sensitive ability and willingness to understand the client's thoughts, feelings, and struggles from the client's point of view. . . . [It] means entering the private perceptual world of the other . . . being sensitive, moment by moment, to the changing felt meanings which flow in this other person or sensing the arising of new dawning sensations, perceptions, or insights. This openness to subtle change is essential for "inviting the new" into the flow of experience. It may mean sensing meanings of which he or she is scarcely aware. (p. 142)

Relational mindfulness is the ground of the therapist's ability to invite a patient into a new or subtle shift in the direction of the therapeutic inquiry.

Relational mindfulness practice supports clarity and subtlety of perception. For example, after I returned from a 5-day relational meditation retreat, one of my (J. L. S.'s) patients came into the office and immediately began to speak. However, my attention was drawn to the movement of her hands. She was expressing her grief with the wringing of her hands, each hand comforting the other. The mindfulness retreat had sharpened my awareness of body sensations and feeling states, and I saw and felt in a direct, visceral way how this patient expressed her loneliness and her yearning for contact. Relational mindfulness practice had opened my heart and mind to receive her nonverbal cues more vividly—with greater awareness, compassion, and understanding—than would have ordinarily occurred.

Important new brain research on empathy is revealing what may be occurring when we see another person in pain. Social pain overlap theory (SPOT) suggests that both physical and psychological pains are registered in similar regions of the brain (Eisenberg & Lieberman, 2004). Social neuroscientists such as Jean Decety (2011), Tania Singer and Claus Lamm (2009), and Christian Keysers (2011) are beginning to map how our brains register the experience of another person, how we come to know and to understand the other, and where in the brain empathy and compassion are likely to occur. For example, Decety (2006) has studied the patterns of activation in the brains of an observer and those of a person in pain, revealing a great deal of overlap as well as important differences. The person in distress shows more limbic activity and sensorimotor localization, whereas the observer demonstrates more frontal lobe activity. The observer's ability to know and "be with" another's pain, while adding other higher-order executive functions, seems to be a good description of empathy. In clinical practice, the therapist needs to register in her or his body the experience of the other's pain, knowing that it is not his or her own pain, and then to bring other qualities such as care, compassion, equanimity, and emotional intelligence to the encounter.

Empathy is always an ongoing, relational process, what Surrey and Jordan (2012) call *mutual empathy*. The therapist is working to "see" and to "know" by attuning and adjusting to what the patient is seeing. As the therapist moves toward the patient's experience, giving and receiving microcommunications, the therapist reads and misreads the patient's cues until the patient feels seen and heard. Eventually, emotional and somatic resonance creates the experience of actually being joined, of not being alone.

Jordan and colleagues (1991) note that "being with" is an antidote to the suffering of isolation and disconnection that are at the core of so much suffering in modern culture. Reconnection is a central healing factor of the relational–cultural theory developed at the Jean Baker Miller Training Institute at Wellesley College (Surrey & Jordan, 2012). The movement out of exile and into connection with the rest of humanity, especially when we suffer, is one way to understand the healing power of empathy and compassion.

MINDFULNESS OF RELATIONSHIP-IN-RELATIONSHIP

Miller and Stiver (1997) describe attunement to the therapy relationship as the clinician's primary task. For example, the mindful therapist can be aware of the texture of the relationship, the intensity of connection, the sudden or subtle shifts into disconnection, the sense of collaboration or division, the struggles for power and control, and the dance of safety and danger. In one couple's therapy session, I (J. L. S.) asked the husband if he felt a change in the relationship when he made a comment his wife perceived as critical. He described feeling the texture of the relationship change abruptly from "smooth" to "sandpaper." Attending to the relationship can help move the discussion from "he said, she said" to how the two are meeting or moving together, to what is happening in the space between them. This shift in focus can be a great relief to patients in couple therapy as well as to clinicians engaged in individual psychotherapy.

Miller and Stiver (1997) also describe the power of mutually empathic and mutually empowering relationships to challenge and disrupt past relational images constructed from traumatic or chronic disconnections. They emphasize the importance of honoring the strategies of disconnection in protecting vulnerability that we all develop in our relational lives to varying degrees. The therapist's awareness of, and freedom to loosen, the grip of her or his own personal and professional strategies of disconnection are crucial for the patient's parallel work.

Daniel Siegel (1999) studied the role that attuned and resonant relationships play in brain development. Secure attachment supports neural and personality integration through contingent communication, coherent narrative, repair of disconnections, and the soothing of negative mind–body states and the amplification of positive states. Early attachment experiences have the power to shape the brain and relationships over a lifetime, but, fortunately, new relational experiences can support and propel healthy development at any age. Cozolino (2010) describes how the healing power of relationship can transform disorders of attachment by rewiring the brain. The therapy relationship provides a secure and stable base that, over time, can facilitate these changes.

Effective therapists develop this capacity to stay present and connected to self, other, and the relationship. Through the practice of staying with difficult emotions and experiences, relational mindfulness is cultivated and sustained, and there is less identification with any particular emotional state. It becomes possible to remain present and balanced, yet fully engaged, in challenging moments in therapy, without resorting to judgmental diagnostic labeling (e.g., "She is clearly a borderline"). Equanimity grows over time and difficult moments in therapy are perceived less as a threat and more of an opportunity to "be with" and "stay with" a patient.

Rogers (1980) and Norcross (2001) describe the importance of unconditional positive regard in the therapy relationship. Genuine acceptance, respect, affirmation, and relational warmth have a positive influence on therapy outcome. Practicing the *brahma viharas* (wholesome attitudes or states of mind such as friendliness, compassion, empathic joy, and equanimity—see Chapter 4 and the Appendix) is a fruitful extension of relational mindfulness practice. Giving and receiving these qualities in psychotherapy can bring joy, inspiration, and emotional freedom to the difficult work of being with the emotional suffering of our patients.

Stephen Porges (2011a) has extensively researched the vagus nerve and discovered that under conditions of safety and tranquility, the vagus nerve inhibits the fight–flight–freeze response. In conditions of safe, quiet, relaxed verbal exchange, with access to a branch called the *smart vagus* (i.e., ventral vagus), we can engage in social behaviors like eye contact, touch, and empathy. We can "recruit the neural circuits that enable us to express the wonderful aspects of being human, such as mindfulness" (Porges, 2011b). It appears that mindful relationships activate the smart vagus and maximize the potential for psychological change.

Practicing Mindful Co-Meditation: Mindfulness of Self, Other, and Relationship

This exercise can best be led by a trained therapist in a workshop setting. Participants should find partners and sit on chairs or cushions. Each pair of partners decides who will be the first speaker, and thereafter maintain silence, except as instructed by the leader. The leader uses a meditation bell to signify the beginning and end of periods of practice.

- To begin, both partners close their eyes and practice mindfulness internally, focusing on breathing in and breathing out. (3 minutes)
- Then they open their eyes, maintaining a soft, relaxed gaze; no need to fixate or stare. Participants are invited to notice the arising of different emotions, thoughts, and judgments. Also, notice any discomfort that might arise while remaining with one's breathing.
- Now, the first speaker practices authentic, mindful speaking while his or her partner practices deep mindful listening. The speaker responds to the questions: "What is here now? What are you aware of arising in this moment?" Participants are reminded to pause, again and again, and notice what is present. The speaker is invited to stay with what he or she sees, hears, or feels in the body and to align his or her speech with actual experience. (8 minutes)
- Meanwhile, the listener practices deep mindful listening, "being with" the speaker moment to moment . . . simply receiving and accepting what is being spoken.
- Then the listener reflects back what he or she heard, saw,

or noticed while listening, and the speaker relates his or her experience of being seen and heard. They may discuss, for example, how this experience differs from internal mindfulness practice. (6 minutes)

- Then the partners switch roles—the first speaker becomes the listener, and the first listener becomes the speaker. Repeat the previous steps.
- At the end of the exercise, the participants are invited to express gratitude, *in silence,* to their co-meditation partners for sharing this exercise, allowing well-wishes for one's partner's to arise in the heart. Soon thereafter, those wishes can be expressed verbally and participants are encouraged to receive them as well.
- Finally, participants are invited to rest in the flow of shared care and friendship. (3 minutes)

RELATIONAL PRACTICE IN BUDDHIST PSYCHOLOGY

Since most of our lives are lived in relationship, we continually experience interpersonal contact that vibrates an inner web of conditioned reactions. We are interactive and interreactive creatures; conditioned reactivity in one triggers the patterns of reactivity in the other, impacting and influencing each other in an ongoing dance of interreactivity. Just as the truth of sensory discomfort rests on the fact of our sensitivity to a stimulating physical environment, the truth of interpersonal suffering reveals us as sensitive psychological creatures in a complex and stimulating social environment. Humans are essentially relational.

We are wired for relationships, and our survival depends on relationships to live. We must rely on others for safety, comfort, and love as children and throughout our lives. We form bonds of attachment that impact all future relationships, and we're shaped not only by our own suffering as human beings, but also vicariously by the suffering of others. To be human and relational is to be touched by the sorrow, lamentation, grief, and despair that spring from participation in the web of life and our shared biological limitations, including the inevitability of sickness, aging, and death.

Out of this flux we learn to construct an "I," a sense of self as a vehicle for managing sensory input and participating in social life. This strategy inevitably creates a sense of separation between oneself and others. As adults, we struggle mightily between our yearning to break down the self–other duality and take refuge in relationships (Surrey & Jordan,

2012) while at the same time seeking safety by withdrawing into the illusion of a separate, independent self. Western culture is obsessed with the centrality and primacy of the individual and the defining of self and other in hierarchical and stratified relationships. These social constructions of race, class, gender, sexual orientation, etc., further influence our intimate relationships.

A Buddhist analysis of interpersonal suffering goes beyond our contemporary psychologies, which posit "healthy attachment" or "mutuality" as a remedy for relational suffering. The First Noble Truth of Buddhism (see the Appendix) declares that suffering is built into the human experience. There is a universality of *interpersonal* suffering as we constantly seek security in an uncontrollable, contingent world. In relational meditation practice, we can directly experience interpersonal suffering with the healing capacities of mindfulness and compassion. By awakening together, we can support each other in finding pathways to greater ease and well-being. Paradoxically, recognizing the inevitability of suffering can lead us on the path to emotional freedom—the end of suffering, directly experienced and released through relating mindfully with one another.

RELATIONAL MINDFULNESS PRACTICE

The guidelines for Insight Dialogue, a relationally engaged meditation practice, support relational mindfulness practice and are immediately applicable to clinical practice. At the same time, these guidelines provide access to very subtle levels of mindfulness and point the way toward the possibility of a deep emotional and psychological liberation that goes to the very roots of interpersonal suffering. Even mature clinicians who begin practicing Insight Dialogue may discover depths of relational awareness currently unimaginable.

The Insight Dialogue approach grew out of solitary retreat practice within the Theravada Buddhist tradition. Co-meditation is introduced as an extension of silent meditation. The initial practice is an opportunity to observe the emotional obstacles that arise when we engage in an intimate face-to-face encounter. Thereafter, pairs of participants practice deep listening and authentic speaking as they contemplate a variety of wisdom teachings together. Over perhaps 5–10 days, deep insights into the nature of mind (impermanence, the illusion of a separate self) begin to arise and qualities of awakening are often experienced, such as energy, joy, and tranquility (see Chapter 4).

GUIDELINES FOR INSIGHT DIALOGUE

The following are the instructions for Insight Dialogue, a relational practice developed for mindfulness meditation practitioners in general, which can be adapted for training clinicians at all levels of experience. These guidelines are first offered by a meditation teacher or practitioner and then become internalized.

Pause

The invitation to *Pause* refers to both a temporal pause from habitual automatic thoughts and responses and the return to an attitude or remembering of mindfulness (*awareness* of *present experience* with *acceptance* and *compassion*). The Pause allows for awareness of the changing vibrations of self, other, and the relationship and for loosening identification with and clinging to strong emotional reactions and past mental constructions (see Chapter 4). This is a reminder to cultivate and sustain mindfulness, moment to moment, to notice when our attention has drifted and what has taken it away, and to return it again and again to observing thoughts and feelings, with freshness and curiosity. In a verbal exchange, Pause is especially helpful for encouraging mindfulness before speaking, during speaking, and after speaking. The spaciousness of the silence underlying speech brings depth and mindfulness to what may become automatic and patterned by the therapist role. The Pause can initially feel disruptive in challenging comfortable habits and ways of being.

Relax

The guideline to *Relax* invites us to calm our bodies and minds and to accept and receive whatever sensations, thoughts, and feelings are present. This guideline invites tranquility, but because the moment of interpersonal contact is often not serene, Relax also is intended to cultivate an attitude of acceptance of difficult thoughts and emotions. Relax can ripen into concentration, compassion, and care. The therapist's practice of Relax offers an ease and depth of "being with" that becomes available to the patient through the intimacy of relationship. Siegel's (1999) description of the therapist soothing negative states and amplifying positive states is relevant here.

Open

When we Open, we extend mindfulness beyond the boundaries of mind and body to the so-called *external* world. In relational practice, Open is the spacious extension of meditation into the relational moment and into mutuality. The reminder to return to openness and wider awareness can be a direct way of working with the closing down or closing off of relational awareness. *Open* serves as a reminder that shutting down into internal awareness alone and losing the thread of relational awareness is antithetical to the commitment to be present for the other and the intention to "be with." Mindfulness of the flow of this ongoing movement of expanding and shrinking can be known and maintained, serving as a guide for the therapist to the ever-changing qualities of relational movements and support in a deepening empathic connectedness with the patient. The practitioner of relational meditation can become familiar with, and fluent in, the movement between mindfulness of internal phenomena, external phenomena, and both simultaneously. In this way, the therapist is less likely to get lost in self or other; empathy may arise with external mindfulness, while the internal awareness of the body can remain grounded and stable.

Trust Emergence

The guideline to *Trust Emergence* invites the therapist (and through his or her connection, the patient) to release past history and agendas, to soften the attitude of authoritative certainty, and to allow for the knowing that is emerging in the present moment. In relational practice, the arising of new insight is often co-emergent—neither in one person nor the other alone, but in the relationship procreated between them. Trust Emergence supports the quality of mutual discovery and offers both the therapist and the patient the invitation to investigate and discover, to see together, to sit together at the edge of creative knowing, emerging in its own time and at its own pace, in moment-to-moment awareness.

Listen Deeply

Listen Deeply, a full meditation practice in itself, is an invitation to be mindful of the obstacles to full receptivity and to rest in embodied, non-self-referential deep attunement and resonance. This kind of listening is a foundational practice for clinicians. We practice receptive, whole-bodied listening to speech, words, nonverbal and embodied movements and expressions of the other. At the same time, we remain mindful of internal changing aspects of the listening, seeing, feeling, and resonating with—all qualities of empathic listening. Learning to Pause while listening supports clinicians in offering a depth of attention, concentration, and spaciousness to the relationship. This kind of attention is received by the patient as unconditional acceptance and nonpossessive warmth (Rogers, 1961) One therapist trained in the Focusing method described it as "minimum intrusion, maximum accompaniment" (J. Klagsburn, personal communication, March 8, 2011).

Speak the Truth

The last guideline for insight dialogue invites the practitioner to bring authenticity of presence and speech into the therapy relationship. *Speak the Truth* and *Listen Deeply* are interwoven in relational practice. The therapist also invites authenticity in the patient by speaking the truth him- or herself. The healing factors of genuineness (Rogers, 1961) and congruence (Norcross, 2011) are mutually emergent and mutually co-arising in relationship. Furthermore, the relationship is gradually liberated from fixity, superficiality, impasse, or chronic states of disconnection (subtle or gross) through the practice of authenticity that has mindfulness and concentration for its foundation. Miller and Stiver (1997) describe a pathway into deepening or restoring connection when the therapy relationship has begun to feel stuck, prickly, lifeless, or at an impasse. They remind the therapist that finding "one true thing" (something honest and genuine) that can be said often provides an opening, a return of the possibility of movement and change. Finding this subjective truth and putting it into clear, fresh, relevant language engages one in a rejuvenated relationship with words as carriers of meaning, compassion, and awareness.

FACTORS OF AWAKENING
AND CO-MEDITATION PRACTICE

The Buddha described seven factors of awakening (see Chapter 3 and the Appendix) that emerge naturally with the maturation of mindfulness practice and that can be cultivated directly in relational meditation. They are specifically developed at Insight Dialogue retreats. These factors (mindfulness, investigation of phenomenal experience, energy, joy, tranquility, concentration, and equanimity) are touched, but often not fully realized, in ordinary therapy practice. Cultivation of these factors in relational meditation potentiates their power on the path of awakening together and points to a new depth of relational practice for psychotherapists.

As a practitioner develops the factors of awakening, his or her experience of the therapeutic relationship undergoes significant qualitative shifts. Mindfulness and concentration, together, foster unbroken attention to self, other, and the relationship. With this quality of relational awareness, the practitioner more clearly perceives and more deeply responds to nuances of expression in the client's eyes, voice, and language. Compassion and care grow and are balanced by equanimity. When all the factors are strong and balanced, especially if we are engaged with someone also meditating in this way, we can experience an intimacy that is not based on shared emotional constructions, but rather has a quality of being joined—an unconstructed intimacy of "nothing in the way." The common reference point is no longer the personality and its concerns, but awareness itself.

At the same time, mindfulness facilitates direct apprehension of the impermanent nature of self, other, and all constructs; they become phenomena rising and vanishing, with no central core. The protective fabrications of the personality, even one's identification with the body as self, may drop away, leaving a co-arising experience of bright, simple, peaceful awareness. Such an experience significantly expands the spectrum of what we may have thought possible in relationship. Experiencing the aliveness and peace of an unconstructed, undefended way of being with another will have a profound impact on our everyday lives and on our work as therapists.

In their 2011 comprehensive review of research on the clinical benefits of mindfulness, Davis and Hayes write that there has been no research studying the benefits of the experience of intersubjectivity, or *interbeing*, although the movement out of alienation or separation and into the shared human experience is implicit in the healing power of compassion. Further study of relational mindfulness may help to identify and differentiate specific healing factors and to validate the clinical value of mindfulness in the therapy relationship.

6

Practical Ethics

Stephanie P. Morgan

> It is in everybody's interest to do what leads to
> happiness and avoid that which leads to suffering.
> And because, as we have seen, our interests are
> inextricably linked, we are compelled to accept ethics
> as the indispensable interface between my desire to
> be happy and yours.
> —DALAI LAMA (1999)

*F*rom a Buddhist perspective, ethical training is a critical component of living skillfully and happily (Dalai Lama, 1999; Hanh, 2007).
Although ethics has a place in Western mental health training, it is typically not understood to have the reach and power that it is accorded in
Buddhist traditions. This chapter lays out the central features of Buddhist ethical training, examines the ways in which personally undertaking this discipline can enhance our clinical skills, and explores how
we might skillfully engage with ethical issues in our patients' lives. It is
intended to invite inquiry into a practice that can be of tremendous help
to us, both personally and professionally. More questions are raised than
answered.

In mental health training, ethical discussions have usually focused
on helping clinicians to avoid wrongdoing and stay out of trouble. As
our culture has become more litigious, there has been a commensu-
rate rise in the number of books, articles, and professional presentations about ethics, often under the heading of *risk management*. There

is scant literature, however, addressing how ethical considerations might illuminate the therapy encounter (Monteiro et al., 2010) or enhance our well-being as clinicians (Devettere, 1993).

Why do our psychotherapeutic traditions have such a hands-off stance regarding ethics? In the West, morality has customarily been considered a religious rather than a scientific matter. As psychology and psychiatry became increasingly scientific, issues of morality were deliberately set aside. Additionally, any emphasis on morality was seen as threatening the hallmark value of psychotherapy—an individual's freedom. Yet, in the last two decades, research from the field of positive psychology (Dahlsgaard, Peterson, & Seligman, 2005; Peterson & Seligman, 2004) has demonstrated a correlation between ethical behavior and happiness. Studies point to a bilateral relationship between morality and well-being: happier people act more ethically, and ethical behavior leads to greater happiness (Diener & Kesebir, 2008; James & Chymis, 2004). These findings certainly merit our attention as mental health clinicians. Along similar lines, Buddhist psychology has long recognized that the motivation for moral behavior need not derive from a limiting prohibition, but rather can arise from the understanding that moral behavior increases our happiness and the happiness of others. Ethical action can evolve from something one *should* do into something one *wants* to do.

BUDDHIST ETHICAL TRAINING

This motivation—the desire to enhance our well-being and happiness— is at the core of a Buddhist understanding of ethical behavior. Although the tradition emphasizes ethical conduct as a means to prevent or reduce harm, it also describes how ethical conduct increases well-being. According to Buddhist scholar Andrew Olendzki (2012), *moral health* is seen as an important aspect of a person's overall wellness. Just as behavioral choices impact physical health, ethical decisions impact moral health. Buddhist ethical training is also noteworthy for its emphasis on personal research. In undertaking ethical training, we begin a phenomenological investigation into cause and effect. As Owen Flanagan (2011), a contemporary moral scholar, notes, "Buddhism is the one religion that asks for its truth claims to be verified by research." We examine in our own experience what happens when we act ethically and what happens when we don't.

Additionally, the term *ethical training* aptly conveys the developmental nature of the enterprise—a practitioner is a lifelong learner, developing ever-increasing moral sensitivity and greater capacity to live in alignment with this awareness. From the Buddhist perspective of the interdependence of all things, ethics is the behavioral manifestation of good reality testing. As the Dalai Lama put it, "Due to the fundamental interconnectedness which lies at the heart of reality, your interest is also my interest" (1999, p. 47).

Moral action is cultivated by observing five basic precepts (Aitken, 1984; Hanh, 1998). Rather than prohibitions, these precepts are guidelines for living skillfully. They frame a discipline, which, when undertaken, calms the mind and allows for the development of what Davis (2011) calls *moral sensitivity*. Traditionally, the five precepts have been described as restraint from (1) killing, (2) stealing, (3) sexual misconduct, (4) lying, and (5) using intoxicants. In the last few decades, Zen master and teacher Thich Nhat Hanh (2007) has offered a reformulation of these precepts to address the realities and challenges of contemporary living. In this reformulation, the guidelines for skillful behavior include acts of commission as well as acts of restraint:

1. Restraint from killing—compassionate action, reverence for life.
2. Restraint from stealing—concern for equity, generosity.
3. Restraint from sexual misconduct—skillfulness with sexual energy.
4. Restraint from lying—honest, skillful speech.
5. Restraint from using intoxicants—awareness of consumption.

From a Buddhist perspective, the cultivation of moral sensitivity and skillful moral action are experiential, developmental, and work in tandem. The training requires attention and effort in three dimensions: concentration (Sanskrit: *samadhi*), insight (*prajna*), and moral action (*sila*). Traditionally referred to as the *three-fold training*, these dimensions are interdependent—each one potentiates the other two. Undertaking the precepts creates a calming, settling effect in one's life that aids concentration. Greater concentration leads to more insight, which in turn deepens and refines our understanding of and ability to embody the precepts. *Sila*, or morality practice, pushes and develops our understanding, while also being an expression of our understanding (Olendzki, 2010). We *work it*, so to speak, and *it works us*. Additionally, each of the precepts is understood to represent a continuum, offering the opportunity to attend, practice, and learn with increasing refinement in wisdom and skillful means. Practicing with the precepts involves reflection, intentionality with behavior, and awareness of cause and effect.

This practice involves taking care with a light touch. In discovering that the precepts are actually impossible to keep, we cultivate genuine humility. As Davis (2011) notes, "This experiential approach to morality is as demanding as it is liberating" (p. 12). We undertake the five precepts knowing that we will regularly fail, though as our understanding deepens, we will more often act skillfully. Precept practice opens us increasingly to what we might call our *practice edges*. On these edges, we hone our discernment. We understand more about the causes, conditions, and outcomes of our behavior. We express our willingness to begin again, time after time—much as one does when trying to simply be with the breath in meditation practice.

There is also a kinship between the feedback loop noted in ethical practice and what we observe as a therapy session unfolds: The more we pay attention, the more we notice. The more we notice, the more skillfully we interact with our patients. The more skillfully we interact with our patients, the more rich material arises, which in turn invites even more refined attention. Although this level of attention is challenging, it is also enlivening and adds freshness to our day-to-day work.

ETHICAL TRAINING FOR THE THERAPIST

The starting point for ethical training is observing our own behavior, both inside and outside of our consulting rooms. We will use each of the five precepts as a lens and explore ways that this lens can enhance and refine our clinical work. As the Dalai Lama (1999) says, "It is far more useful to be aware of a single shortcoming in ourselves than it is to be aware of a thousand shortcomings in someone else. For when the fault is our own, we are in a position to correct it" (p. 153). The following are just a few of many ways to explore our conduct in the course of our clinical practice.

First Precept: Reverence for Life

The Hippocratic oath states "First, do no harm." Although this is certainly our intention as psychotherapists, looking more closely, we see that this precept is impossible to keep. My colleague Ed Yeats wisely warns, "We are most dangerous when we are unaware of our capacity for harm" (personal communication, 1995). Working with this precept clinically, we investigate those ways in which our actions can be unintentionally harmful.

Working with Anger

How do we deal with our own anger when it arises in a session? Noticing that anger is present is the first step. If we repudiate this aspect of our experience, we are more likely to be driven by the anger in some way—be it a reduction in empathy, an unskillful response, or a distancing from the patient. In working with a patient who had a pattern of cancellations, I found that I became slower than usual in returning his phone calls for rescheduling. In becoming aware of my own enactment, it became possible to bring the issue into the treatment for mutual exploration.

Subtle Forms of Mistreatment

It can be useful to step back from our caseload and examine the quality of care that we are bringing to each of our patients. We each have our own standards with regard to punctuality, responsiveness to phone calls, how we end sessions. Wherever your bar is set, are there any patients with whom the bar is a bit lower? Becoming aware of those individuals whose appointment time we might more readily shift, or with whom we're comfortable being a few minutes late, focuses our attention on these less-than-caring behaviors, enabling us to bring more wholehearted attention. In our sloppiness, we may be exploiting a patient's goodwill or reenacting a subtle form of neglect familiar to him or her. Again, the wonderful aspect of working with this first precept is that it invites us to examine our behaviors on this more subtle level, increasing coherence between our intentions and our actions.

Making Mistakes

One of the hard truths about doing psychotherapy is that we make mistakes. The existential therapist James Bugental (1987) distinguishes *realistic* from *neurotic* guilt. In realistic guilt, we experience a creative discomfort when we acknowledge a mistake and learn from it. He challenges us to be aware that while we are probably better at our craft today than we were years ago, we are likely less capable now than we will be in another year. This is the spirit of humility in which we work with precepts in Buddhist practice. As my colleague Nancy Cahan put it, "You mop up and learn what there is to learn" (personal communication, 2011). An experience during my training illustrates this understanding:

I was seeing a retired seamstress who was very appreciative of my time and attention. She started bringing me little hand-sewn gifts. I thanked her and tried to explain that the gifts were unnecessary. The gifts kept on coming: a cloth glasses case, a fabric tissue box. I discussed the dilemma in supervision and was coached to set a limit, my supervisor advising that it was unethical for me to continue to receive her gifts. She heard me and stopped bringing me gifts, but unfortunately, she stopped bringing herself as well, dropping out of treatment. In naively sticking to the "letter of the law," I abandoned its spirit. Had I been more seasoned, I would have found a way to work with this dilemma, surrendering to a process that would have been more murky, but also more mutual and respectful.

As Schwartz and Sharpe (2010) suggest, "Moral skill and will, like technical skill, are learned by practicing the craft" (p. 271).

Second Precept: Money and Equity

What Are We Being Paid For?

In attempting to be fair to both our patients and ourselves, we might ask, "What are they paying us for?" Perhaps we can all agree that one thing our patients are paying us for is skillful attention. We intend to provide our attention, yet we have, as Joan Halifax (1993) says, "wayward minds and forgetful hearts" (p. 144). When we work with this precept, we undertake not to rob our patients through our inattention. Time is precious. Think of your hourly rate and divide by 50, if you do a 50-minute hour. So if your fee is $100, a patient is paying $2 per minute. If we're off doing our grocery list, our patient is not getting full value. While our inattention might also be pointing to other factors in the treatment, this reflection adds another dimension to our awareness. Again, working the precept is not about indicting ourselves; it is about looking carefully at our motivations, our behaviors, and cause and effect.

There are other ways that we can exploit our patients' time. Do we ask more questions when someone is talking about content in which we are particularly interested for our own ends? Working with this precept challenges us to be more aware of the motives behind our curiosity. We can bring mindful attention to the questions we ask and why we ask them. If we are asking out of idle curiosity or to satisfy a particular interest of ours, it is more equitable to exercise restraint. A colleague told me he once asked his therapist, "Is that question for me or for you?"

A similar issue arises with gratifying content. When a patient is entertaining or funny, we love to sit back and enjoy the ride. When someone falls in love, we delight in hearing all of the intoxicating details. Again, these are delicate and nuanced issues for our discernment. Our delight isn't necessarily problematic and people so want to be enjoyed. Both of these dynamics can be just the right medicine. But we want to be tracking what is going on within ourselves and noticing our motives in the moment.

Fees

This second precept concerning equity also provides a lens we can bring to our fees. Getting paid for the work we do is essential and appropriate. Payment and the boundaries around time enable us to sit with patients in a way that is, as philosopher Paul Russell said, "free of need." The value of this can't be overestimated. A person is paying to be in a relationship where we need nothing of him or her and have no need for our patient to be anything for us. Yet within the complicated territory of fees and payment, working with this second precept involves:

- Viewing our work as an ecological system, wherein higher fees can enable us to provide some services for lower fees. In social work training, the tradition of pro bono work is a hallmark of the profession. Working with this precept involves practicing generosity with our time and effort.
- Knowing what side of the road we're on and our leanings and vulnerabilities with regard to money. Are we too concerned with money? Are we insufficiently attentive to these issues? If we are unaware of our tendencies, they will play out in the treatment.
- Examining our monetary dealings with third-party payers and the tax collector. Do we have a consistent standard across the board or do we rationalize different standards?

Third Precept: Skillfulness with Sexuality

This precept refers to restraint from any sexual involvement with our patients. Bringing more refinement to this area involves recognizing the power of sexual energy and committing to developing compassion and wisdom around it. As therapists, it is a great gift to our patients to be loving and safe to love. By *safe to love* I mean that our patients can have their full range of feeling, which might include love and desire.

Awareness helps us stay steady and receptive to this full range of expression, while at the same time not leaving our seat.

In working with this precept, we attempt to refrain from using our patients for our own gratification. If we find ourselves doing something unusual with our apparel or in any other way in anticipation of seeing a particular patient, it might indicate the need for further attention to our motivations. Does our behavior point to some hunger, absence, or dimension of feeling in our own life that merits attention?

A lovely female college student who was in therapy shared that her middle-age therapist exclaimed, "You look so much like my girlfriend in college!" She recounted this because she felt it was off, but doubted her own response, since she generally felt trusting and helped by her therapist. This behavior, while not a flagrant boundary violation, points to the ways in which, if we are not conscious, our own sloppiness with sexual energy can diminish our patients' trust. Working with this precept involves taking care with our feelings and impulses.

Flirtatious Energy

This precept also raises the question of how we relate to flirtatious energy. Flirtatious energy can represent so many different things, in and out of the therapy hour. Is it a celebration of life and vitality? Is it a deadened and habitual way of relating? Is it an avoidance of pain that deserves attention? Is it a veiled form of aggression? For many of us, our reflexive comfort or discomfort with sexual energy can inhibit our awareness and investigation. We might disengage by either reflexively shutting down or participating with less awareness. Navigating these waters wisely takes attention and practice.

Playfulness can be life-affirming. I've noticed that there are instances when I've been working with someone over time and then one day I simply see him in a fresh way, as more attractive. Becoming aware of this new energy is often a harbinger of the person feeling better—less depressed, or less anxious.

If the flirtatious energy feels like a defense against underlying vulnerability, a gracious acknowledgment can be skillful. For example, "While I am complimented that you are flirting with me, perhaps your heart needs a different kind of attention." When the flirtation feels deadened or deadening, there might be underlying hostility. In trying to effectively respond to this form of flirtation, we often feel tied-up and uncomfortable. At such times, the introduction of an existential perspective can be helpful. I sometimes find a way to bring up aging or death. Working with a powerful CEO in his 60s, I was repeatedly struggling, feeling powerless and ineffective in the face of his antics. One day, I simply stated, "You know, we're both growing old." This existential truth had a great settling effect and grounded our connection in something real.

Fourth Precept: Skillful Speech

The fourth precept, skillful speech, probably has the most ramifications for psychotherapy. What we say or don't say is a central feature of the therapy encounter. Most importantly, our trustworthiness is paramount to the therapeutic power of the relationship.

Honesty

Joseph Goldstein, a wise and senior *vipassana* meditation teacher, once said that if we undertook this precept completely, it would be a full practice—meaning that it would cultivate sufficient awareness and discernment to bring enlightenment. We lie in little ways all the time. Precept practice directs us to look in the mirror. What do we rationalize on a tax return? How impeccable are we in our dealings with insurers? When we are less than honest with our patients, what are the implications?

Bare honesty advances our work. I remember a moment from my own treatment. I was looking down, talking about something, and happened to look up and sensed that my therapist's attention had wandered. I asked, "Where'd you go?" She responded, "Not far." I loved her response because I felt fully met in that moment. Her honesty enriched the closeness and authenticity in our relationship.

When we can step up and acknowledge our missteps, it often brings both discomfort and greater intimacy. Months ago, I had a phone appointment set up at a time when I don't usually work. I remembered hours later. As I prepared to call my patient, I considered the multiple ways I could put a spin on what had occurred. Of course, none felt very satisfactory because none was true. I called her and said, "Jean, I completely forgot." We make our very best attempts and when we fall short, this precept invites us to be truthful about things, just as they are. In the context of responsible treatment, people can usually forgive our fallibility. Certainly there are times in which bare honesty is not appropriate and can be hurtful. But the motivation for our little white lies is more often reflective of what Steven Pinker (2008) describes as "a nasty tendency to put self on the side of the angels" (p. 58).

Restraint from Frivolous Speech

Working with the precept of skillful speech also includes an examination of frivolous speech—talking that is unnecessary and can diminish the richness of a moment. At times, the texture of a silence is best left undisturbed, as a shared silence can give birth to a deepening of expression. When we are fully available to accompany a patient in silence, we might be helping him or her find freedom in just simply being.

At the beginning and end of the hour, we are more prone to fall into reflexive patterns of speech. We want to convey warmth, yet this might be more effectively conveyed in eye contact, fully taking the person in as we greet him or her, rather than through a more socially conventional "chatty" greeting. While a person is sometimes freed to ease into the session via friendly conversation, we want to be conscious of what motivates our talking. Similarly, the end of a session can be an occasion for greater care with speech. There are times when I've gotten up and seen the person to the door in a manner that isn't in keeping with the affect of the session we've just had, when I've fallen into a less present, socially conditioned way of saying good bye. Practicing skillful speech supports us in extending our attention to the transitional interactions that are part of the therapy encounter.

Disclosure

Meditation teachers often advise that skillful speech requires that we ask two questions: (1) Is it honest? (2) Is it skillful? We've been looking at honesty. Exploring disclosure takes us into the question of skillfulness. Will the information be helpful and is it a good use of the patient's limited time with us? So often, when we disclose in an unbidden way, it reflects what Joseph Goldstein (2010) refers to as "the irresistible, pregnant-with-conceit desire to say, 'Here I am'." Such comments rarely add to our patient's experience.

Although there are no hard and fast recipes with regard to disclosure, leaning toward restraint gives us space and time to be aware of our motivations and to consider consequences. Certainly, when an absence of disclosure contributes to a lack of reality testing, it may be harmful to be silent. In addition, there are times when a client asks us a question and a straightforward answer helps him or her experience mutuality and respect in the relationship. When we are in doubt about whether to disclose, we also have a third option, which is to share our process of consideration.

Fifth Precept: Mindful Consumption

This precept is about restraining from the use of any substances that cloud the mind and, I might add, heart. Clearly, if we are struggling with substance abuse, there is a level of pain in our lives that will hamper our capacity to sit fully with someone else.

More broadly and subtly, this precept pertains to all that we consume. It opens us to examine what we ingest with each of our senses. As the adage goes, "We are what we eat." We do our best work when we take care of ourselves. In addition to the healthfulness of the food we eat, we can investigate the material we read, the media we take in, the degree to which we are nurturing our full selves. As we look closely in this area, we can see the impact that mindful consumption can have on our clinical work as well as our overall well-being.

We all have times when we are struggling with life's circumstances and feel depleted. We notice that we are not as fully present or that we are seeking something to provide additional stimulation within the therapy hour. We might find ourselves asking more questions or becoming overly active in a manner that isn't responsive to our patient, but rather is an attempt to rouse our own energy. Or we might look to our patients for that which we should seek elsewhere. As Warkentin (1972) commented, "If we are not taking care of our hearts, we offer our patients but an empty hand" (p. 254). Heart care is challenging within the vicissitudes of our daily lives. It might be that we need to feed on rejuvenating music, quiet, time in nature, or nurturing friendship. In working with this precept, we look at cause and effect, both when we are taking care of ourselves and when we are not. Years ago, a colleague was back at work after having been away for a weeklong meditation retreat. He reported that one of his patients (who didn't know about the retreat) looked at him in the middle of the session and said, "You're listening differently."

When working with patients who are very challenging, we might need to take extra care, such as having some free time available before or after the session. Having a wise and inspiring book available in our offices to read for a few moments can also be nurturing. Mindful walking between sessions, even for 5 minutes within the office, can similarly be an invaluable support to refreshing our energy and intention.

The Benefits of Precept Practice

We have considered specific ways in which the consideration and practice of the five ethical precepts can inform our clinical work. There are broader and deeper implications as well. As we actively engage this lens of examination and practice, there is a growing integrity that informs how we sit with someone. Precept practice:

- Supports us in the development of trustworthiness. We trust ourselves more and are less afraid, more fully available to engage with our patients.
- Cultivates genuine humility because we are intimately aware of our own failings, our own practice edges.
- Grounds our interventions in respect and mutuality. While we are aware that our patient is walking a different path, we are also aware of our own daily footsteps and the fact that the same earth is under our feet.
- Fosters fuller presence, less encumbered by anxiety and concerns. We are freer to attend to the person in front of us.
- Nurtures confidence in our capacity to grow in wisdom and compassion. The more we practice, the more we notice, the more we understand.

ETHICAL ISSUES WITH OUR PATIENTS

"I want to know how to live." This was the stark statement of a middle-age man at a critical juncture in his life, reflecting on the barren ground of a marriage ended, a life deconstructed. He wasn't asking for advice; rather he was defining himself in the moment with this simple admission. His declaration is an apt entrée into this last section of the chapter. *How* we live, how our patients live, has powerful impact on the trajectory of our lives and how we feel about ourselves, others, and life.

How do we hold moral considerations regarding our patients' lives? Psychotherapy has traditionally been described as value-neutral. As we sit in our offices, doing the trench work of our guild, we know that this is not true. Our interventions are continually informed by value judgments about what is more or less helpful. Most of us are not shy about suggesting that it is more helpful for a depressed person to exercise than to watch TV, or for an anxious person to work with fear rather than to organize life around avoidance. This sort of guidance, which might have been seen as inappropriately directive and value-laden years ago, is now part of care standards because of data demonstrating the importance of behavioral choices. The current attention given to gratitude practice is another example. Clinicians don't advise patients to start gratitude journals from a stance of moralizing superiority, but rather because research shows that this intervention can help people feel better. Accumulating findings that values and behavior bear on well-being make ethics a relevant therapeutic issue.

Certainly, it is not our role to sit in judgment. The sanctity of a relational space where a person is met with consistent acceptance and positive regard is a foundation of psychotherapy. And we can't possibly know sufficient details of another's circumstance to adequately judge his or her actions (Dalai Lama, 1999). However, therapists need not skirt the exploration of ethical issues with patients for fear of seeming like morality police. Buddhist psychology and more recent positive psychology research highlight the risks here, as both disciplines find alignment with ethical values and practices to be essential for happiness. Ethics define the quality of care that we take in relationship with others and ourselves. When we turn a blind eye to the examination of ethical issues, we ignore a powerful source of suffering and a powerful resource for well-being.

Uncertainty

Ethical issues take us into uncertainty. Often the path of ethical action is uncharted, formulaic responses are unskillful, and we are challenged to refine our discernment. Ethical teachings in both Western psychotherapeutic and Buddhist meditation traditions point out that because of the unique features of circumstance and social interaction, we're often faced with a situation for which our guidelines and rules are inadequate (Bond, 2000; Dalai Lama, 1999; Pope & Vasquez, 2011; Schwartz & Sharpe, 2010; West, 2002). We are charged to find a way *with* the demands of the situation that avoids the extremes that the Dalai Lama (1999) refers to as "crude absolutism and trivial relativism" (p. 28).

Considerations

Although there is no roadmap for how to engage with our patients in these matters, there are considerations that can aid us. As discussed earlier, our personal work with ethical precepts helps us to be understanding and humble as we examine these issues. Being intimately aware of our own growing edges, we are more able to approach our patients in a genuinely respectful way. We need to be clear about our motivations. If we are feeling critical, angry, or challenged, we are wise to make use of supervision or collegial support to regain our balance and empathy before addressing an issue. We need to factor in the quality of our connection, the degree to which we have a working alliance.

Timing is also important. Often at the outset of treatment, we might hear something that concerns us, but sense (or are told) that it is too early to address the matter. Sometimes the patient then goes underground with the material and we feel we cannot bring it up. An option in these circumstances is to respectfully acknowledge that the person does not want to explore something at the moment, but enlist his or her permission to discuss it later. For example, a woman who had just started treatment came into the third session saying that she was late, partly because she had had difficulty waking up. She then looked me in the eye and said, "I realize that I don't want to talk about my Ambien use, because I don't want you to touch my Ambien." I took in her words and then inquired, "May we put a little flag there for now?"

Grounding in Direct Experience

In his book on ethics, the Dalai Lama (1999) states: "Ethical conduct is not something we engage in because it is somehow right in itself. . . . A meaningful ethical system divorced from the grounding of our experience of suffering and happiness is hard to envisage" (p. 147). The central challenge in helping our patients work with ethical issues is finding a way to foster this sort of direct, moving experience. As discussed earlier, mindfulness practice can increase moral sensitivity, and this sensitivity can lead to skillful action that supports greater mindfulness. Although we might wish that all of our patients would begin meditation, many will not.

What else can we do to nurture ethical mindfulness? How can we foster engagement with and learning from direct, lived experience rather than dwelling on ideas about experience? We might suggest at the beginning of a session to take a moment to simply arrive and breathe together, facilitating deeper contact. We might also suggest this in moments when a patient seems particularly caught up in a story line or distant from feeling. The respectful inquiry, "May we take a moment together to pause and check in with how you are doing in this moment?", can deepen the patient's access to his or her direct experience. For some individuals, an invitation to check in with body sensations can help access the pulse of the moment.

We can further facilitate deeper contact by suggesting that our patients journal about one or all of the following questions:

- What things do you do that distance you from your deeper self?
- What things do you do that put you more in touch with your deeper knowing?
- What things did you do or not do that contributed to your suffering this week?
- What things did you do or not do that contributed to your happiness this week?

Note that both acts of restraint as well as acts of commission are included. We are trying to facilitate more mindfulness, more direct contact with lived experience, rather than dwelling in ideas about experience. As Jake Davis (2011) notes, "The practice of mindfulness can also give us an embodied and experiential way of knowing which ways of acting feels right" (p. 1). We are doing whatever we can to help our patients find this pathway to deeper knowing.

Harmful Behavior

As therapists, we are mandated to try to stop homicidal and suicidal behavior and to report child or elder abuse and neglect. Yet there is a vast continuum of harmful behaviors that can negatively impact a person's life that we're not mandated to address. If we turn away from these destructive behaviors, we may inadvertently collude with our patients' sense of impotence and hopelessness in the face of harmful action.

Addictions are one of the clearest examples of this phenomenon, and professional guidelines charge us to address them. In Alcoholics Anonymous (AA) peers can ask, "How's that behavior working for you?" The question includes both challenge and respect. At times, we clinicians may claim the moral high ground of restraint from being judgmental, when in fact we're colluding with our patients in denying an elephant in the room. Perhaps we do this to avoid discomfort, or worse still, to perpetuate a status quo in which the patient is deluded into thinking he or she is "working on issues," as we continue collecting our hourly fee.

I am humbled by the experience of seeing a patient for a decade while his or her addiction intensified despite consultations, AA meetings, and endless exploration. There are no easy answers and each situation is different. Do we take a hard line and make treatment conditional upon a person "working the program"? Such a black-and-white stance eliminates the leverage of a good treatment relationship in the recovery process. On the other hand, we need to stay awake to the pull of being inducted into denial and minimization. We want to avoid getting lulled into what Pope and Vasquez (2011, p. 2) refer to as an "ethical sleep" in which we avoid responsibility for addressing difficult issues. Some questions to consider:

- What is the trajectory of the treatment?
- Is the person thinking and feeling more or less about his or her situation?
- What is happening with regard to the person's work and relationship life? Are things improving or getting worse?

Wisdom may lead us to a middle path: to practice complete acceptance of the person in our office while not shying away from examining the causes and effects of actions. To paraphrase Marsha Linehan (2009), "Love the person, take issue with the behaviors."

Bearing Witness

Working skillfully involves not doing harm by abandoning, while at the same time being honest and engaged with the harmfulness that we witness. A young man who grew up in an abusive alcoholic family initially entered treatment for social anxiety but revealed over time that he had a gambling addiction. He was also aware that his growing professional success was viewed as disloyalty by his family, and he felt conflicted about doing well. After buying a home (his family never owned one), he reflected that he was trashing it, not keeping it neat as he had his rental unit. With characteristic humor he quipped, "I want to make sure I don't feel too good about my life." I asked him if this was also one function of his gambling. He was initially angry at the question, but the following week took up the issue.

A former patient returned to treatment saying that he wanted to leave his marriage of 25 years because he had found his "soul mate," a coworker with whom he was having an affair. I remember starting to deaden in the session. I didn't want to appear judgmental, yet in my silence, I was becoming disengaged. Upon noticing this deadening in myself, I reconnected with my breathing as a way of staying alive in the moment. I then recalled with him that when I last saw him a few years earlier, he had used these very same words to describe another woman with whom he'd had a brief affair. He didn't really want to hear this from me in the moment. Yet it deepened our conversation.

What is the practice edge here? It involves active surrender. We accept our impotence (meeting once or twice a week, trying to interrupt a behavior that is being practiced and reinforced daily). We try to move from impotence *against* a behavior to engagement *with* a behavior. We step up to be someone real in our patient's life who will speak the truth without the rage of a hurt spouse, and who will be accepting without the shared denial of a drinking buddy.

Honesty lacking compassion leads to judgment. Compassion lacking honesty leads to collusion. Neither judgment nor collusion is helpful. Our practice is to watch the constant oscillation, remaining engaged. It is hard. This is where our personal mindfulness practice is particularly helpful. It is a demanding, middle-path course. Some reflections can help us stay present and act skillfully:

- Are we *managing* our patient rather than *connecting* with him or her? Sometimes we only become aware of this stance as someone is leaving a session. Our patient is leaving and yet we have the distinct sense that he or she had never fully arrived. If we feel this dilemma and don't know how to resolve it, we can speak to it. Sometimes the simple statement, "I'm feeling more distance between us . . . what is your experience?" can be the first step in reestablishing connection.

- Are we talking too much? Are we talking *at* our patient rather than *with* him or her? If so, what is this about? Usually, there is very little that we can say that hasn't already been said. Our words are most useful if they can foster a new or fresh experience.

- Have we been killed off by our patient's deadening and unskillful behavior? Returning to our own breath and experiencing our aliveness directly can help us reengage.

- Are we listening *at* our patient rather than *with* him or her? By listening *at* a person, I mean that we are not really listening in the sense of breathing him or her in, such that we are moved or affected by what he or she is saying. In such moments, it is often the case that our patient is not listening to him- or herself either. We've handled our sadness, anger, or fear about repeated destructiveness by moving away. Noticing this is the first step in getting back to something that is *real*.

- If we are feeling tied up or beset with a dilemma about what would be skillful in a moment, we can speak to it with our patient. Acknowledging it as a shared dilemma empowers both parties.

- Are we reticent to talk about a case with a colleague or in supervision? If so, why? Is shame being induced rather than explored in the treatment? It is freeing to remember that there are no easy answers. An additional set of eyes and ears is always helpful.

In this chapter I have tried to give a brief introduction to the richness and vast trajectory of Buddhist ethical training. Undertaken personally, it can enrich our lives and enhance our clinical skills. The phrase *Buddhist ethical training* might sound like an arid discipline. But embodied, it is both a challenge and delight. This practice, which can be endlessly refined over a lifetime, opens us to a deeper sense of aliveness, interconnectedness, and meaning. Ethical practice is both the seed and the expression of our growing understanding that our happiness and the happiness of all beings are inextricably intertwined.

Part III

Clinical Applications

*M*indfulness practices are being successfully implemented in an ever-widening array of interventions to treat virtually every type of patient. While some principles apply across clinical situations, treatments are most effective when tailored to meet the needs of individuals. This part, organized by disorders and populations, provides frameworks for applying mindfulness under varying conditions.

Chapter 7 examines therapist training, how to introduce mindfulness exercises into treatment, and how to select practices or modify them for the needs of particular individuals. Chapter 8 explores the common characteristics of depressive disorders and how mindfulness practices are suited to their treatment, along with a discussion of mindfulness-based cognitive therapy, an approach that is demonstrably effective in treating depression. In parallel fashion, Chapter 9 explores the nature of anxiety and how mindfulness can serve as its antidote, including a detailed description of a mindfulness and acceptance-based behavioral approach. Chapter 10 addresses the stress-related medical disorders that mindfulness practices were first employed to treat in the West, and illustrates how these practices can be particularly effective when combined with both psychodynamic exploration and rehabilitation aimed at regaining normal life activities. Chapter 11 goes on to explore the use of mindfulness practices to treat trauma, considering how our habitual attempts to escape pain can lock us into posttraumatic suffering, and how traumatic experience can be transformed when viewed through the lens of dependent origination. Chapter 12 then looks at pain avoidance from another perspective, outlining how our instinctive attempts to feel good can trap us into self-perpetuating addictive cycles. Finally, Chapter 13 explores how mindfulness practices can help us become more attuned to children as both therapists and parents, and introduces a number of mindfulness practices that children themselves can try.

7

Teaching Mindfulness in Therapy

Susan M. Pollak

> Don't turn your head.
> Keep looking at the bandaged place.
> That's where the Light enters you.
> —RUMI (1995, p. 139)

*T*eaching mindfulness in therapy is more art than science. The mindfulness-based clinician takes a complex web of factors into consideration, including the patient's clinical needs, life circumstances, cultural and religious background, and willingness to develop new habits, as well as the therapist's own mindfulness experience, the treatment alliance, and timing. Previous authors discussed the importance of mindfulness in helping clinicians remain present and compassionately engaged in the therapy relationship. This chapter explores how to introduce and teach mindfulness exercises in psychotherapy.[1]

The clinical usefulness of mindfulness techniques has been demonstrated for a broad range of psychological disorders (see Chapter 1). Yet for many clinicians, the idea of bringing mindfulness practices into therapy can feel overwhelming or intimidating. Where to start? Which practices to use? How to avoid harm? Are there patients who should avoid

---

[1]For a comprehensive exploration of this topic, see the companion volume, *Sitting Together: Essential Skills for Mindfulness-Based Psychotherapy* (Pollak et al., in press).

mindfulness exercises altogether? This chapter attempts to demystify the process, offering a roadmap with the goal of making these practices accessible to clinicians from all theoretical orientations. It includes informal and formal meditation instructions, vignettes illustrating clinical applications, and suggestions for how to use various practices. Although the therapist's own meditation experience is invaluable, it may not be necessary to have decades of meditation or retreat experience in order to effectively introduce mindfulness to patients suffering from a wide variety of disorders.

MINDFULNESS-BASED TREATMENT PROGRAMS

As mentioned in Chapter 1, there are four well-established, empirically supported, multicomponent, mindfulness-based treatment programs that have been adapted to treat a wide range of clinical conditions. These programs are mindfulness-based stress reduction (MBSR; Kabat-Zinn, 1990), mindfulness-based cognitive therapy (MBCT; Segal, Williams, & Teasdale 2002), dialectical behavior therapy (DBT; Linehan, 1993a, 1993b), and acceptance and commitment therapy (ACT; Hayes et al., 1999; Hayes, Strosahl, & Houts, 2005). (For more details, see Baer & Krietemeyer, 2006.)

Jon Kabat-Zinn created MBSR out of his personal practice of Zen, insight meditation, and yoga to treat chronically ill patients at a university hospital. It is the most widely used, structured, mindfulness training program and occurs over an 8-week period. MBCT was adapted from MBSR by research clinicians who skillfully integrated elements of cognitive-behavioral therapy (CBT) to treat recurrent depression. Marsha Linehan, also a Zen practitioner, developed DBT to treat borderline personality disorder, especially suicidal, substance-abusing patients. DBT is based on radical acceptance and skills training, including mindfulness skills. Finally, ACT evolved out of the work of Steven Hayes and colleagues, who noticed that problems are created and perpetuated by how we relate to them, primarily through our use of language. The focus of ACT is on living a valued life rather than on removing negative thoughts, feelings, and behaviors. Acceptance, committed action, and mindfulness are antidotes to how we make problems worse by resisting unpleasant experience. These programs offer an abundance of mindfulness exercises that can be brought into individual therapy by skilled clinicians.

THERAPIST CREDENTIALS

As more and more clinicians incorporate mindfulness into their practices, expectations for therapist training and personal mindfulness practice are being hotly debated—and expectations vary widely. The Center for Mindfulness at the University of Massachusetts Medical School offers MBSR teacher certification with a host of requirements, including daily meditation practice and attendance at four silent meditation retreats (see details at *www.umassmed.edu/cfm/certification/index.aspx*). MBCT therapists are required to have a daily formal and informal meditation practice, be qualified mental health practitioners, participate in a training program, and receive ongoing peer supervision (Segal et al., 2012). DBT and ACT clinicians are not expected to have a personal meditation practice to be qualified therapists because formal meditation, although often encouraged, is not emphasized in those programs.

Given this diversity of approaches, a helpful guideline is that a therapist should, at minimum, have practiced and experienced what he or she teaches (Davis & Hayes, 2011). Mindfulness is not just a technique; it's a lifelong endeavor to embody awareness, compassion, and ethical behavior in one's life. As Jon Kabat-Zinn put it, *"The teaching has to come out of one's practice.* There is simply no other way" (cited in McCown et al., 2011, p. xviii, original emphasis). Shapiro and Carlson (2009) recommend a regular mindfulness practice in addition to learning principles of Buddhist psychology, such as how we create and alleviate suffering.

One of the many benefits of developing our own meditation practice is that it helps us gain confidence in using mindfulness under a variety of circumstances and with different states of mind. This personal understanding and knowledge can guide and facilitate skillful interventions with patients. On the other hand, to introduce some mindfulness-based techniques, such as listening to ambient sounds in the environment or feeling the breath in the body, we need only a modest amount of instruction, supervision, and practice. In short, the question of how much training is necessary may rest on how much mindfulness we want to bring into our clinical practice.

MOTIVATION

In order to experience the many benefits of mindfulness, patients must be open to the idea of mindfulness and be willing to practice. Cultivating mindfulness, like learning an instrument or embarking on a fitness regime, requires time, commitment, and discipline. Emotional pain and suffering often provide this motivation—the gift of desperation. Many patients enter treatment during a time of crisis, or "creative hopelessness" (Hayes et al., 1999), and as a result are open to learning new ways of relating to their problems. To ensure a good match between mindfulness practice and the individual patient, it's important to carefully explore the patient's emotional pain and understand what he or she wants and values.

Mindfulness practice is not for everyone. Some patients don't want to venture from traditional talk therapy; others may feel uncomfortable with silence and introspection. Is the patient willing to explore his or her own experience even if it involves temporary discomfort? Is he or she willing to allow things to be as they are? Does the patient want a quick fix? Receptivity to new ways of *being with* emotional pain and suffering are important precursors to effective mindfulness-oriented therapy.

Many patients are inspired by the research evidence that supports the mindfulness approach to therapy. Sara Lazar's work (Lazar et al., 2005; see also Chapter 15) on cortical thickening from mindfulness meditation; Stefan Hofmann's meta-analysis of mindfulness-based interventions on anxiety and depression (Hofmann et al., 2010); Norman Farb and colleagues' (2010) study on deactivation of the default mode network with mindfulness practice, and Zindel Segal and colleagues' (2010) favorable comparison of MBCT to pharmacotherapy are all compelling studies that can enhance a patient's willingness to practice. Dan Siegel (2010c) has found that teaching patients about brain mechanisms provides a helpful understanding about what happens during situations of emotional distress, which can enhance their motivation to try practice mindfulness-based practices.

HOW TO INTRODUCE
MINDFULNESS PRACTICES IN THERAPY

Mindfulness practices should never be forced, even if the clinician believes they would benefit the patient. A good way to start is to present mindfulness practice as an "experiment" (Gunaratana, 2002) and a collaboration in which both clinician and patient keep an open mind and are willing to try different practices in order to find a good fit. Although it can be difficult to explore mindfulness alone, there is comfort in practicing in the safety of a trusting therapeutic relationship. As the writer Anne Lamott (1993) put it, "My mind is a bad neighborhood I try not to go into alone" (p. 84)—a metaphor that speaks to both patients and practitioners alike.

When introducing mindfulness practice, it's not necessary to delve into Buddhist philosophy. Simply say something like this: "There is good research on this approach, and I think it might help. Are you willing to try it here with me as an experiment? I will do this with you and we can stop at any time." If a patient decides that mindfulness practice is not something he or she wants to explore, there need be no guilt or pressure about that choice.

Careful attention to language is also important. Some patients may recoil from the word *mindfulness*, associating it with Buddhism or New Age philosophy. Carmody (2009) suggests presenting mindfulness exercises as *attention training*, finding that this wording is more palatable to many people. Along these lines, Segal and colleagues (2002) originally called their work *attentional control training*, and Kabat-Zinn (1990) introduced mindfulness by calling it *stress reduction*.

Modifications

Just as a skilled exercise or yoga teacher will offer modifications to make a practice accessible to different students, it is important to know and offer meditation variations to fit the needs of an individual patient. For example, people with a history of asthma, respiratory illness, trauma, and anxiety often do not feel comfortable with the practice of following the breath, which is frequently the first mindfulness practice taught in meditation classes. These patients may find it easier to start with the practice of listening to sounds in the present moment.

Different individuals often have a preference for meditations that emphasize auditory, kinesthetic, linguistic, or visual objects of attention. It may be that a person's way of learning, processing information, and functioning in the world (Gardner, 1983) correlates with his or her meditation practice preference. Hölzel, Lazar, and colleagues (2011) note that different personality types may be attracted to different mindfulness-based practices, and this preference may influence their response as well as the benefits they derive from various practices. Rather than seeing a preference for one practice over another as resistance, therapists can be sensitive to and understanding of individual preferences. Finding the right fit can enhance willingness to practice and the potential for successful outcome.

Homework

Research has shown that because the benefits of meditation are dose-dependent (Segal et al., 2012), homework assignments can increase its effectiveness. Home practice is encouraged in the multicomponent, mindfulness-based programs mentioned earlier, but not necessarily in formal sitting meditation. Practice does not need to be onerous—in fact, it can be pleasant. The Zen master Thich Nhat Hahn was asked by a student how to practice mindfulness. He replied, "Do you want to know my secret? I try to find a way to do things that is most pleasurable. There are many ways to perform a given task—but the one that holds my attention best is the one that is most pleasant" (Murphy, 2002, p. 85). Meditation teachers suggest that even 1 minute of practice can be useful, especially for those who are just starting. For patients willing to devote more time to practice, 30 minutes has been shown to produce significant brain changes (Hölzel et al., 2010). Although existing data on changing neural pathways reflect changes from formal practice, informal practice during the course of daily life is useful to help patients manage everyday challenges of living. The goal is to design a user-friendly practice that is pleasant and not burdensome. Framing it as a daily *mini-vacation*, a *time in*, or as *time just for you* can help.

Basic Mindfulness Techniques

In 2009, the Dalai Lama spoke at a Harvard Medical School conference on compassion and wisdom in psychotherapy. One of the codirectors of the conference asked His Holiness to lead a brief meditation. The Dalai Lama laughed and said, "I think some of you may want just one single meditation—a simple one, and 100 percent sort of positive. That, I think, impossible" (Siegel, 2011, p. 26). He elaborated by noting that there are a multitude of states of mind that lead to suffering and therefore a multitude of practices to work with them skillfully.

Deciding which practices to suggest to a given patient requires both clinical skill and familiarity with a range of techniques. The goal is to create a practice that is attuned, relational, and responsive to the needs in the present moment. To begin, we can consider a number of simple, fundamental practices.

As discussed in Chapter 1, three types of mindfulness meditation practice are (1) concentration, (2) mindfulness per se, and (3) compassion (Salzberg, 2011). Research by Brewer, Worhunsky, and colleagues (2011) and others suggests that these practices activate overlapping, yet different, regions of the brain.

Most meditation teachers begin with concentration practices (focused attention) as a way to steady and calm the mind. These practices involve learning to focus on an object of attention (such as the breath, sounds, or other body sensations) and trying to stay with it. When the mind wanders, it is gently and kindly brought back to the object of attention. Hölzel and colleagues (2011) consider attention regulation to be a "building block" that facilitates other meditation practices. Concentration is in itself a practice that can be explored and developed over years (Rosenberg, 1998) for the benefit of calming and steadying the mind.

Once there is some comfort with concentration practice and the individual has learned to gather and steady attention, we can then expand the focus to begin practicing mindfulness per se (open monitoring). In concentration practice, we gently return the mind to the object of attention each time it wanders. In mindfulness practice, we get curious about what has distracted us and captured our attention, and attend to the rising and passing of all phenomena in experience. Mindfulness is not about emptying the mind or escaping from problems; it is about finding new ways to relate to our difficulties and our often chaotic minds. If the content of what is arising becomes overwhelming or too intense, it is fine to return to the breath or other object of attention for a while. A return to concentration can provide a refuge and an anchor when difficult material arises.

If we are in significant pain or feeling overwhelmed, compassion practice can be especially useful. It can be an effective counterpoint to self-criticism and self-loathing. This practice involves embracing who we are in an awake, accepting, and openhearted way, bringing kindness and acceptance to even the most difficult experiences. Researchers are finding that compassion plays a key role in decreasing emotional reactivity and thus in symptom reduction (Kuyken et al., 2010). As we learn to respond with kindness in moments of pain and distress, acknowledging our imperfections, we learn to accept others as well. Key components of compassion practice are discussed more fully in Chapter 4 (see also Germer, 2009; Gilbert, 2009b; Neff, 2003; Salzberg, 1995). Some researchers even theorize that compassion underlies the effectiveness of mindfulness-based programs such as MBSR (Davis & Hayes, 2011) and MBCT (Kuyken et al., 2010).

DESIGNING AND SELECTING EXERCISES

The basic principles of the mindfulness techniques are outlined in Chapter 1. When teaching them to patients, it's important to emphasize that they are complementary to one another and work synergistically. And as meditation teacher Christina Feldman (2001) points out, these practices appear deceptively easy: "Mindfulness is neither difficult nor complex, remembering to be mindful is the great challenge" (p. 167).

Concentration Practices

Although many meditation teachers begin developing concentration by attending to the breath, in a clinical population this often is not the easiest starting point. Focusing on the inner, as opposed to the outer world, may stir up uncomfortable affect. For patients with a history of anxiety or trauma, beginning with the simple practice of "just listening" or "mindfulness of sound" is usually a gentler and safer introduction to practice.

Sounds

The following exercise has been refined and used in my clinical practice for many years. If this is a patient's first foray into mindfulness practice, it is best to keep it short and simple, practicing for 3–5 minutes. This exercise can also be done for extended periods of time.

Just Listening

- Start by sitting comfortably, finding a relaxed posture that you can hold for a few minutes. Eyes can be open or gently closed. As you settle into the chair, see if you can get in touch with your essential dignity.
- Let yourself be in the room, feel the chair you are sitting on, and allow yourself to listen to the sounds around you. Don't worry about naming or judging them, just listen.
- Let yourself listen with your entire being. Open to sounds in front of you, behind you, above you and below you. No need to create a story about them—let them come to you. Just notice the sounds.
- Allow the sounds to arise and pass away. No need to grasp—let them come and let them go. If your mind wanders, don't worry, just return to the sounds in the present moment.

Alison had a history of sexual abuse and posttraumatic stress disorder (PTSD). Although she had read about the benefits of mindfulness meditation, she became agitated when she tried to feel her breath. She was willing to try another technique. "Just listening" was a good way for Alison to stabilize, calm, and come into the present moment. When she began to feel overwhelmed by memories of the past, listening to the hum of her air conditioner or the noise of street traffic was enough to help Alison anchor her awareness in the moment and in her present life, so different from rural home where the abuse had occurred. With practice, as Alison focused on the sounds of her hard-won new life, her flashbacks and PTSD began to diminish.

As Williams and colleagues (2007) note, even a moment of mindfulness can change things. Heroic measures are not required—"it may simply involve a shift in the way we pay attention" (p. 71). By creating greater awareness of the present moment, without judgment, with warmth and compassion, we can break the cycle of intrusive, ruminative thoughts that can perpetuate anxiety, depression, and PTSD. Although "just listening" is a formal meditation practice, it can be adapted as an informal practice as well. Patients can listen to sounds as they walk, sit on a bus or a subway, or wash dishes. For Allison, when a disturbing memory would interrupt her day, she learned to treat it as "street noise," allowing it to arise but then fall away, not getting caught in the story.

No practice is ideal for everyone, however. For patients with a hearing impairment, mindfulness of sounds is not a good place to start. War veterans and those who have witnessed violence are likely to be triggered by loud sounds. This practice can be modified to include more neutral sounds, such as white noise from a machine.

Body Sensations

Focusing on the body as a way to calm the mind is a technique that has been practiced for thousands of years and is also at the heart of yoga (Iyengar, 1966). Meditation techniques that concentrate on the body are a direct and effective way to redirect attention away from the obsessive thought stream, where we are constantly worrying about the future or caught up in regrets about the past. Shapiro (2009) theorizes that by attending to bodily experience in an open way, we learn to "reperceive" our situation and become "less identified with it and better able to see it with clarity and objectivity" (p. 558). In her view, this process of disidentification mediates change.

The following practice, taught by many mindfulness meditation teachers, is a favorite technique of patients who want to reconnect safely with their bodies without arousing intense emotions. I first learned it from Tara Brach. It is an introductory practice and can be done for just a few minutes, or if the patient is comfortable, for a longer periods.

Mindfulness of Hands

- Start by sitting in a comfortable position, eyes either open or slightly closed. Let yourself feel the support of your chair.
- Let your hands rest in your lap. Begin wiggling your fingers and gently moving your hands. Become aware of this movement.
- Rotate your wrists. Clench and unclench your hands. Start to feel your hands, noticing sensations, pulsations, and vibrations within them.
- Feel your hands from the inside out. If you like, allow the muscles to soften. Become aware of each finger, the palms, the backs of your hands.
- See what it is like to fully inhabit your hands. Allow your attention to rest as fully as possible in your hands.

Zachary had dropped out of college feeling overwhelmed by his mother's recent death after a long and painful illness. It was hard for him to concentrate, and he became worried about his health. He began to obsess about his own death. Zachary had always been anxious, but now he had trouble sleeping and hated to be alone. He was spending most of his time shut in his room playing computer games and had developed carpal tunnel syndrome.

As Zachary practiced bringing his attention to his hands and allowed the muscles to soften, he found that his whole body began to relax. His jaw unclenched, his shoulders dropped, and his breath slowed. At times his body shook with grief, but it felt safe to Zachery and even a relief to grieve in therapy, not to bear the sadness alone. As he learned to accept his loss rather than escape from it in computer games, Zachary developed a renewed interest in spending time with friends. After a few months of this grief work and mindfulness practice, he returned to school, finding that his carpal tunnel symptoms had lessened.

A variation of this practice can also be done with the soles of the feet (Singh, Wahler, Adkins, & Myers, 2003). Working with the extremities of the body rather than moving into the core often makes people feel safer. I have found that this practice is therefore a good entry point for people with anxiety, trauma, and depression. However, for people who have severe dissociation, even this practice may be problematic. For example, when asked to focus on his hands, one patient became overwhelmed and confused about who owned the hands. When practices exacerbate symptoms or cause disorientation, it's best to try another approach.

Breath

Most meditation teachers begin with the practice of feeling or following the breath, for good reason. The breath is always with us, and constantly changing. It is (for most people) neutral, unburdened with negative associations, and doesn't require us to believe in any particular dogma or system of thought. For patients who are high-functioning and relatively well integrated, this can be an excellent practice. However, as mentioned above, the breath can be problematic for those with anxiety or a history of trauma or dissociative disorders.

I first learned this brief, simple, direct practice from meditation teacher and therapist Trudy Goodman.

Just Three Breaths

- Start by sitting comfortably, finding a posture that is relaxed and upright. If you like, you can close your eyes or keep them partially open, softly focusing on a spot on the floor a few feet in front of you.
- Feel your natural breath. There is no need to hold, alter, or control it.
- Notice the sensations as you inhale and then gently notice the sensations as you exhale.
- Feel the next full inhalation as well as the next full exhalation. If the mind wanders, don't worry, this is what all minds do, just bring your attention back without judgment or criticism.
- Bring your attention to the third and final breath, feeling the sensations of the natural inhalation and feeling the sensations of the natural exhalation.

Anna was a busy emergency room nurse in a large metropolitan hospital. She came into treatment to help decrease her stress and find some calm in the midst of her frantic job. Anna didn't have the time for extended, formal meditation but wanted to find a better coping strategy than overeating when she was upset. We tried *Just Three Breaths* as a way to help her navigate the demands of her work. She found after a few weeks of practice that just noticing that she was breathing helped her remain calm, focused, and composed in stressful situations. She used this technique while sitting in the nurses' station writing notes and even when hurrying through the hospital corridors.

Making contact with the breath or body offers a way to shift one's attention from preoccupations or frantic thoughts and worries. When we shift perspective, we can find a different relationship to our concerns, creating a little more ease and spaciousness. Meditation teachers often call this *clear seeing*. By shifting the focus from our thoughts to our breath, we begin to establish a new vantage point, analogous to what psychodynamic approaches call an *observing ego* (Kerr, Josyula, & Littenberg, 2011).

Mindfulness Practices

The next exercise offers a good transition to mindfulness practice because it incorporates elements of concentration (in the hub of the wheel) as well as the open monitoring and spirit of investigation that characterize mindfulness practice per se. I learned the practice from Daniel Siegel, who popularized it in his book *Mindsight* (2010b). This is a condensed and simplified version.

The Center of the Wheel

- Start by sitting comfortably in a dignified posture. Notice the sensations of sitting in chair. Eyes can be closed or softly open.
- Take a few breaths, letting go of any burdens you might be carrying. Stay with your breath, the sounds around you, or the sensations in your hands for a few minutes until you can focus and gather your attention.
- Picture an image of a wheel and bring your attention to the hub. Then expand the image to include the spokes going out to the rim of the wheel.
- Now place yourself in the hub of the wheel. Give yourself a few moments to feel anchored and steadied.
- Place the things in your life that may be upsetting or distracting you on the rim of the wheel. The distance between the hub and the rim is up to you. Allow as much space as you need—a few feet or yards, or even a football field. Give yourself a few moments to find the space you need. Allow yourself this respite.
- When you're ready, see if you can venture out on a spoke and begin to investigate one of the items on the rim. Start with something that is manageable, not the most difficult problem that you face.
- See what arises as you begin to bring your attention to this issue. What do you notice in your body? What emotions arise? If you start to feel overwhelmed, return to the hub and allow yourself to steady and ground. Experiment with going back and forth between the hub and the rim. Go slowly.

Marianne was overwhelmed by the details of her life. She was recently divorced and had three young children. She knew that there would be budget cuts at the school where she taught, and she worried about losing her job. Both her parents had died recently and her home was filled with their belongings. Marianne felt that the walls were closing in on her. She entered treatment feeling depressed and exhausted, complaining that she couldn't keep up with the mail, the bills, the lesson plans, and the kids.

Although we experimented with a number of different practices, the center of the wheel soon became Marianne's favorite. It gave her a sense that she could find some calm in the midst of her chaotic life. It was an especially useful practice for her at night, when she would wake up thinking of all the things she had to do, feeling that there was no one to help her.

As she practiced, she became more and more able to focus on completing one task at a time, staying in the moment rather than multitasking and panicking that she wasn't getting enough done. The practice helped her find some peace of mind and clarity. Whenever she started to feel overwhelmed, she would return to the hub of the wheel, find her breath, and reestablish being in the moment and taking things one at a time. To help her function during the day, we added the informal practice of saying, "Just this moment, nothing more."

Once a patient is able to settle the mind, perhaps through listening, awareness of the body, or breath awareness, the next step is opening up to present-moment experience with curiosity and compassion. Concentration practices function as a soothing touchstone, so that the patient can return to them if the investigation gets too intense or overwhelming. This helps titrate and manage difficult emotions. As we train the mind, developing friendly curiosity, we continue to cultivate an attitude of nonjudgmental openness toward experience.

The next practice, originally taught as a Zen koan, is a narrative exercise. It can be a natural transition from talk therapy to mindfulness practice. It was originally designed as a way to work with anger and anxiety. I first learned this practice from the meditation teacher George Bowman.

What Is This?

- Start by sitting comfortably, finding a position you can maintain without stress or strain.
- Take a few moments to ground or anchor your attention with one of the concentration practices.

- Next bring your attention to what you may be experiencing right now. It could be anger, fear, self-doubt, worry, or sadness.
- Begin to notice what you are feeling with a warm curiosity. If you like, put a hand on your heart, noticing whatever is present with kindness, interest, and without judgment or criticism.

Janet was a student who suffered from severe and debilitating anxiety. Many days she was unable to leave her house or attend classes, which further increased her worry about her anxiety. When Janet woke up each morning, she would check to see how anxious she was, which only exacerbated her distress. As we worked with this practice, Janet began to notice what anxiety felt like in her body, but not to add to her fears. Instead of getting caught in an inner dialogue about what might happen, she simply noticed what she was feeling and put a hand on her heart because she was suffering, asking kindly, "What is this?"

By not magnifying what she was feeling, and by finding a new way to be with her body's sensations and by bringing some kindness to her suffering, Janet found that what she was experiencing was uncomfortable, but not unmanageable. She could be with anxiety and work with it rather than seeing it as something that need stop her life.

Compassion Practices

A number of different practices can be used to cultivate compassion (see Chapters 1 and 4). Many begin by cultivating loving-kindness, using statements such as the following:

Loving-kindness Phrases

May I be free from inner and outer harm.
May I be free from suffering.
May I be healthy.
May I be peaceful.
May I live with ease.

Jerry was living in New York City on 9/11. He was always "nervous" and joked that he came by it honestly, as his mother was fanatical about dirt and his father was a hypochondriac. Jerry had never really felt safe and was always checking to see if there was someone following him when he walked down the street. Things became worse when Jerry had his own child, as he feared that his son might also be harmed, would eat something poisonous, or become ill. Jerry stayed away from subways and buses, and even refused tickets to a baseball game due to a fear of crowds. Jerry's wife had finally had enough of his worries, compulsive cleaning, and concern about germs. She insisted that he seek help.

In therapy, mindfulness practice helped Jerry realize just how much distress he was "adding on" to benign situations. He learned to settle his body, be in the moment, and not assume that disaster was impending. Yet it was the loving-kindness phrases that really helped Jerry learn to soothe himself and establish a sense of inner safety. Jerry realized that his mother was so worried about contamination, she had rarely held or comforted him, and his father was too self-involved to notice if Jerry was distressed. As he practiced loving-kindness meditation, Jerry became more resilient and courageous. After months of work, Jerry was delighted to report that he had taken his son to a Red Sox–Yankees game, and even though he felt distressed at times, he and his son had thoroughly enjoyed the day.

The essence of mindfulness is not that we change our lives, but that we learn to bring kindness and gentle attention to what the poet Rumi called "the bandaged places." This radical, counterintuitive perspective on emotional healing is difficult to share with others unless we first have a personal practice of mindfulness meditation—a practice that can provide a foundation for conducting mindfulness-based psychotherapy. Teaching mindfulness techniques to patients is a creative enterprise of adapting core mindfulness practices to the unique characteristics of each patient in his or her world, embedded in a therapeutic relationship.

8

Depression

Finding a Way In, Finding a Way Out

Thomas Pedulla

It is only by going down into the abyss that we
recover the treasures of life. Where you stumble,
there lies your treasure.
—JOSEPH CAMPBELL (1995)

What do you see in a patient struggling with depression?

If you're an epidemiologist, you see part of a growing public health problem, a pandemic that represents the fourth greatest burden to society among all diseases—and is projected to move up to become second by the year 2020 (Murray & Lopez, 1998).

If you're a psychopharmacologist, you see someone who has a biologically based illness that disrupts the neurotransmitter system, and who requires medication.

If you're a psychotherapist, you might see someone who's experiencing a pathological reaction to the loss of a loved object (Freud, 1917/1961c), or who is stuck in a pattern of maladaptive thinking (Beck, 1972; Burns, 1999), and who needs psychodynamic, cognitive-behavioral, or some other type of talk therapy in order to heal.

Depending on the lens through which you look, depression can be seen and treated in a variety of ways. It can also appear in different shapes and forms. It can be unipolar or bipolar, chronic or episodic, mild to severe. It can exist by itself or together with another disorder.

This chapter draws on recent research and my own clinical experience to explore how mindfulness can transform the way therapists and their patients understand depression, no matter which form it takes. It will also discuss how this new understanding can be part of a multipronged approach with the potential to bring relief to those who suffer from this often complex disorder.

TAPPING THE POWER OF MINDFULNESS

Mindfulness is both a trait (part of one's disposition) and a state (a quality one can cultivate) that makes depression less likely to occur, and makes it less severe when it does. Recent studies have shown that dispositional mindfulness protects against depression because it is associated with affect regulation and self-acceptance (Jimenez, Niles, & Park, 2010); those who score high in mindfulness are less likely to allow negative cognitions to develop into depressive affect (Gilbert & Christopher, 2009); and mindfulness can reduce the negative self-judgments that fuel rumination and deepen emotional distress (Rude, Maestas, & Neff, 2007).

In addition to this inoculation against depression offered by dispositional mindfulness, formal mindfulness training may increase the ability of depressed individuals to experience positive emotions and to appreciate pleasant activities in daily life—factors that protect against depression (Geschwind, Peeters, Drukker, van Os, & Wichers, 2011). Formal mindfulness training also improves affect regulation among participants with mood disorders (Ramel, Goldin, Carmona, & McQuaid, 2004); reduces self-reported rumination, depression, and psychological distress among adults experiencing such symptoms (McKim, 2008); and lowers participants' emotional reactivity during and after watching sad films (Farb et al., 2010).

Mindfulness-based approaches such as acceptance and commitment therapy (ACT; Hayes et al., 1999; Strosahl & Robinson, 2008) and mindfulness-based cognitive therapy (MBCT; Ma & Teasdale, 2004; Segal et al., 2002; Teasdale et al., 2000; Williams et al., 2007) continue to show promise. Two recent randomized controlled studies have shown MBCT to be as effective as antidepressant medication in preventing depressive relapse, and more effective than medication in reducing residual symptoms and improving patients' quality of life (Godfrin & van Heeringen, 2010; Kuyken et al., 2008).

How Does Mindfulness Help?

Turning toward the Pain

A number of mechanisms may be responsible for the effectiveness of mindfulness-based treatments. For example, mindfulness may help patients face emotional pain and suffering by cultivating qualities such as affect tolerance and self-acceptance (see Chapters 3 and 4). By learning to face pain directly, patients change their relationship to it. Instead of reacting in habitual ways—hating it, ruminating about it, or pushing it away—they can begin to open to it, become curious about it, even accept it by degrees. Paradoxically, such acceptance often leads to positive change.

Conversely, what we resist is often perpetuated. Why? Because resistance is a way of holding on, and results in tightening and contraction. By bringing mindfulness to emotional pain and suffering, depressed patients can learn to stop resisting it and start letting it go— or as some prefer to say, *letting it be*. Once they do this, they're better able to respond to it skillfully instead of reacting to it automatically. "The depressed patient, regardless of the form of the depression, is turning away from his or her experience" (Morgan, 2005, p. 133), and mindfulness functions as a sort of redirection *toward*, an antidote to this turning away. Turning away from pain is understandable and nearly reflexive. The problem is that in turning away from pain, the patient also turns away from life. The pain is alive, and turning away from it results in withdrawal, shutting down, and disconnection from experience—conditions often at the heart of depression.

Through mindfulness, patients can make contact with their pain, and in the process, with their sense of aliveness. Even if the patient starts with something small, like bringing attention to the tension at the back of his or her neck, it can create the confidence to go further and look more deeply, especially when encouraged by a therapist who provides a safe environment, support, and a willingness to bear witness to this difficult process. In the words of Jon Kabat-Zinn (2002):

> The meditation orientation is not about fixing pain or making it better. It's about looking deeply into the nature of pain—making use of it in certain ways that might allow us to grow. In that growing, things will change, and we have the potential to make choices that will move us toward greater wisdom and compassion, including self-compassion, and thus toward freedom from suffering. (p. 35)

Finding a Way In

Upon close examination, we can break down the experience of depression into three components: emotions, thoughts, and physical sensations. *Emotionally*, depression predominates, along with feelings of worthlessness, guilt, helplessness, and a loss of pleasure. In the realm of *thinking*, depression may be marked by rumination, poor concentration, indecisiveness, a loss of hope, and thoughts of suicide or death. Depression is often manifest *physically* in changes in appetite and weight, changes in sleep patterns, diminished energy, and psychomotor retardation or agitation.

Why break depression down in this way? For many patients, it helps turn depression from a large, vague, frightening conglomeration—an 800-pound gorilla—into something smaller and more manageable, something to which they can begin to bring a measure of mindfulness. Although it is difficult, sometimes even impossible, to be mindful of *depression*, one can more easily be mindful of tightness in the jaw, fear in the heart, or the thought that says "I'm a loser." In other words, deconstructing depression in this way helps us find a way *in*. And finding a way in is the first step toward finding a way *through*.

Mindfulness as Part of a Multi-Pronged Approach

First, it should be noted that mindfulness alone is seldom enough for effective treatment of depression. Even the most ardent mindfulness-based clinician knows that mindfulness tools and techniques work best when they're part of a comprehensive approach that starts with a thorough history taking and a careful exploration of current issues that are creating distress, including an assessment of the risk for self-harm. Wise treatment will likely include perspectives and methods drawn from broad clinical training. One might suggest physical exercise, social activities, and other behavioral interventions that have been shown to alleviate depression. If the patient isn't already taking medication, one should also consider if a psychopharmacological evaluation would be appropriate.

Meditation and Medication

In the not-too-distant past, it was common for meditation teachers and practitioners to be skeptical about—or even hostile toward—psychotropic medication, perhaps due to the Buddhist precept against the use of intoxicants that cloud the mind. Another source of caution is that people may use medication to avoid their pain, foreclosing on an opportunity for psychological and spiritual growth. But when the pain is too great, no growth is possible. More recently there is a growing acceptance among meditation teachers and mindfulness-oriented clinicians that judicious use of medications such as selective serotonin reuptake inhibitors (SSRIs) can actually help support a patient's meditation practice. This is especially true when depression is severe and includes significant neurovegetative symptoms such as lack of energy, difficulty concentrating, appetite loss, and sleep disturbance. If the patient doesn't have the energy to get out of bed or concentrate for more than a few seconds, he or she is not going to be able to practice mindfulness effectively, if at all. In fact, trying to do so may exacerbate feelings of worthlessness and failure and actually deepen the depression. Psychologist and meditation teacher Sylvia Boorstein (2012) says, "When the pain of depression or anxiety is confusing to the point of overwhelm, appropriate medicine can rescue the mind from painful self-preoccupation" (p. 19). And B. Alan Wallace (2012), a Buddhist scholar and former monk who decries what he sees as our culture's overreliance on medication, also agrees that "in cases of very severe depression, antidepressants help to restore enough emotional balance so that people can benefit from other forms of treatment such as mindfulness-based cognitive-behavioral therapy" (p. 31). Clearly, medication can be an important first step that brings the patient to the point where he or she can start taking charge of recovery—and start some type of mindfulness practice. The mindful path through depression is fundamentally pragmatic, and remaining mired in a treatable depression is not in service of overcoming suffering.

Which Treatment Approach Is Best?

Chapter 1 of this book described the differences between mindfulness-*informed* treatment—therapy that is guided by the psychotherapist's theoretical understanding of mindfulness and personal practice—and mindfulness-*based* treatment—in which the therapist also teaches mindfulness skills to the patient. Both have value. The remainder of this chapter describes a continuum of care from mindfulness-informed to mindfulness-based treatment, drawing on case material to illustrate how each approach can be applied to depression.

MINDFULNESS-INFORMED APPROACHES TO DEPRESSION

Clinicians know the challenge of sitting with depressed patients. We want to help, but our efforts to empathize and our well-intended interventions are often rejected or simply fail. In the face of the patient's hopelessness and despair, it is easy to fall prey to these same feelings ourselves.

This is when our own mindfulness practice can help. Perhaps we notice ourselves turning away from the patient's—and our own—pain. It can be subtle: a glance at the clock, a thought about the upcoming weekend. These are signs that we've begun to abandon our patient, just as the patient may have already abandoned him- or herself. If we can be mindful of this movement, we can encourage ourselves to return, to *turn toward* and *be with* what is happening. We can start by bringing mindfulness to our breath or the sensations of our body against the chair. We can then expand the mindfulness to include whatever feelings might be present. And we can invite our patient to do the same.

> Robin, a woman with a history of major depression, came into a session complaining that lately she'd been waking up with a feeling of heaviness and was afraid she was slipping "down the rabbit hole" again. I asked her to describe the feeling and to see if she could locate it in her body. She said that it was in her chest and felt like a weight pressing down on her. I encouraged her to stay with it, and asked if this feeling were familiar. She shared a memory of herself as a child sitting at the dinner table, crying because she wanted something, but being ignored by her parents and siblings. We both knew this was a common experience in her childhood: feeling disconnected and emotionally abandoned in her large, chaotic family. She went on to say that she'd been feeling that way in her relationship with her partner and that they needed to talk. The heaviness in her chest became lighter.

Although there was no formal mindfulness practice involved, Robin was able to *turn toward*, bringing mindful attention to the physical sensations connected to her experience of depression. This led to an emotional opening both in terms of her history and in the current circumstances of her life. It also suggested that there is something she can do as an adult that she couldn't do as a child: put her feelings into words and have a dialogue with her partner.

Mindful Co-Exploration

In mindfulness-informed psychotherapy, we engage in a process of mindful co-exploration with the patient. As in any effective treatment relationship, we seek to establish a holding environment (Winnicott, 1965) in which the patient feels accepted for who he or she is, and we maintain that environment by bringing mindfulness to the ups and downs of the relationship. Then, together with the patient, we bring our joint attention to the patient's experience as it unfolds moment by moment. Stephanie Morgan (2005) describes this attention as "characterized by awareness, present-centeredness and acceptance" (p. 135). She also suggests three questions we can ask our patients that capture the spirit of this endeavor:

1. What is happening right now?
2. Can you stay with what is happening?
3. Can you breathe *into* what is happening, or can you breathe *with* what is happening right now?

Vipassana meditation teacher Narayan Liebenson Grady (personal communication, October 18, 2011) adds a fourth question that captures the sense of inner freedom mindfulness can create:

4. Is it possible to make space for this?

It is useful to begin the exploration with the body for several reasons. First, physical sensations are more tangible than thoughts and feelings and are usually easier to access. Second, bringing attention to physical sensations helps people get "out of their heads," which is especially useful for those who tend to ruminate. Finally, the body anchors attention in the present moment, for the body is always in the here and now. Even if physical sensations trigger thoughts about the past, as they did for Robin, it's possible to learn to experience these thoughts as mental events happening in the present.

Thoughts Are Not Facts

As most therapists and patients know, negative thoughts feed depression. These thoughts are often automatic and inaccurate, especially when one is already depressed. In traditional cognitive therapy, we help patients identify these *cognitive distortions* (Beck, 1976) and replace them with thoughts that are more rational, realistic, and hopeful. This can help patients gain some distance from their thoughts as well as some mastery over them, which can enhance self-esteem, improve mood, and lead to positive behavioral change.

In mindfulness-informed treatment, the focus is slightly different. Our effort, first and foremost, is to help the patient see thoughts as just thoughts, not as facts. The content of the thought is not so important, and changing it is not necessary. Drawing on our own mindfulness practice, we can sometimes guide the patient to see a negative cognition as "just a thought," and then redirect his or her attention away from the thought stream to the feelings that are beneath it.

> Karen, a high school teacher, had just finished another academic year and reported that she was depressed. "I keep thinking that I did a lousy job this year, that I'm just no good as a teacher." This was inconsistent with what she had been reporting to me during past the year, when she generally seemed to have confidence in her ability to meet the challenges of her work. I pointed this out to her and asked how it felt when she experienced the thought "I'm no good." Instead of focusing on the thought, I suggested that she bring attention to her bodily experience. She was able to identify a familiar "knot" in her stomach. When I asked her to breathe into the knot and see if there was an emotion associated with it, she said, "It feels sad," and her eyes began to tear up. We explored the possibility that her negative thoughts, instead of being an accurate assessment of her skills as a teacher, were arising out of this feeling of sadness, and that the sadness was perhaps a response to the end of the school year, to being left behind by her students, just as she had been left behind by other important people in her life.

Questions that can help direct the process are:

- Can you see that as just a thought? (Instead of saying to yourself, "I'm no good," can you say, "Having the thought that I'm no good"?)
- Can you remember a time when you didn't think this way?
- Can you move below the level of thought into your feelings and physical sensations?

Of course, in Karen's case, the thought that she was no good wasn't *just* a thought because she believed it to be so, and exploring it with mindfulness led to some important therapeutic insights and associations.

Cultivating Self-Acceptance and Self-Compassion

By engaging in mindful co-exploration with our patients and encouraging them to examine their thoughts, we help them turn toward the source of their pain and suffering. Implicit in this movement is an attitude of acceptance, of being willing to see and feel what is there to be seen and felt. But sometimes this attitude of self-acceptance and self-compassion can be cultivated more directly.

> "I'm really down on myself," said Jack. "I feel like such a loser." Jack was once again ruminating about being an underachiever, about working as a waiter when he wanted to be a musician. Although classically trained, he loved jazz, and he couldn't decide which to focus on. "Either way," he said, "I'm not practicing enough, and I'm scared of performing, so maybe I should just drop the whole thing." This was familiar territory in our work together. We both knew that Jack was the product of a strict, religious family. We also knew that his musical training had been at the hands of harsh teachers who demanded perfection. Not surprisingly, he had a tendency to be self-critical. I reminded him of this and asked him if there were some way he could be kind to himself while he was having these negative thoughts.

Rather than challenging the negative thoughts or the painful feelings underneath them, sometimes it's important to help the patient hold his or her experience with a sense of compassion. Some questions that can facilitate this shift are:

- How are you relating to your pain?
- Given your history and your temperament, can you understand why you are feeling the way you do?
- Can you have some compassion for yourself as you go through this difficult time?

Here, we are beginning to see a difference between pain and suffering. In Buddhist psychology, pain is inevitable but suffering is not. *Pain* is the initial experience of being stung by a bee or laid off by an employer. It hurts. There's no way around it. *Suffering* is what we create when we resist or deny that pain, reacting to it with thoughts such as "This isn't fair!", "Why did this happen to me?", "I can't stand this!", "What's wrong with me?", or "It's my own damned fault."

In most cases, depression isn't caused by the initial experience of pain. Depression is what happens when people react to that pain by shutting down, turning away, ruminating about it, blaming themselves, and getting lost in the suffering that results.

MINDFULNESS-BASED APPROACHES TO DEPRESSION

Although still relatively new, the mindfulness-based treatment of depression is rapidly evolving and now covers a wide range of approaches and techniques. The common feature is that the therapist teaches mindfulness skills to the patient, who is encouraged to practice those skills during the clinical hour, at home, or both. In this section, we first consider mindfulness-based approaches in individual psychotherapy and then discuss MBCT, one of the most popular and well-researched group programs for depression.

The Importance of the Therapist's Own Practice

Most clinicians who practice mindfulness-based psychotherapy agree that in order to bring mindfulness effectively into the therapeutic relationship, the therapist must have his or her own mindfulness meditation practice. This is important in mindfulness-informed approaches, and it is absolutely essential in more intensive mindfulness-based approaches. Although mindfulness skills may initially seem simple to learn and practice, integrating mindfulness to the point where it becomes a way of being in the world—and part of one's therapeutic presence—requires practice. For most people, getting to this point means spending a lot of time on the meditation cushion. Unless one is personally willing to engage in the practice over time, one probably shouldn't attempt to teach more rigorous mindfulness skills or conduct mindfulness-based psychotherapy. To illustrate this point, the developers of MBCT (Segal et al., 2012) make an analogy with swimming instruction:

> A swimming instructor is not someone who knows the physics of how solids behave in liquids, but he or she knows how to swim. It is not just an issue of credibility and competence, but of teachers' ability to embody "from the inside" the attitudes they invite participants to cultivate and adopt. When we started this work, we believed that it was unreasonable to expect all instructors to have experienced such mindfulness practice, or even to have practiced before. We have changed our minds about this. (p. 79)

In other words, teaching formal mindfulness practice is not just about giving instructions. It's about the way you say hello and sit in your chair, the way you respond to questions, conflicts, and everything else the patient brings to the therapeutic encounter. The contribution of practice to the therapist is described in detail in Chapter 3.

Tailoring the Approach to the Individual

There are almost as many ways to conduct mindfulness-based psychotherapy as there are therapists and patients. What's most important is finding an approach that is tailored to the patient's temperament, level of interest, and level of experience. If, for example, the patient has no preexisting interest in mindfulness practice, the therapist may choose to start with a mindfulness-informed approach and later introduce mindfulness skills that the patient might find useful.

> When Melissa first came to see me, her head was spinning. In couple therapy, her husband recently confessed to having had an affair with a coworker, and she didn't know what to do. She was clearly angry at him, but blamed herself for "being duped." She was feeling badly about herself because she was unemployed and had no sense of direction in her career. "I need to do something about that, too," she said. She bounced from topic to topic, story to story. After listening to her for several weeks, I suggested that before figuring out what to *do*, it might make sense to learn how to simply *be* with things as they are. I told her about mindfulness practice, how it involves shifting from the *doing mode* to the *being mode*, and how that shift can sometimes open up the space for new possibilities to emerge. Although skeptical, she said she was willing to give it a try, and I taught her a mindful breathing practice. After a few minutes, we stopped. The silence in the room was palpable. She opened her eyes, looked at me, and for the first time was able to hold my gaze for more than a second or two. She seemed calmer, and she said that the exercise helped her get in touch with her body, and that this felt like a good place to start.

Even though she had never meditated before, Melissa's first experience with it was positive. And when she opened her eyes, she could begin to envision a new way of relating to her difficulties. Our next task would be to determine how interested she was in developing her mindfulness skills, and how much time she might be willing to devote to mindfulness practice outside of our sessions.

If, on the other hand, the patient already has a meditation practice and is seeking mindfulness-based treatment, then the emphasis isn't on teaching mindfulness skills, but on utilizing those skills, deepening them, and applying them to the experience of depression. With such patients the therapist can begin simply by suggesting sitting together in silence for a few minutes at the start of each session.

Many patients fall somewhere in the middle. Perhaps they've dabbled with meditation, but they've never practiced on a regular basis. Maybe they've heard that mindfulness could help, but they don't know where to start. For such individuals the challenge is generally threefold: (1) finding the right practice, (2) finding ways to integrate it into the session, and (3) helping the patient integrate the practice into his or her life.

Finding the Right Practice

Expecting depressed people to devote 20 minutes or more per day to formal meditation practice may not be realistic, so it's best to start small, recommending a brief exercise such as the three-minute breathing space (Williams et al., 2007). Many patients like to begin each session with such an exercise. It not only gives them a chance to settle down and bring some attention to their inner experience, but also provides a way to transition from a doing mode to a being mode (Segal et al., 2002), from the busyness of their daily lives to the sacred space of the therapeutic hour. Here is an adaptation of the exercise.[1]

The Mini Mindfulness Break

- Sit in an upright position with the feet flat on the ground and the body in an upright but relaxed posture. Allow the eyes to close if that feels OK. If not, just look down at the floor a few feet in front of you.
- Bring awareness to the body–mind and acknowledge any strong sensations or energy you find. Briefly name the experience, if you can (by saying to yourself something like "tightness in the lower back," "feeling anxious," or "obsessing about yesterday's conference call").
- Redirect your awareness to the sensations of breathing, focusing on the abdomen rising and falling with each in- and outbreath. As best

---

[1]This exercise is adapted from Williams, Teasdale, Segal, and Kabat-Zinn (2007). Copyright 2007 by The Guilford Press. Adapted by permission.

you can, make the breath your exclusive object of attention, staying
with it for at least a minute or two. When your attention wanders,
put aside whatever caused it to wander and gently bring it back to
the breath.
- Staying connected with the breath, gradually expand your field of
  awareness to include the whole body, so there's an awareness of the
  breath sensations together with other sensations in the body.
- Continue expanding the field of awareness by adding sounds and
  the experience of hearing. Just notice sounds as they arise and pass
  away.
- When you're ready, open the eyes and bring this expanded
  awareness to the next thing you think, feel, say, or do.

Concentration and Mindfulness Practices

The breath can be used to build concentration (focused attention), in
which case the focus is narrow and the emphasis is on one-pointed attention; or it can be used to cultivate mindfulness per se (open monitoring),
where the focus is wider and the emphasis is on noting the changing
nature of experience (see Chapters 1 and 7). Either way, the breath serves
as an anchor, an object that keeps the awareness grounded in the present
moment. Used since ancient times as a focus of meditation (Rosenberg,
1998), the breath literally keeps us alive from moment to moment and
has the benefit of being completely portable and readily available. And
while it usually operates in the background of our awareness as part of
our autonomic nervous system, we can also bring conscious awareness
to it with relative ease, helping to bring body and mind together (Bien,
2006).

But some patients either aren't drawn to the breath or find it problematic. For these individuals, other body sensations can be an alternative. Some people prefer a body scan, in which the attention is directed
through different parts of the body, and some do better by focusing the
attention on the touch points—areas where the body comes in contact
with the chair, the floor, and itself. Bringing mindfulness to the body has
the added benefit of taking attention away from thoughts, which can be
useful for patients who tend to ruminate.

Other objects, such as sounds, can also serve as anchors. Although
it is beyond the scope of this chapter to provide a complete guide to
the relative advantages of different meditation objects, and to all the
differences between concentration and mindfulness practice, it's generally wise to give patients a chance to practice with a variety of objects
in order to determine which ones are most useful. For more on this

topic, see Pollak and colleagues (in press), Salzberg (2011), and R. Siegel (2010b).

Loving-kindness and Compassion Practices

Another valuable set of practices for treating depression involves the cultivation of loving-kindness (Salzberg, 2002) and self-compassion (Germer, 2009). In these exercises, one wishes oneself and others well by repeating certain phrases, such as *May I be happy. May I be peaceful. May I be free from suffering.* (See Chapters 1 and 7.)

These practices can be a powerful antidote to the negative thoughts and feelings that both feed and result from depression. Although this claim makes sense on an intuitive level, the latest research is beginning to support it as well (e.g., Boellinghaus, Jones, & Hutton, 2012). A recent scholarly review outlines some of the ways the "upward spirals" of positive emotions generated by mindfulness and loving-kindness meditation may counteract the "downward spirals" of negativity experienced by depressed patients (Garland et al., 2010).

Integrating Mindfulness into Psychotherapy

After a patient has found practices that help him or her to cultivate mindfulness, the question becomes: How do we incorporate this practice into our work together? Again, there are many possible approaches, and the key is flexibility. Perhaps we start our sessions by sitting together in silence, practicing mindfulness of breath. Or maybe we take a *mini-mindfulness break* when things become overly frightening or confusing. Or we could agree to do a guided meditation in order to shift attention away from ruminative thinking to sensations in the body.

Once mindfulness practice has been established, it also gives the therapist and patient a common frame of reference, and it will subtly change the therapist's questions. For example, if a patient is describing an argument with his or her spouse, the therapist might ask:

- Were you aware of your breath at all during the argument?
- Can you bring attention to your breath as you remember the experience now?
- Does this change your experience in any way?

As we incorporate mindfulness into our clinical practice, it's helpful to remember that we are therapists, not meditation teachers; our

expertise is in our clinical training. Listening deeply to our patients'
stories remains our most important task and a crucial part of the healing we hope to facilitate. So sometimes we simply listen—redirecting
a patient's attention to his or her breath at the wrong moment can be
experienced as an empathic failure. Conversely, such redirection, when
it is helpful, can enable a person to create some space around the pain
and, in the process, change his or her relationship to it. Knowing when
to just listen and when to bring in a mindfulness-based intervention is an
art, not a science. Fortunately, our own mindfulness practice can inform
our choices by keeping us attuned to the flow of the session (see Chapter
5). The following case illustrates a number of ways mindfulness and
psychotherapy can be integrated in the treatment of depression.

> Roger was a 34-year-old divorced father of a young son. After
> his divorce became final, he sank into a deep depression. Feeling
> suicidal, he contacted a psychiatrist, who prescribed an SSRI and
> began meeting with him weekly. This alleviated some of his symp-
> toms, including the suicidal thoughts. But after a year, he still wasn't
> feeling great, and was unhappy about the weight gain he attributed
> to his medication. He had been reading about meditation, thought a
> mindfulness-based approach might help, and so was referred to me.
>   "My life's a mess," was the first thing Roger said after I showed
> him into my office. Dressed in sweatpants and a T-shirt, he was
> walking with crutches due to recent surgery on his leg. He told me
> that he was in a car accident as a teenager that had left one leg badly
> injured, and he'd undergone a series of operations over the years
> to repair the damage. Currently on medical leave, he was anxious
> to get back to work. He was also filled with feelings of loneliness,
> unworthiness, and a wish to be in a healthy, intimate relationship.
> Since his marriage had ended, he had been in several short-term
> relationships, all of which ended painfully. When I ask about his
> goals, he said he wanted to "be in a relationship and find inner
> peace," but added that these goals are, in his experience, "mutually
> exclusive."
>   Roger was raised by an alcoholic single mother who struggled
> to make ends meet. He never knew his father and never felt loved
> by his mother, who was preoccupied with her own problems. The
> injury to his leg just added to his sense of being defective and unlov-
> able. But Roger also had strengths. A good student, he had landed a
> job after college with a startup software company. As the company
> prospered, so did he, and he was doing well financially. His career,
> along with his commitment to be a good father to his son, were
> important sources of self-esteem.

Although Roger said he was interested in meditation, he hadn't done any formal practice. So after listening to his story for several weeks, I taught him a basic mindfulness of breathing exercise, suggested we start each session with a *mini mindfulness break*, and encouraged him to practice at home.

The early results were mixed. Roger said he found it difficult to practice because his mind was "too active" and "too full of negative thoughts." Like many beginners, he had ideas about what meditation *should* feel like, and he was disheartened when his own practice didn't measure up. Not surprisingly, he also brought his self-critical tendency to his mindfulness practice. He often thought, "I just can't do this" or "What's wrong with me?" Hoping to counteract these negative thought spirals, I taught him a loving-kindness practice—but he said he just couldn't imagine sending himself such kind wishes.

Meanwhile, Roger continued to ruminate about his inability to be in a relationship, often experiencing the same negative thoughts in this challenging area of his life. "It's hopeless," he said. "Maybe I should just give up."

Through it all, I relied on my own mindfulness practice to help me bring some equanimity and acceptance to Roger's frustration and hopelessness, and to the similar emotions I often felt as I sat with him. I tried to stay connected to his pain—and to my own—and not give up on him or on the hope that he could find a different way to relate to his experience. Eventually, I told him about the MBCT groups I co-facilitate with a colleague and suggested he sign up as a way to deepen his practice. He readily agreed, and it was a turning point in his treatment.

The Power of Mindfulness Meets the Power of the Group

MBCT (Segal et al., 2002) is a treatment for recurrent depression that has been shown to be effective in a number of randomized controlled trials (Kuyken et al., 2008; Ma & Teasdale, 2004; Teasdale et al., 2000). Based on the mindfulness-based stress reduction (MBSR) program developed by Jon Kabat-Zinn (1990), MBCT incorporates elements of cognitive therapy that target the negative thoughts associated with depression. The developers describe it as "80% meditation, 20% cognitive therapy" (Law, 2008). The program introduces a variety of mindfulness techniques, provides opportunities for discussion, and includes homework intended to help participants establish a daily mindfulness practice. The goal is to help participants apply mindfulness to the moment-to-moment experience of depression so that they can relate to painful thoughts, feelings, and bodily sensations with more acceptance and ease instead of self-defeating defenses such as rumination and denial.

MBCT seems especially effective in reducing rumination. For many depressed patients, rumination is an attempt to use critical thinking skills to solve emotional problems, and in the process, to close the gap between where they are and where they want to be. But instead of moving them forward, rumination keeps them stuck. And the more they struggle, the deeper they sink:

> Rumination invariably backfires. It merely compounds our misery. It's a heroic attempt to solve a problem that it is just not capable of solving. Another mode of mind altogether is required when it comes to dealing with unhappiness. (Williams et al., 2007, p. 45)

Roger ruminated a lot, which is one reason I believed he could benefit from participating in an MBCT group.

Finding a Way Through

Initially, Roger's experience in the group was far from positive. In fact, in our individual session after the first group meeting, Roger told me he was thinking about dropping out because it "just feels weird." But he decided to stick with it and make the homework a priority, practicing at least 30 minutes a day. After several weeks, he reported that "something has clicked" and that he finally understood what mindfulness is:

> "It's like everything's turned upside down, but in a good way. I feel like I can just be aware of all these thoughts and feelings without taking them so seriously. I'm also starting to rethink what it means to be happy. Maybe being in a relationship isn't the answer after all."

Roger completed the group and continued his daily practice. He also began taking classes at a local meditation center and even went on a short retreat. In our individual sessions, Roger was more positive and confident. It was clear that a transformation had begun. When he said he wanted to try going off his SSRI, his psychiatrist and I both supported him. He soon lost some weight, joined a gym, and signed up for an online dating service. A few months later, he said he was ready to stop therapy because he was just too busy with his job, his son, his life. It was time to move on.

How Does It Work?

A recent study (Kuyken et al., 2010) suggests that MBCT is an effective treatment for depression because it not only enhances mindfulness and self-compassion among participants, but also reduces reactivity to negative thinking. The following factors may also contribute to its effectiveness:

1. *It helps people establish a daily practice.* Research has shown that regular meditation practice has positive effects on brain structure and functioning (Davidson, 2004; Hölzel et al., 2008; Lazar et al., 2005).
2. *It helps people integrate practice with daily life.* Through exercises such as the three-minute breathing space and homework that brings mindfulness to daily activities, MBCT shows participants that mindfulness is not just a formal practice reserved for the meditation cushion, but a way of relating to life.
3. *It reduces rumination.* By shifting attention away from thoughts toward other aspects of experience, it takes some of the power out of endless negative thinking (Williams et al., 2007).
4. *It helps people deconstruct depression.* By breaking depression down into thoughts, feelings, and bodily sensations, MBCT gives people a way in, and eventually a way through, their depression.
5. *It helps people disidentify with symptoms.* When patients recognize that their thoughts, feelings, and other symptoms are part of the territory of depression, they can more easily see them as impermanent and impersonal.
6. *It helps people respond, not react, to their symptoms.* Once they see their symptoms for what they are, participants are better able to respond appropriately, instead of reacting in habitual, self-destructive ways.
7. *It offers group support and validation.* By giving participants a chance to work together with others who are struggling with similar issues, MBCT reduces the stigma, shame, and isolation of depression.

Of course, many of these factors apply not only to MBCT, but also to mindfulness-informed and mindfulness-based treatment in general.

Depression remains a challenge to the patients who suffer from it and the therapists who treat them. Although many patients who participate in mindfulness-based treatment improve significantly, others are either not interested in this approach or try it but do not seem to benefit. Until research can identify which patients are likely to benefit from MBCT and other mindfulness-based approaches, we therapists must continue to rely on our own clinical judgment and feedback from our patients. Because patients respond differently to different forms of treatment, we best serve them by developing competence in the use of a variety of interventions and verifying *with our patients* that treatment is headed in the right direction (Horvath et al., 2011). In this respect, the use of mindfulness-based interventions is no different from the use of any other approach: We ask our patients if they would be open to learning about mindfulness practice, assess how well it is working, and be prepared with alternatives approaches. At the very least, we can always use our own mindfulness practice to remain as fully present to them as possible, to help them feel connected and more alive, even in the midst of their pain.

9

Anxiety

Accepting What Comes and Doing What Matters

Lizabeth Roemer
Susan M. Orsillo

> When we simply experience fear just as it is—without
> our opinions, judgments, and reactions—fear is not
> nearly so frightening.
>
> —EZRA BAYDA (2005)

*A*nxiety and fear are natural human responses. We experience
fear when confronted with immediate threat or danger, such as when
we step out into the street and hear the sound of screeching brakes as a
bus hurtles toward us. Our bodies experience a fight-or-flight response,
with our heart rate increasing, palms sweating, and blood rushing to our
limbs so that we can take immediate action to escape threat and keep
ourselves safe. In the face of actual danger, this is an adaptive response.
However, these same panicky sensations can arise in the absence of
a true threat, elicited by the memory of a past event or an imagined
future peril, preparing us to fight or flee when no clear action is needed.
Furthermore, fully engaging in life often requires us to approach real
threats, such as accepting a career challenge when we could fail or taking a social risk when we might be rejected. In these situations, our
biological predisposition to avoid danger and seek safety may not be the

optimal responses. We naturally experience anxiety when we anticipate a potentially threatening situation: feeling apprehensive, worrying about possible negative outcomes, and feeling on edge or on guard. These responses can also be useful; sometimes they help us plan for potential difficulties and consider ways to minimize possible harm or loss. Yet, when anxious apprehension or worry becomes a rigid habit, we can lose touch with the present moment, and constant preparation for future threats can erode our quality of life.

Although fear and anxiety are natural, inevitable responses to life, the messages they send to us can be confusing. We feel the urge to escape danger, when no clear threat is present. We feel compelled to control the future, despite the fact that many aspects are beyond our control. Thus, it is not surprising that we often respond to our own fear and anxiety with judgment and criticism, seeing our thoughts and emotions as a sign of weakness or flaws that will prevent us from living a peaceful and fulfilling life.

Although we can learn to respond to situations, thoughts, and feelings with apprehension, judgment, and avoidance, we can also learn to cultivate a mindful, compassionate, and accepting response to our experience. The practice of gently turning toward anxious feelings and sensations, with kindness and compassion, while continually bringing attention back to the present moment even when it repeatedly wanders to imagined, feared future events, can help to counteract learned anxious responses and promote life satisfaction. Learning to accept whatever internal experiences arise (e.g., sensations of panic, thoughts of others' judgments, worries about the future), rather than trying to suppress or avoid them, can paradoxically reduce distress and hasten recovery from anxious episodes. These strategies can help us to move from withdrawing and restricting our lives to approaching and broadening them.

Drawing from Buddhist and behavioral traditions, mindfulness- and acceptance-based behavioral therapies have been developed to help people learn these new ways of responding in order to reduce symptoms of anxiety and improve quality of life. In this chapter, we briefly review the empirical evidence for these approaches, including our own work in this area. We then present an evidence-based conceptual model that can guide mindfulness- and acceptance-based behavioral approaches to treating anxiety, along with an overview of our own integrated approach to treatment, with illustrative examples.[1]

---

[1] Readers interested in a more detailed description of this approach to therapy are directed to Roemer and Orsillo (2009) for a therapist guide, and Orsillo and Roemer (2011) for a self-help manual.

EVIDENCE FOR THE EFFICACY
OF MINDFULNESS- AND ACCEPTANCE-BASED
TREATMENTS FOR ANXIETY

Cognitive-behavioral treatments include some combination of the following approaches: teaching about the nature of anxiety; helping people to monitor and increase awareness and understanding of their own anxious responding; encouraging exposure to feared stimuli (either external, such as social situations, or internal, such as panic-related sensations); and identifying and questioning anxiety-related thoughts and beliefs. These interventions have been established as efficacious treatments for all anxiety disorders (generalized anxiety disorder, panic disorder with and without agoraphobia, social anxiety disorder, posttraumatic stress disorder, obsessive–compulsive disorder, and specific phobias [Hofmann & Smits, 2008]). However, not everyone who receives these treatments responds to them, and some treatments have high dropout or refusal rates.

In the past decade, interest has developed in exploring the potential efficacy of mindfulness- and acceptance-based treatments for anxiety disorders.[2] Although research on these approaches is still in its early stages, results have been promising. A recent meta-analysis indicated that mindfulness-based treatments are associated with significant, reliable reductions in anxiety and depressive symptoms across studies of a wide range of presenting problems (Hofmann et al., 2010). Specifically, mindfulness- and acceptance-based therapies have been found to yield significant reductions in anxiety symptoms among individuals[3] diagnosed with social anxiety disorder (SAD; Dalrymple & Herbert, 2007; Koszycki, Benger, Shlik, & Bradwejn, 2007; Kocovski, Laurier, & Rector, 2009; Piet, Houggard, Hecksher, & Rosenberg, 2010), generalized anxiety disorder (GAD; Craigie, Rees, & Marsh, 2008; Evans et al., 2008; Roemer & Orsillo, 2007; Roemer et al., 2008), and

---

[2]Treatments such as mindfulness-based stress reduction, mindfulness-based cognitive therapy, and acceptance and commitment therapy all fall into this category of treatments due to their shared focus on teaching clients to relate to their internal experiences differently (with mindfulness and acceptance, rather than aversion or avoidance). Despite this overarching similarity, these treatments vary in terms of their emphasis on formal mindfulness practice, amount of practice included, and inclusion of exposure and other behavioral elements.

[3]Studies were included in this review if they focused on individuals who met criteria for a principal diagnosis of one anxiety disorder and they had a large enough sample to determine statistically significant changes in symptoms.

obsessive–compulsive disorder (OCD; Twohig et al., 2010). Preliminary evidence also suggests that these treatments significantly improve quality of life among individuals with GAD or SAD (Craigie et al., 2008; Koszycki et al., 2007; Roemer & Orsillo, 2007). However, only two studies thus far have demonstrated significant improvements over a comparison condition (Roemer et al., 2008; Twohig et al., 2010), and no studies have found these therapies to be more efficacious than established efficacious treatments for the target disorders.[4] However, two recent studies found these therapies to yield comparable effects to established efficacious treatments (acceptance and commitment therapy [ACT] for a sample of mixed anxiety disorder clients [Arch et al., 2012]) and our acceptance-based behavior therapy for GAD (Hayes-Skelton, Roemer, & Orsillo, in press). Also, some studies of mindfulness-based interventions have yielded smaller effects than studies of cognitive-behavioral therapies for the same disorders (e.g., Craigie et al., 2008; Evans et al., 2008; Koszycki et al., 2007; Piet et al., 2010). It may be that treatments are more efficacious when they incorporate elements of cognitive-behavioral treatments (e.g., Arch et al., 2012; Dalrymple & Herbert, 2007; Roemer et al., 2008; Twohig et al., 2010), rather than focusing solely on mindfulness-based elements; however, more research is needed to clarify whether this is, in fact, the case. Nonetheless, given the established efficacy of cognitive-behavioral treatments for anxiety disorders, incorporation of some type of exposure or other behavioral approach strategies, self-monitoring of anxious responding, and psychoeducation about anxiety is clinically indicated at this point in our knowledge.

In our own research with people who meet criteria for GAD, we have found that an integrative acceptance-based behavioral treatment that draws from evidence-based cognitive-behavioral treatments for GAD (Borkovec, Alcaine, & Behar, 2004), as well as acceptance-based behavioral therapies (ACT [Hayes et al., 1999]; mindfulness-based cognitive therapy [MBCT; Segal et al., 2002]; dialectical behavior therapy [DBT; Linehan, 1993a]), significantly reduces symptoms of GAD and comorbid depression, with a trend toward improvements in other comorbid disorders (Roemer et al., 2008). We see clients who present with a wide range of additional diagnoses (e.g., social anxiety disorder, panic disorder, major depressive disorders), as well as complex lives that add to their worry and stress. For the remainder of this chapter, we share what we have learned

---

[4]Twohig and colleagues (2010) found that acceptance and commitment therapy was more efficacious than progressive muscle relaxation, but progressive muscle relaxation is not an efficacious treatment for OCD.

from this work, others' work in this area, and our own experiences with anxiety to help readers design effective, individualized therapies for clients with anxiety disorders and other anxiety-related challenges.

AN EVIDENCE-BASED MODEL OF ANXIETY AND ITS DISORDERS: A MINDFULNESS, AND ACCEPTANCE-BASED, BEHAVIORAL APPROACH

Humans are complex, multifaceted creatures who vary greatly in their biological makeup, their habitual way of responding to people or situations, the experiences they have had in their lives, and the contexts in which they live. Yet, in the midst of all of this variation, certain consistent themes emerge that can provide a foundation for understanding, and eventually helping, people. Buddhist psychology provides one resource for understanding why people suffer and how to reduce suffering, and Western psychological theory provides another. It is particularly encouraging when disparate sources of wisdom provide overlapping perspectives. Our approach is influenced by the advice of Teasdale, Segal, and Williams (2003), who emphasize the importance of developing a clear conceptual, evidence-based model that can be used to inform the application of mindfulness to a particular clinical presentation. Here we describe the model that guides our treatment.

Neuroscience and learning theory highlight the function of fear and anxiety in promoting the survival of our species. Yet, as noted above, we can develop habits that leave us stuck in an endless cycle of avoiding situations that are not life-threatening and imagining potential catastrophes without generating any solutions. Both Buddhist and Western psychological theory emphasize the ways that humans can develop stuck habits of mind, consistently responding with certain types of thoughts and believing them—due, in part, to their incessant repetition. The more our minds travel down these paths, the more well worn they become, so that our thoughts increasingly slip into familiar patterns. Often these habitual thoughts carry with them suggestions to avoid potential threat, yet following these suggestions may keep us stuck rather than safe.

Reacting to Internal Experiences with Distress, Criticism, and Judgment

One of the most formative, consistent findings to emerge in the field of anxiety disorders is that the experience of anxiety or fear, in and of itself (e.g., sensations of panic, worrisome thoughts, catastrophic images, recurrent painful memories), does not cause an anxiety disorder. Instead, it is our reactions to these symptoms, or our *reaction to our reactions* (Borkovec & Sharples, 2004), that exacerbates their intensity and duration, causes distress, and interferes with our quality of life. For instance, people who report a high sensitivity to anxiety (i.e., who view the physiological sensations of anxiety as threatening) are more likely to develop panic attacks and panic disorder (Ehlers, 1995); trauma survivors with negative attitudes about emotional expression (e.g., "I think getting emotional is a sign of weakness") experience increased posttraumatic stress symptomatology (Joseph et al., 1997); and those who worry excessively report worrying about their own worry (Wells, 1999). Anxiety can also lead to a *narrowed focus* of attention (both external and internal) toward potential threat (Cisler & Koster, 2010). Moreover, anxiety often elicits negative judgments and criticisms ("I'm so weak!" "Other people don't worry the way I do"), which can, in turn, increase anxiety.

All of these reactions can lead people to become *entangled with* (Germer, 2005a) or *hooked on* (Chödrön, 2007) their experiences of anxiety, so that the anxiety comes to seem self-defining and all-encompassing. Instead of viewing anxiety as a response that is elicited in a particular context, we may come to define ourselves as *anxious*, fusing our identity with these experiences. This makes it much harder to see the ways that thoughts, feelings, and sensations naturally arise, change, and pass over time. When anxious sensations and thoughts seem frightening, defining, and unrelenting, they naturally lead people to want to escape and avoid them.

Rigidly Trying to Avoid Internal Distress

Trying not to think about, feel, or remember something distressing is entirely natural. At times, we all attempt to put something stressful out of our minds so that we can focus on what is in front of us, distract ourselves from painful memories so we feel less distressed, or control physical sensations that are making us uncomfortable. Yet, studies show that rigid, repeated efforts to put thoughts, feelings, sensations, or memories out of our minds (i.e., *experiential avoidance*; Hayes et al., 1996) are often unsuccessful and can actually entangle us more deeply in the very experiences we are trying to escape (Gross, 2002; Levitt, Brown, Orsillo, & Barlow, 2004; Najmi & Wegner, 2008). Consider a time when you really needed to fall asleep, but you were wide awake. Simply willing yourself to feel drowsy often backfires.

Avoiding Rather Than Approaching

Emotions are partly adaptive because they are linked to action tendencies. When we experience fear, we are prompted to avoid or escape whatever we perceive as a threat. However, fully engaging in life requires us at times to override our action tendencies. For example, in order to ask someone out on a date or give a public presentation, we have to be open to the possible risk of rejection or criticism. When fear and anxiety are viewed as dangerous responses, intensified and sustained through our efforts to control them, we may be unwilling to take any actions that could elicit them. Although avoiding potential threats is often immediately comforting, this stance can lead to chronic pain and suffering by maintaining fears and distress, and limiting contact with the rewarding and meaningful aspects of life.

Many anxiety disorders are associated with strong, obvious patterns of avoidance: People with social anxiety may avoid speaking in class; people with agoraphobia may avoid crowded, public places; those with posttraumatic stress disorder may avoid reminders of their trauma. Sometimes avoidance is more subtle. People with GAD can seem extremely busy, yet refrain from engaging in personally meaningful activities that could elicit discomfort, such as pursuing challenges at work or opening up to emotional intimacy (Michelson, Lee, Orsillo, & Roemer, 2011).

A Mindful Solution

If our habitual internal and behavioral responses to anxiety interfere with our ability to live a meaningful and satisfying life, we can free ourselves from these patterns by changing our relationship with, and reactions to, that anxiety. Expanding our awareness of experience, noticing reactions as what they are and allowing them to be, developing kindness and compassion toward ourselves, and intentionally choosing to engage in activities that matter to us are alternative ways of responding that can be cultivated through mindfulness practice (Kabat-Zinn, 1994). Thus, integrating mindfulness with cognitive-behavioral strategies may be a useful antidote to chronic, habitual anxiety.

A MINDFULNESS- AND ACCEPTANCE-BASED BEHAVIORAL APPROACH TO TREATMENT

Our approach to treatment focuses on helping clients (1) develop a new relationship with their internal experiences (one that is broad rather than narrow, compassionate rather than critical and judgmental, and decentered—that is, seeing thoughts objectively rather than as all-encompassing truths—rather than entangled); (2) cultivate willingness rather than trying to avoid experience; and (3) engage in actions that matter to them rather than habitually avoiding.

Mindful Assessment

Treatment begins with an assessment of how anxiety looks and feels for the client (thoughts, feelings, sensations, and behaviors associated with anxiety; contexts in which anxiety occurs; antecedents and consequences to anxious responding), how the client typically responds to—and tries to cope with—distress or pain, and what changes he or she would like to see to improve quality of life. We also think it is critical to understand how the client and his or her family understand anxiety and ways of dealing with it. Drawing from our model and the client's individual experiences, strengths, and resources, we develop a shared conceptualization of the development and maintenance of the client's current challenges that informs a treatment plan aimed at helping the client live a more enriching, fulfilling life, even in the face of anxiety.

From the beginning, the language we use to discuss thoughts, feelings, sensations, and memories associated with anxiety cultivates a sense that these are specific responses that come and go, rather than defining characteristics of the client. By describing specific sensations ("I notice tension across my shoulders," "My heart feels like it's pounding out of my chest"), thoughts ("I have the thought that I'll never succeed at anything," "I find myself thinking that people are mad at me"), and behaviors ("I play video games for hours," "I don't answer my phone"), we begin to break down the seemingly all-encompassing experience of anxiety into more manageable pieces. This deconstruction initiates a process of decentering, an important aspect of mindfulness, which helps to reduce entanglement with these experiences.

Modeling acceptance and compassion, we share with clients how the challenges with anxiety that they describe make sense within a broad social–cultural context and within their specific learning histories. We also explain how learning new skills, such as mindfulness, may help them address these problematic, habitual patterns of responding; promote more flexible, intentional action; and decrease the distress and interference they are experiencing in response to anxiety. Some clients connect to aspects of this explanation immediately and tentatively express hope for treatment. At times, understandably, clients are skeptical that anything will help them change such ingrained patterns of responding. We validate their concerns, refrain from arguing or trying to convince them otherwise, and ask if they are willing to try things out for a few weeks and see if they notice any improvements. If not, we can revisit our plan and explore other options. This sets the stage for a constant theme throughout treatment of trying things out, paying attention, and seeing how they go, rather than assuming that therapists or clients know in advance what will or will not be helpful. Mindfulness skills help with this observation and eventually promote attunement to one's own experience, rather than (or perhaps in addition to) one's fears.

Learning

A central element of treatment is providing information that can help clients more fully understand, and importantly, have compassion for their own experiences. We teach clients about the nature of anxiety and the ways in which responses to anxiety may paradoxically increase distress and decrease satisfaction. In this way clients can begin to observe whether these general principles apply to their own lives. Our methods include didactic instruction (supported by handouts), experiential demonstrations (e.g., demonstrating the paradoxical effects of thought suppression), and exploration of examples from the clients' own lives. Although simply learning about these concepts rarely leads to dramatic change, it does begin the process of loosening the cycle of anxiety, judgment, criticism, and avoidance, and can help clients begin to feel compassion for themselves as their anxious cycles get underway.

We are careful to convey new information within a context of compassion, validating both the humanness of our clients' responses and the difficulty associated with changing established patterns of responding. Like Linehan (1993), we see explicit, consistent validation as an important active ingredient in therapy. For instance, when Myra criticized herself in session for feeling anxious during a difficult conversation with her mother, her therapist responded by validating that anxiety was a natural reaction associated with self-disclosure. Over time, Myra was able to have more compassionate responses on her own, which actually lessened the intensity of the anxiety she felt disclosing her feelings to her mother. The therapeutic relationship is a crucial vehicle for new learning, helping clients relate differently to their own internal experiences because we do.

It can be helpful to teach people about the function of emotions. Clients with anxiety disorders have understandably come to see emotional responses as problematic. Yet primary emotions, such as sadness, anger, and fear, provide important information (Greenberg & Safran, 1987; Mennin & Fresco, 2010). Often anxiety or worry occur when other primary emotions are present but are being avoided or ignored. Learning to notice our emotional experiences can give us access to the information that these primary emotions provide, which can in turn help to guide us in living more satisfying lives.

However, emotions sometimes communicate distorted or inaccurate information. We teach clients to distinguish between *clear* emotions, which occur in direct response to the situation at hand, such as feeling sad after a loss, and *muddy* emotions, which are distorted in some form and provide less clear information. We suggest that emotional responses that are confusing, exceptionally long-lasting, and that seem more intense than warranted by the situation may be muddy. Emotions can become muddy because (1) we aren't taking good care of ourselves (e.g., poor sleep, poor eating, not exercising); (2) we are worrying about the future or ruminating about the past, rather than responding to the present moment; or (3) we are reacting to emotions with judgment and/ or attempts to avoid. Mindfulness can help us notice when our emotions are muddy and also can help us clarify what we are feeling.

Another aspect of emotions that can be confusing is their close connection to action tendencies. Often people try to avoid certain thoughts and feelings because they believe they need to act on them. For example, a client may feel that he has to leave a social event early because he is anxious or that she must decline an invitation because she is feeling sad. Although fear is associated with the urge to escape, and sadness with the urge to withdraw, we can still behave in ways that are inconsistent with how we feel. For example, someone can feel anxious, have the urge to avoid, and still attend a dental appointment. Often clients are able to react less negatively to their own emotions when they are able to recognize that they can choose actions without having to directly control or change their internal responses. This understanding allows greater flexibility in responding. Emotions (and thoughts) can be just what they are, not the actions they call to mind.

Noticing

Both Buddhist psychology and learning theory highlight the importance of increasing our awareness in the present moment. Noticing what arises in a given instant provides an opportunity to relate differently to internal experiences and to make choices about how to act in a particular context. Most of us habitually fail to notice most of what happens in the present moment. Instead, we multitask, daydream, worry, or engage in efforts to distract ourselves from discomfort. In doing so, we miss a great deal of information, including data about our own experience, preferences, and choices, as well as the consequences that follow choices.

For decades, cognitive-behavioral approaches to treating anxiety have emphasized the importance of self-monitoring. In our view, the process of writing down one's thoughts, physical sensations, feelings, and behaviors is a type of mindfulness exercise. It involves turning toward experience, noticing that experience as what it is, not what it says it is, and gaining some distance or perspective on the experience (decentering) by writing it down.

We have clients begin by monitoring their most prominent anxiety symptoms (e.g., panic, worry, social anxiety), noting the context in which they occur and their intensity. We gradually expand instructions so that clients increase their awareness of (1) specific thoughts and emotions, (2) their reactions to these reactions, (3) their efforts aimed at avoiding internal experiences, and (4) their chosen behaviors and actions.

> Tony's first attempt at monitoring suggested that his response to most situations was anxiety. After learning about clear and muddy emotions and practicing mindfulness, he began to notice that he felt sad and angry at times, often in response to conflict with his partner. He also began to notice that he often tried to distract himself from thinking about his relationship by worrying about the maintenance and upkeep of his house. As Tony's mindfulness practice developed, he was able to notice these patterns as they emerged. He also became more willing to acknowledge the full range of his responses, allowing himself to experience them rather than distracting himself, and to consider possible actions. Tony noticed that his sadness and anger were not as frightening as he feared, and he found that the less he fought his feelings, the more tolerable they seemed. As Tony learned to allow and pay attention to his full range of emotions, he became more willing to engage with his partner and resolve some of the conflicts they had been experiencing. His worrying became less frequent and less intrusive over time.

Practicing

In a sense, those of us who struggle with worry or anxiety have been practicing anxiety, panic, or worry for years. Learning new ways of responding and establishing new habits are possible, but they also require a commitment to practice. We encourage clients to establish a *formal* practice in which they set aside time to regularly engage in mindfulness.

We introduce clients to a variety of formal practices varying in length and focus, building on previously practiced skills. Typically, we begin with mindfulness of breath and eating, then mindfulness of sensations (hearing, physical sensations), mindfulness of emotions and thoughts, cultivating self-compassion, and noticing the transience of internal experiences (Mountain Meditation [Kabat-Zinn, 1994]). This order can be flexibly adapted to meet the needs of the client. (An example of an exercise we use repeatedly to cultivate self-compassion is presented below; other exercises are available at *www.mindfulwaythroughanxietybook. com.*) Although we encourage clients to try each new practice for at least a week, our goal is to promote flexibility and personalization. Thus, we do not prescribe a particular practice regimen, and instead encourage clients to set aside as much time as they can, stressing that committing to some brief practice is better than not practicing at all.

Inviting a Difficulty In and Working with It through the Body[5]

- Before you begin this exercise, think of a difficulty you're experiencing right now. It doesn't have to be a significant difficulty, but choose something that you find unpleasant, something that is unresolved. It may be something you are worried about, an argument or misunderstanding you've had, something you feel angry, resentful, guilty, or frustrated about. If nothing is going on right now, think of some time in the recent past when you felt scared, worried, frustrated, resentful, angry, or guilty, and use that.
- Noticing the way you are sitting in the chair or on the floor. Noticing where your body is touching the chair or floor. Bringing your attention to your breath for a moment. Noticing the inbreath . . . and the outbreath. . . . Now gently widening your awareness, take in the body as a whole. Noticing any sensations that arise, breathing with your whole body.
- When you are ready, bringing to mind whatever situation has been bringing up difficult emotions for you. Bringing your attention to the specific emotions that arise and any reactions you have to those emotions.
- And as you are focusing on this troubling situation and your emotional reaction, allowing yourself to tune in to any *physical sensations* in the body that you notice are arising . . . becoming aware of those physical sensations . . . and then deliberately, but gently, directing your focus of attention to the region of the body where the sensations

---

[5]This exercise is adapted from Williams, Teasdale, Segal, and Kabat-Zinn (2007). Copyright 2007 by The Guilford Press. Adapted by permission.

are the strongest in the gesture of an embrace, a welcoming . . . noticing that this is how it is right now . . . and *breathing into that part of the body* on the inbreath and breathing out from that region on the outbreath, exploring the sensations, watching their intensity shift up and down from one moment to the next.

- Now, seeing if you can bring to this attention an even deeper attitude of compassion and openness to whatever sensations, thoughts, or emotions you are experiencing, however unpleasant, by saying to yourself from time to time, "It's OK. Whatever it is, it's already here. Let me open to it."

- Staying with the awareness of these internal sensations, breathing with them, accepting them, letting them be, and allowing them to be just as they are. Saying to yourself again, if you find it helpful, "It's here right now. Whatever it is, it's already here. Let me be open to it." Softening and opening to the sensation you become aware of, letting go of any tensing and bracing. If you like, you can also experiment with holding in awareness both the sensations of the body and the feeling of the breath moving in and out as you breathe with the sensations moment by moment.

- And when you notice that the bodily sensations are no longer pulling your attention to the same degree, simply return 100% to the breath and continue with that as the primary object of attention.

- And then gently bring your awareness to the way you are sitting in the chair, your breath, and, when you are ready, opening your eyes.

Each new mindfulness practice is introduced at the beginning of session. Clients and therapists engage in the practice together and then the client is encouraged to share his or her observations. In discussing practice, we help clients to apply their observations to their presenting problems and the kinds of changes they want to make. For instance, Ahn expressed anger after practicing mindfulness of breath because she was breathing "wrong" and couldn't keep her focus. After congratulating Ahn for noticing how busy her mind was, the therapist asked whether similar worries, judgments, and evaluations arose when Ahn was preparing her lecture or meeting with the parent of one of her students. Ahn was encouraged to cultivate a compassionate stance toward herself (e.g., "How hard it must be to work effectively when my mind is so busy and critical") and to practice acknowledging where her mind went and gently guiding it back to the present.

Sometimes clients experience physical sensations of anxiety during their practice and express the concern that practice is making them worse. We predict that this may happen ahead of time and encourage clients to notice these sensations as they arise, label them as what they are, and allow their awareness to expand around the sensations. During a practice, Layla noted:

> "My chest feels tight and my heart is pounding. I'm having the thought that I can't breathe. I feel like I have to stand up and run out of the room. I'm having the thought that I'm a failure at this, just like everything else. The thoughts are coming so fast and forcefully. . . . I can also notice that I am still breathing. I can feel air coming into my throat and my chest moving, even though it still feels tight. I notice that even though everything in me wants to run, I can still sit here, noticing my breath. I am feeling uncomfortable, and I am noticing that that isn't all of my experience, even in this moment."

This is a powerful realization. Layla finds that she is able to continue doing something that matters to her (in this case, formal practice) even while she experiences distressing sensations and thoughts and a strong urge to escape. Successful treatment for panic disorder involves intentionally experiencing physical sensations without escaping (called *interoceptive exposure* by Craske & Barlow, 2008); if clients are experiencing panic, we incorporate these kinds of interoceptive exposure exercises to ensure that they are practicing directly with their feared sensations.

Clients may also want to try movement practices. In our treatment, we use mindful progressive muscle relaxation, in which clients notice sensations associated with tensing and releasing their muscles. We like this as an early practice because it gives clients who are easily distracted by worry a concrete focus. Clients also find walking or yoga meditations to be useful, such as taking a step with each half breath and noticing the sensations of walking.

Informal practice is also encouraged throughout treatment, with clients beginning by bringing mindfulness to mundane tasks such as washing the dishes or brushing teeth, and moving toward mindfulness during more challenging situations such as a difficult discussion with a family member. This application of skills to living is an essential part of treatment—we want to help clients take the skills of mindfulness "off the cushion" and into their lives (Hanh, 1992). Eventually this will help them be able to engage in meaningful actions even when they are experiencing fear or anxiety. Layla can translate her experience in formal practice to being able to talk to someone new, even though her heart is pounding and she feels like running away.

Doing What Matters

Developing the skills of mindfulness, paying attention in any given moment, noticing emotional responses, and reducing reactivity may naturally lead people to engage more fully in their lives, given that habitual reactivity and avoidance were reducing this engagement. However, because of the prominence of avoidance in anxiety disorders, we have found it useful to explicitly focus on behavioral engagement in therapy (drawing from methods described in ACT [Hayes et al., 1999; Wilson & Murrell, 2004]). Asking clients to articulate their personal values helps to shape a direction for therapy. Most clients present to treatment with the unattainable goal of being anxiety-free; instead, we encourage clients to identify the actions they would take if anxiety and avoidance were not holding them back.

Early in treatment, we ask clients to first write about how anxiety has interfered with their lives and then how they would like to be living, focusing specifically on three domains: relationships, work/school/household management, and self-nurturing and community involvement (see the example writing instructions). Once clients have articulated their values, we have them begin to monitor opportunities to act consistently with their values that are taken or missed each week. Clients are encouraged to use their newly developed skills of mindfulness to become aware of and address obstacles, and to bring awareness to their actions.

Clarifying Values in Relationships[6]

- Set aside 20 minutes during which you can privately and comfortably do this writing assignment. In your writing, we want you to really let go and explore your very deepest emotions and thoughts about the topic. You may want to take several minutes to practice mindfulness before you start, so that you can approach this task with openhearted awareness.
- As you write, try to allow yourself to experience your thoughts and feelings as completely as you can. Pushing disturbing thoughts away can actually make them worse, so try to really let yourself go. Bring your mindfulness practice to the exercise so that you can accept and allow any reactions you have and continue to clarify what matters to you most. If you cannot think of what to write next, repeat the same

---

[6]This exercise is adapted from Orsillo and Roemer (2011). Copyright 2011 by The Guilford Press. Adapted by permission.

thing over and over until something new comes to you. Be sure to write for the entire 20 minutes. Don't be concerned with spelling, punctuation, or grammar; just write whatever comes to mind.

• You may notice that you often have thoughts about why you cannot be the way you would like to be in your relationships. This is natural, and we will explore these obstacles at other times. So, for this particular exercise, see if you can notice these thoughts as they arise and gently turn your attention back to how you would like to be if you were not experiencing the obstacle so that you can really explore what matters to you.

• Choose two or three relationships that are important to you. You can either pick actual relationships (e.g., "my relationship with my brother") or relationships you would like to have (e.g., "I would like to be part of a couple," "I would like to make more friends"). Briefly write about how you would like to be in those relationships. Think about how you would like to *communicate with others* (e.g., how open vs. private you would like to be, how direct vs. passive you would like to be in asking for what you need and in giving feedback to others). Think about *what sort of support you would like* from other people and *what sort of support you can give* without sacrificing your self-care. Write about anything else that matters to you in your relationships with others.

In traditional exposure exercises, clients are encouraged to approach feared sensations, memories, or contexts, often using a fear hierarchy so that they are able to learn nonfearful associations with cues that are lower on the hierarchy first. Mindfulness can be used to complement these types of exposures—clients are encouraged to remain present and aware, noticing everything that arises, as it arises, while remaining in contact with the feared situation, memory, or sensation. Mindfulness may, in fact, enhance the new learning that occurs during these exposures (Treanor, 2011), although more research is needed to determine if this is the case.

Clarification of values can help to provide motivation for exposures and can help the client select a broader range of behavioral actions, with an aim of increasing a sense of meaningful engagement in life, rather than diminishing fearful responding (although fear and anxiety are likely to naturally decline as more behavioral engagement occurs). For example:

Troy experienced panic attacks whenever he was in a crowd, and as a result he avoided approaching many situations that were important to him. He spoke poignantly about how much he would like to attend his son's football games and share that experience with him, the way Troy's father had done with him when he was young. Therapy focused on teaching Troy to relate to his sensations of panic differently, so that they felt less overwhelming, by developing mindfulness skills. Then Troy began to attend scrimmages, using his skills when panic sensations arose. Finally, he attended a game. Although he noticed sensations of panic while he was there, he also noticed his son's wide smile when he heard his father cheer after a particularly key block. Troy didn't miss a game for the rest of the season.

An Ongoing Practice

G. Alan Marlatt's seminal work in relapse prevention (e.g., Marlatt & Donovan, 2007) has taught us the importance of recognizing that even change itself, like all things, is impermanent. Although we can learn and strengthen new habits of approaching rather than avoiding, our old habits remain etched in our neural circuits (e.g., Hermans, Craske, Mineka, & Lovibond, 2006). Old patterns of responding may emerge during times of stress or transition, or simply because our practices have ebbed over time, seeming less needed.

Toward the end of treatment, we spend time reviewing what clients have found useful and help them consider how they might maintain the changes they have made. Clients are provided with a notebook of the handouts and exercises they have used throughout treatment, and we encourage them to review these materials when they notice that their anxiety or stress level is increasing, or that their lives are beginning to narrow again. We encourage clients to maintain some type of consistent mindfulness practice to keep developing their skills, and also so that they will notice when muddy emotions, reactivity, and avoidance begin to reemerge in their lives. Drawing from Marlatt's work, we emphasize the importance of seeing these inevitable experiences as *lapses*—or opportunities to practice—rather than as relapses. We all experience such events. All we can do is notice them and then recommit ourselves to practicing in ways that help us to maintain a meaningful engagement in our lives.

10

Psychophysiological Disorders

Embracing Pain

Ronald D. Siegel

> What you resist, persists.
> —ANONYMOUS

*N*obody likes pain, and people go to great lengths to get rid of it. Although some physical discomfort is inevitable, a remarkable variety of medical disorders are actually maintained by our attempts to feel better. Mindfulness practice can help to resolve these conditions and enrich our lives in the process.

The first structured program that taught mindfulness to patients was designed for the management of chronic pain (Kabat-Zinn, 1982). Over subsequent decades, mindfulness-based programs have been used to treat a wide variety of pain syndromes, including fibromyalgia (Goldenberg et al., 1994; Grossman, Tienfenthaler-Gilmer, Raysz, & Kesper, 2007; Kaplan, Goldenberg, & Galvin-Nadeau, 1993; Sephton et al., 2007), chronic low back pain (Mehling, Hamel, Acree, Byl, & Hecht, 2005; Morone, Rollman, Moore, Li, & Weiner, 2009), chronic pelvic pain (Fox, Flynn, & Allen, 2011), and arthritis (Pradhan et al., 2007; Zangi et al., 2012). In the early years, encouraging outcomes were frequently reported, but studies often lacked control groups or randomized designs (e.g., Kabat-Zinn, 1982; Kabat-Zinn, Lipworth, & Burney, 1985; for reviews, see Baer, 2003; Grossman et al., 2004). Although more recent studies still have some methodological limitations, they tend to be better controlled (e.g., Cramer, Haller, Lauche, & Dobos, 2012; Rosenzweig et al., 2010; Wong et al., 2011; see Veehof, Oskam, Schreurs, & Bohlmeijer, 2011, for a review). Overall, more recent studies typically demonstrate that mindfulness practice yields modest benefits in reducing pain intensity for patients with chronic pain and more significant benefits in improving other quality-of-life measures (Veehof et al., 2011). As I argue shortly, the benefits of mindfulness meditation in reducing pain intensity are increased when integrated into a more comprehensive rehabilitation program, rather than when applied in isolation.

Medical applications of mindfulness have grown, and the practice has now been successfully integrated into the treatment of a wide range of other physical disorders with psychological components, including psoriasis (Kabat-Zinn et al., 1998), irritable bowel syndrome (Garland, Gaylord, Palsson, et al., 2011; Gaylord et al., 2011; Kearney, McDermott, Martinez, & Simpson, 2011), insomnia (Gross et al., 2011; Ong, Shapiro, & Manber, 2009; Yook et al., 2008), sexual dysfunction (Brotto, Basson, & Luria, 2008; Silverstein, Brown, Roth, & Britton, 2011), hot flashes (Carmody et al., 2011), and heart disease (Tacon, McComb, Caldera, & Randolph, 2003).

MIND–BODY MEDICINE

The distinction between mind and body, so familiar in Western discourse, is misleading. Subjective mental states are influenced by physical factors such as medications, exercise, and diet. Conversely, a host of physical disorders is influenced by psychological factors. The most common are *psychophysiological* disorders, in which persistent mental distress creates changes in tissues, in turn causing symptoms. Examples include headaches, gastrointestinal distress, dermatological disorders, and musculoskeletal pain of all sorts. Because these disorders are often maintained by a mix of medical, psychological, and behavioral factors, clinicians have needed to evolve flexible, integrative interventions that attempt to address all of these elements. It turns out that psychophysiological disorders are particularly well suited to treatments that incorporate mindfulness.

One such intervention is the Back Sense program—an approach my colleagues and I developed that integrates cognitive, psychodynamic, behavioral, and systemic interventions along with explicit teaching of mindfulness practice for the treatment of chronic back pain (Siegel,

Urdang, & Johnson, 2001). The program goes beyond the use of mind-fulness for pain management, drawing on evolving innovations in reha-bilitation medicine and psychology to resolve the disorder fully for many people. Patients can participate in the program by following a published self-treatment guide[1] or through treatment with a mental health or reha-bilitation professional.

This chapter discusses the program as an illustration of how mind-fulness practice can be fruitfully combined with other psychotherapeutic and rehabilitative interventions to treat psychophysiological disorders. It explores the benefits of formal mindfulness practice, as well as how principles derived from mindfulness practice—such as relaxing control, tolerating discomfort, staying with negative emotions, and returning attention to the present—can inform treatment. We will also see how the approaches used to treat chronic musculoskeletal pain are supported by recent neurobiological research, and how they can readily be adapted to treat a wide range of stress-related health problems.

An Evolutionary Accident

Until relatively recently, medical professionals typically believed that most chronic back pain was caused by an unintended consequence of evolution. This view, presented to countless patients, suggests that our spines became vulnerable when our ancestors stood up to walk on two legs. The increased pressure on spinal structures supposedly leads to damage over time that accounts for the epidemic of back trouble among modern humans.

To the surprise of doctors and patients alike, accumulating evidence now points instead to a cycle of psychological stress, muscle tension, and fear-based avoidance of activity as the true cause for the vast majority of sufferers (Leeuw et al., 2007; Picavet, Vlaeyen, & Schouten, 2002; Siegel et al., 2001; Vlaeyen & Linton, 2000). A different evolutionary accident is the more likely culprit, and mindfulness can help us to respond to it effectively.

Fight or Flight

All mammals share an ancient, sophisticated, highly adaptive emergency response often called the *fight-or-flight* system. When a mammal is threat-ened, its sympathetic nervous system and hypothalamic–pituitary–adrenal

---

[1] *Back Sense: A Revolutionary Approach to Halting the Cycle of Chronic Back Pain* (Siegel et al., 2001).

(HPA) axes are activated, resulting in increased epinephrine (adrenaline) in the bloodstream and corresponding physiological changes (Sapolsky, 2004). Respiration, heart rate, body temperature, and muscle tension all increase—the better to fight an enemy or flee from danger.

Let's look at how this process usually works. Imagine that a rabbit grazing in a field spots a fox. It freezes, hoping not to be noticed, while becoming vigilant and physiologically aroused in preparation for running away (rabbits aren't big fighters). If the fox wanders off without seeing the rabbit, soon the rabbit's parasympathetic nervous system becomes active, and its physiology returns to a resting level. This system works wonderfully for rabbits and undoubtedly has contributed to their survival.

Imagine now that the rabbit possessed a highly evolved cerebral cortex like ours, allowing for language and complex symbolic, anticipatory thought. Once the fox left, the rabbit might begin to think: "Will he return? Will he find my family?" Even after the immediate danger has passed, the rabbit could find itself thinking about the fox—not to mention whether it can save up enough carrots for retirement and other concerns. All such thoughts would continue to activate its fight-or-flight system, which would remain stuck in the "on" position.

Though admittedly oversimplified, this is what happens to us. Our capacity for symbolic, anticipatory thought, although extraordinarily adaptive in allowing us to construct complex civilizations, is ill suited to coexist with our mammalian fight-or-flight system. Rather than our transition to walking upright, it appears that *this* evolutionary accident is responsible for the epidemic of chronic back pain as well as a host of other psychophysiological disorders. Virtually every physiological change brought about by the fight-or-flight system can cause or exacerbate a stress-related symptom if the system remains continuously active. As we will see, mindfulness practice can be very salutary, interrupting this overactivation of our emergency response system.

The likelihood that stress-related symptoms will become chronic is increased dramatically if we misinterpret these symptoms when they arise. Before we introduce mindfulness practice into treatment, it is therefore important that patients be well grounded in the most accurate possible understanding of what causes their distress.

BAD BACK?

Let's return to the problem of chronic back pain. Most patients, and until recently most health care professionals, have naturally assumed that persistent back pain must be due to damage to the disks or other structures of the spine. After all, if we cut our finger, we see blood and feel pain. We automatically surmise that back pain functions similarly, even if the injury isn't visible to us.

Many research findings question this assumption. They point to a lack of correlation between the condition of the spine and the presence of pain. Education about these findings is a necessary part of effective treatment programs, for the research helps to alleviate patients' concerns (and consequent anxiety) about being damaged or fragile. For example:

- Approximately two-thirds of people who have never suffered from serious back pain have the same sorts of "abnormal" back structures that are often blamed for chronic back pain (Jensen et al., 1994).
- Many people continue to have pain after "successful" surgical repair. There is little correlation between the mechanical success of repairs and whether or not the patient is still in pain (Fraser, Sandhu, & Gogan, 1995; Tullberg, Grane, & Isacson, 1994).
- People in developing countries who do "backbreaking" labor and use ergonomically primitive furniture and tools have the lowest incidence of chronic back pain—not what we would expect if damage to the spine were the culprit (Volinn, 1997).

Along with this data questioning the assumption that damage to the spine causes chronic back pain, we find many studies implicating psychological factors. For example:

- Psychological stress, and particularly job dissatisfaction, predicts who will develop disabling back pain more reliably than physical measures or the physical demands of one's job (Bigos et al., 1991).
- Patients with back pain show significantly increased muscle tension in their backs when placed in an emotionally stressful situation, whereas other pain patients do not (Flor, Turk, & Birbaumer, 1985).
- Chronic back pain is unusually prevalent among people with trauma histories or who live in stressful situations, such as war zones (Beckham et al., 1997; Linton, 1997; Pecukonis, 1996).

THE CHRONIC BACK PAIN CYCLE

Taken together, these sorts of findings suggest that psychological factors, rather than structural abnormalities, are often the cause of chronic back pain. This occurs through a cycle that has many parallels with the dynamics of anxiety disorders, described in Chapter 9. Its core components are irrational fear, increased psychophysiological arousal, misinterpreted symptoms, and behavioral avoidance. Here is a typical example of how it unfolds:

> Last winter Robert's back started to hurt after shoveling snow. He had experienced pain like this before, which usually resolved within a few days. This time, however, it persisted and began to run down his leg to his feet. Robert began to worry. He had been enjoying working out at the gym to stay in shape and relieve stress. Now he stopped exercising and called his physician.
>
> Robert's doctor heard his report of sciatic (leg) pain and became concerned, suspecting nerve impingement in his spine. A magnetic resonance imaging (MRI) scan indicated a bulging disk, and his doctor suggested that Robert take anti-inflammatory medication and avoid activities that might further dislodge the disk.
>
> Prior to his injury, Robert had been having a difficult time at work—the company wasn't doing well, and his boss had been extremely tense. He felt stressed before his back problem began, but now became even more anxious and agitated. Robert began to fear that he might never get better.

Robert was becoming caught in the *chronic back pain cycle* (Siegel et al., 2001). This cycle can begin with an injury from an accident or overuse, or can seem to appear "out of the blue," without a clear physical precipitant (Hall, McIntosh, Wilson, & Melles, 1998).

Once pain has persisted longer than expected or reached high levels of intensity, fear becomes a factor. Because chronic back pain has become an epidemic in industrialized countries, virtually everyone has had contact with someone who has suffered with it. The prevalence of MRIs, with their ability to reveal random variations in spinal structure in great detail, contributes to fear by presenting patients with images of a decaying spine.

Fear and worry about one's back has several negative effects. Like Robert, most people respond by abandoning physical activities that previously helped to reduce stress and keep their muscles strong and flexible. Distressing thoughts coupled with this inactivity lead to anxiety, frustration, and anger, all of which further arouse the fight-or-flight system. This arousal, in turn, contributes to muscle tightness, at the same time that the muscles are deprived of the natural movement that previously helped to keep them relaxed. A cycle of pain–worry–fear–tension–pain accompanied by disability becomes established.

Fear not only adds to pain by increasing muscle tension, it also actually amplifies the pain sensations themselves. We have known for decades that the experience of pain is not simply proportionate to the degree of disturbance to tissues (McGrath, 1994; Melzack & Wall, 1965; Shankland, 2011). People experience a given stimulus as far more painful if they are frightened than if they feel safe (Beecher, 1946; Burgmer et al., 2011; Robinson & Riley, 1999). Thus, concern about pain contributes to pain cycles not only by tensing muscles, but also by amplifying the sensations of pain that the tight muscles produce. As we will see shortly, mindfulness practice, by altering our attitude toward pain, can help muscles relax and also influence our experience of pain by changing our relationship to it (Brown & Jones, 2010, 2012).

Yet another component of the chronic back pain cycle involves mistaken attributions. Once a person becomes worried about back pain, he or she will struggle to figure out which movements or positions seem to make it better or worse. Once such a relationship is observed, every time the person engages in the activity presumed to be problematic, he or she becomes more anxious and tense. Increased pain usually follows, reinforcing the belief that a given action is hazardous. This conditioned reaction, termed *kinesiophobia* (fear of movement), has been shown to be a better predictor of back pain chronicity and disability than medical diagnosis (Crombez, Vlaeyen, Heuts, & Lysens, 1999; Leeuw et al., 2007; Picavet et al., 2002; Waddell, Newton, Henderson, & Somerville, 1993).

The parallels between the chronic back pain cycle and the anxiety disorders described in Chapter 9 are evident. They all result from overactivity of the fight-or-flight system. They also all involve future-oriented maladaptive fear responses, experiential avoidance, and false assumptions about the nature of the problem. Mindfulness can help to counteract these processes by increasing tolerance of discomfort and decreasing identification with worrisome thoughts.

THE RECOVERY CYCLE

Recovery from the syndrome requires interrupting the pain cycle. This process involves three basic elements, all of which can be supported by mindfulness practice: (1) *cognitive restructuring*, (2) *resuming full physical activity*, and (3) *working with negative emotions*. Interventions can be individually tailored, placing more or less emphasis on each element, depending on which aspects of the pain cycle are most salient for a given patient.

Before beginning treatment, all patients should undergo a thorough physical examination to rule out rare but potentially serious medical causes for their pain. These disorders, which include tumors, infections, injuries, and unusual structural abnormalities, are now long established to be the cause of only a very small percentage of chronic back pain cases (Bigos et al., 1994; Chou et al., 2007; Deyo, Rainville, & Kent, 1992). A physical evaluation is needed to avoid overlooking a treatable medical disorder, to facilitate cognitive restructuring, and to grant trustworthy permission to resume activity.

Mindfulness and Cognitive Restructuring

As long as patients believe that their pain is due to structural damage in the spine, they react to it with fear and avoid activity associated with the pain, thus perpetuating the pain cycle. Because the pain can be intense, it is often difficult at first for most patients (and many clinicians) to believe that muscle tension could actually be causing it.

Patients can be presented with key research studies questioning the connection between back pain and structural damage, followed by an explanation of how the chronic back pain cycle functions. This is particularly necessary before patients will embrace a mental exercise such as mindfulness to treat a seemingly physical problem. Many patients are concerned that our addressing psychological factors means that we think that their pain is imagined, or "all in my head." They may also fear being accused of malingering. Clinicians need to emphasize that the pain is caused by changes in the body and is, in every way, real.

Once patients have learned about the chronic back pain cycle, basic mindfulness practices (see Chapters 1 and 7) can be introduced to help interrupt it by increasing pain tolerance, reducing aversion reactions, disentangling from negative thoughts, and facilitating work with difficult emotions. Although the effect is gradual, mindfulness practice can increase the cognitive flexibility that is needed throughout treatment. By observing the arising and passing of thoughts without following or judging them, patients become less identified with their content. Patients can also see that thought is socially influenced—they notice that their mind is full of ideas picked up from doctors, friends, and others. They come to observe that it is not events themselves, but our interpretation of events, that determines our reactions. Direct *experience* of this truism helps pain patients entertain the idea that assumptions about structural damage, and even medical diagnoses, are changeable constructs, not objective conclusions about reality.

Mindfulness practice also supports the ability to observe the interplay among pain, fear, and behavior in one's own experience. Most of the time patients are unaware of the role that thoughts and emotions play in their pain. With mindfulness practice, this awareness can be heightened.

> Cathy had been suffering with back pain for years. Despite the fact that doctors had never found anything more than a mild disk bulge, she was sure that she had a "bad back" and was in constant danger of reinjuring herself. She avoided sitting for more than a few minutes, convinced that her body couldn't tolerate the pressure this put on her spine.
>
> Mindfulness practice was easy at first. She began lying down, was able to follow her breath, and dealt well with the challenges of a busy mind. The practice became difficult, however, when she tried it in a chair. Cathy noticed that her attention was constantly moving toward her lower back, monitoring it for pain. She wanted to get up as soon as she experienced a twinge. Cathy also began to see that her urge to change position was motivated more by fear than by the intensity of pain itself. She saw her mind "budget" her chair time, thinking that if she already hurt after 5 minutes, she'd never be able to sit for 20. She saw a kaleidoscope of fearful thoughts appear, followed by anxiety, increased muscle tension, and more pain.

This use of mindfulness can dovetail well with cognitive-behavioral self-monitoring. For example, I sometimes ask patients to keep a pad with them and make a mark each time they notice themselves having an anxious thought about their back. Most people abandon the exercise after a few hours, as they realize that they're constantly having such thoughts. Patients can also be asked to complete inventories such as the Beliefs about Pain questionnaire[2] (Siegel et al., 2001), the Tampa Scale of Kinesiophobia (Kori et al., 1990), or the Fear-Avoidance Beliefs Questionnaire (Waddell et al., 1993), which help them to notice hitherto unacknowledged assumptions about their condition. These interventions work well with mindfulness practice to increase awareness of negative emotions and cognitions, thereby making the mechanism of the chronic back pain cycle more plausible.

---

[2]This and other Back Sense inventories can be obtained without charge from *www.backsense.org.*

Using Mindfulness to Resume Activity

The second step of the recovery process, *resuming full physical activity*, serves many functions. It is an exposure and response prevention treatment for kinesiophobia and fears of disability. Instead of avoiding activity in response to fear, the patient enters into activity and attempts to open to, or befriend, the fear that results (see Chapter 9). It is also a physical exercise for muscles that have become short and weak, as well as a means of reducing psychological stress.

Patients are asked to create a hierarchy of activities they've abandoned, rating each activity as *pleasant, neutral,* or *unpleasant,* and *easy, moderate,* or *difficult* to resume, using the Lost Activities Inventory (Siegel et al., 2001). They are instructed to begin with those activities that they imagine would be the most enjoyable and the least difficult or frightening to pursue. This selection is designed to make the process self-reinforcing and to keep anxiety at a tolerable level.

When patients initially resume relinquished activities, their pain usually increases. This is both because tight, weak muscles are painful to use at first and because of the increased anxiety that results from challenging a phobia. Mindfulness practice can help patients move through this difficult step.

Pain Does Not Equal Suffering

There is a famous talk attributed to the Buddha, often called the *story of the two arrows* (or two darts), in which he describes our typical response to pain:

> When touched with a feeling of pain, the uninstructed run-of-the-mill person sorrows, grieves, and laments, beats his breast, becomes distraught. So he feels two pains, physical and mental. Just as if they were to shoot a man with an arrow and, right afterward, were to shoot him with another one, so that he would feel the pains of two arrows. (Bhikkhu, 2012c, p. 1)

This ancient realization—that the experience of pain is followed immediately by a response of aversion and suffering—is readily observed in mindfulness practice. One of my patients expressed it in a succinct mathematical formula: *pain × resistance = suffering*. This insight, verified in patients' own experience, can allow them to move forward in resuming activity:

> Beth had been disabled several times by excruciating sciatic pain. She had spent thousands of dollars on ergonomic automobile seats,

workstation chairs, and top-of-the-line orthopedic mattresses. Whenever the pain would return, she'd become despondent, desperately trying to identify its source. She hoped that she could keep it at bay if she were sufficiently careful.

Beth's brother was going to be married soon, and she very much wanted to be at the wedding. Unfortunately, she was terrified by the prospect of the plane trip, sure that several hours trapped in an airline seat would cripple her. We decided to use mindfulness practice to help her prepare.

Beth began by sitting in an ordinary chair, following her breath. After about 10 minutes, she was invited to bring her attention to the sensations in her leg. She was asked to observe the sensations as precisely as she could, to notice whether she felt burning, aching, throbbing, or stabbing. Whenever she had a fearful or distracting thought, she was asked to return her attention to the actual sensations in her leg at the present moment.

At first, the sensations increased in intensity, and Beth was frightened. Over the course of 30 minutes, however, she noticed that the sensations actually became variable. They changed in quality as well as intensity. Thoughts of "I can't stand this" and "I hope this isn't going to set me back" arose and passed.

Beth was asked to see if she could notice how her pain was actually made up of a series of separate momentary sensations, like frames in a movie strung together so quickly as to give the illusion of continuity. She was asked to continue noticing the detail, as she might if watching a sunset or listening to a symphony. Often this was difficult because the sensations were quite unpleasant. Nonetheless, Beth was surprised to find that she could stay with the experience and, by the end, actually felt no more uncomfortable than she had at the beginning.

Several impediments to resuming activity are addressed during this sort of mindfulness practice. First, it becomes possible to see that pain sensations themselves are distinct from aversion responses—negative thoughts and feelings about the pain. These aversion responses constitute the experience of suffering (the "second arrow"). This observation can be enormously freeing because it allows a person to tolerate pain, rather than feel compelled to avoid or alleviate it, thereby allowing for a much wider range of activity.

Second, by bringing attention to the present moment, anticipatory anxiety is reduced. It has often been observed that even in terrible situations, our fear is of the future. For example, when people become conscious following a serious automobile crash, their minds race forward, even if they are bleeding or in pain: "Will I be OK?" "Will my loved ones survive?" By bringing attention to the present, the anticipatory anxiety that is at the heart of most pain cycles (Leeuw et al., 2007) is reduced. This reduction in anxiety lowers muscle tension and reduces the perceived intensity of pain.

Third, mindfulness practice helps people to feel "held." When a person is in pain and has no clear options for relief, he or she often becomes quite distraught. Mindfulness practice reduces the catastrophizing that plays a central role in pain and disability (Cassidy, Atherton, Robertson, Walsh, & Gillett, 2012) and gives patients a structured activity that doesn't feed into the spiral of aversion responses, increased pain, and more aversion. Concentration practice is also calming and fortifying, as the present becomes a refuge rather than a threat. Once patients are less frightened of their pain, they are better able to move forward behaviorally and resume abandoned activities.

Patients may need frequent reminders that uninhibited movement is not dangerous and that they can approach pain mindfully. To extinguish conditioned associations between activity and pain, patients should be encouraged to engage in their chosen activity several times weekly for a few weeks before moving onto the next challenge. They are usually able to observe fluctuations in pain level during this period, despite consistency in activity. These fluctuations help them to realize that the activity itself is not the problem.

Working with Intentions

Many patients are far more concerned about disability than pain per se. Mindfulness practice can help them realize that they need not be disabled by their pain sensations—that sensations need not dictate behavior:

> Michelle was a police officer who loved her work. Her back pain began following an automobile accident that totaled her cruiser. Even though her medical findings were unremarkable, she was unable to sit in a chair for more than a few minutes. She had been given an administrative position, but now her post was about to be eliminated, and she either had to return to regular police work or lose her job. As a competent, can-do woman, Michelle hated the thought of becoming an unemployed single mother.
>
> Michelle was willing to accept that her pain was due to muscle tension, but this did little to lessen her misery. She was introduced to simple breath-focused mindfulness practice and took to it readily

at first. She was able to observe her pain sensations and notice their changing quality. As time went on, however, the pain increased and she began squirming in her chair. "I have to get up," she announced, "the pain is too intense." She was asked to try to stay with the sensations in her back for a few more minutes. When her squirming continued to intensify, she was directed to bring her attention to the sense of urgency to get out of the chair—to focus her mind on the intention to get up itself.

After a few moments, Michelle noticed that she could feel the urge to rise as a tightness or pressure in her chest and neck. She was then asked to try to focus her attention on this area and use *urge surfing* to remain seated (Marlatt & Gordon, 1985). She practiced staying with the urge to move—noticing it grow, reach a crescendo, and then diminish—following a wavelike pattern. Her squirming stopped, and she was able to remain sitting and return her attention to the breath.

This experience had a profound effect. Until now, Michelle had not noticed any gap between her sensations of increased pain and her moving to relieve the discomfort. Observing that the *intention* to rise occurs in between and can be worked with like any other sensation significantly increased her sense of freedom. This gave her confidence that by practicing mindfulness, she could learn to sit for extended periods and resume regular police work.

Strength, Flexibility, and Endurance Training

One way to accelerate the extinction of fear responses to normal activity, as well as to accelerate the return of muscular strength and flexibility, is through structured exercise training. Graded weight lifting, stretching, and aerobic exercises can help move patients beyond their fears that they are structurally compromised (Siegel et al., 2001). Once a person can dead lift 25 pounds, he or she is less likely to fear bending to pick up a child's toy or grocery bag. There is mounting evidence that vigorous exercise, even if it initially exacerbates pain, facilitates recovery (Chou et al., 2007; Guzman et al., 2001; Mayer et al., 1987; Rainville, Sobel, Hartigan, Monlux, & Bean, 1997; Schonstein, Kenny, Keating, & Koes, 2003). As mentioned earlier, many mindfulness-oriented treatments for chronic pain have yielded only modest improvements in pain intensity. These programs would probably be more effective if, in addition to teaching mindfulness practice, they also attended systematically to helping participants overcome their fear of movement.

When patients begin to exercise previously neglected muscles, they usually experience increased pain. Rehabilitation programs often fail at this point. As with the resumption of other activities, mindfulness practice can be used to work with the fear and pain that arise when embarking on a structured exercise program. After developing a degree of concentration by following the breath, patients are instructed to bring accepting attention to the pain sensations associated with lifting weights, stretching, or participating in aerobic activity. This builds pain tolerance and reduces the likelihood that increased pain will cause counterproductive muscle tension.

Using Mindfulness to Work with Negative Emotions

For many patients, learning that their pain is not due to structural damage, seeing for themselves how the chronic back pain cycle operates, and resuming full activity are sufficient changes in their understanding and behavior to free them from the disorder. For others, however, a return to normal activity is not enough. These are generally people for whom emotional difficulties—beyond concerns about back pain—are contributing to persistent muscle tension. Often some combination of psychodynamic exploration and social skills training, supported by mindfulness practice, is helpful.

There is evidence that people who have difficulty acknowledging affect suffer disproportionately from psychophysiological disorders (Schwartz, 1990), that being unaware of feelings can interfere with successful rehabilitation (Burns, 2000; Burns et al., 2012), and that learning to identify and safely express emotion can reduce the frequency of symptoms (Pennebaker, Keicolt-Glaser, & Glaser, 1988). When we are unable to acknowledge or tolerate a thought or feeling, our fight-or-flight system reacts to the threat of it emerging much as it reacts to external dangers. Since life experiences continuously trigger disavowed cognitions and affects, our fight-or-flight system is frequently on overdrive. It's thus no surprise that increasing affect awareness can help to free some people from chronic back pain.

By everyone's account, Eddie was a very nice guy—but he hadn't always been. As a boy he was known for being provocative, and he often got into trouble for fighting.

In adolescence, Eddie turned over a new leaf and became an exemplary citizen. Now as an adult, he rarely argued, and was always well mannered. He often felt sad, lonely, or anxious—but never angry.

Not surprisingly, Eddie was very compliant in following his treatment program. He recognized how frightened he had been about his pain, and he systematically resumed activity, wanting to please his therapist.

Eddie was frustrated, though, that his pain persisted. As it became clear that he was unusually inhibited in recognizing and expressing anger, he was encouraged to discuss things that annoyed him. Although he was able to identify some previously disavowed anger in this way, it was during mindfulness practice that his aggression became most apparent to him. He would notice that when angry thoughts arose, he would quickly talk himself out of them.

Eventually, Eddie recalled that he used to be angry a lot, but had made a conscious decision to stop, since it only seemed to cause trouble. As his therapy and mindfulness practice continued, he was increasingly able to notice and acknowledge a fuller range of feeling. His anxiety lessened, and he consequently experienced much less pain.

Mindfulness practice supports such psychodynamic exploration by both bringing previously unnoticed emotions into awareness, and by helping patients to tolerate them. During mindfulness practice, thoughts, feelings, and memories are free to enter the mind, allowing into consciousness affects and cognitions that we might otherwise not notice. As patients see that emotions arise, are experienced, and eventually pass, they become easier to bear.

CONTROL

Mindfulness practice is full of paradoxes. It is often described as a *goalless* activity, since it involves paying attention to whatever is happening in the moment, including the experience of being distracted from paying attention to what is happening in the moment. Shunryu Suzuki (1973), an influential Zen teacher, suggests: "To give your sheep or cow a large, spacious meadow is the way to control him" (p. 31). This paradox is at work in psychophysiological disorders. It can be seen whenever the overactivation of our fight-or-flight system creates an unwanted symptom because the act of *resisting* the symptom further activates our fight-or-flight system. A person struggling with insomnia finds him- or herself more aroused and awake the harder he or she tries to sleep; the man who fights against erectile dysfunction by attempting to control his body goes limp; *trying* to relax usually backfires. Attachment to symptom reduction perpetuates symptoms.

This insight is particularly valuable for resolving psychophysiological disorders. One mindfulness-oriented approach, acceptance and commitment therapy (ACT), illustrates this mechanism through the metaphor of "Chinese handcuffs," the woven straw tubes into which you insert your index fingers, only to find that the more you try to pull them out, the more tightly the tube grips them (Hayes, 2002b). To work effectively with most psychophysiological disorders, patients must learn to differentiate those areas over which they can exert control from those in which it is counterproductive to try. Generally, we can usefully control our behavior, but not our experience. A student of mindfulness can commit to practicing daily for a prescribed period of time, but cannot control whether he or she will feel relaxed or tense, focused or scattered. Similarly, a patient with back pain can commit to systematically increasing his or her range of activity, and can commit to a program of stretching and exercise, but cannot control whether pain will arise.

The idea that it is counterproductive to try to avoid pain is particularly difficult for most patients to grasp. The torrent of messages we receive from advertisements lead us to feel that if only we would purchase the right remedy, we would never experience discomfort. Conventional treatments for pain reinforce this notion by focusing on pain relief. It can therefore be challenging to accept that relinquishing the goal of alleviating pain is essential for recovery, despite increasing evidence that acceptance is more effective than control as a strategy for dealing with pain (Liu, Wang, Chang, Chen, & Si, 2012; Thompson & McCracken, 2011).

Nonetheless, mindfulness practice can help. By observing that suffering comes from our reaction to pain and learning to watch the coming and going of pleasant and unpleasant experiences, patients are able to cultivate an accepting attitude which ultimately can free them from a chronic pain cycle. They gradually learn to treat the pain as though it's out of their control, like the weather.

TAILORING MINDFULNESS

Many variables go into deciding which mindfulness exercises are most suited to which patients. If patients find a particular exercise too challenging, they won't stick with it. Furthermore, some exercises are can actually be harmful to vulnerable individuals.

Trauma Survivors

We saw above how mindfulness practice can support enhanced awareness and tolerance of affects, and thus help to reduce the chronic tension associated with the effort to keep such contents out of awareness. For individuals who habitually repress painful memories or emotions, however, this can become overwhelming. Since trauma survivors are significantly overrepresented among people with chronic back pain and other psychophysiological disorders (Asmundson, Coons, Taylor, & Katz, 2002; Beckham et al., 1997; Pecukonis, 1996; Schofferman, Anderson, Hines, Smith, & Keane, 1993; Schur et al., 2007; Springer, Sheridan, Kuo, & Carnes, 2007; Yaari, Eisenberg, Adler, & Birkhan, 1999), this vulnerability is frequently an issue in treatment. Such patients often become extremely anxious after a few minutes of following their breath, particularly if they are keeping their eyes closed. In these cases, the ratio between the "holding" effects of the practice and its power to reveal disavowed experience is tilted too far toward bringing contents into awareness.

As discussed in Chapter 7, one response to this sensitivity is to use mindfulness exercises that turn the attention toward the outer, rather than the inner, potentially overwhelming world. Walking meditation in which attention is brought to the feeling of the feet touching the ground often works well and is compatible with the goal of increasing physical activity. Similarly, nature meditation, in which the sights and sounds of trees, clouds, birds, and the like are used as objects of awareness, can cultivate a sense of safety. Yoga exercises that can be practiced mindfully are another good alternative because they combine flexibility training with mindfulness in motion.

MECHANISMS OF ACTION

Now that mindfulness practices are being widely used for chronic pain and evidence is mounting for their efficacy, researchers have begun investigating the mechanisms by which these practices might work. Although results are still preliminary, they are intriguing (see also Chapter 15).

One area of investigation measures the level of mindfulness of patients with chronic pain to see how it relates to factors such as physical, social, cognitive, and emotional functioning, as well as to medication use. Although there are many challenges to reliably measuring mindfulness (such as the fact that a person needs some degree of mindfulness to notice if the mind is wandering [Grossman, 2011]), data suggest that higher levels of mindfulness indeed correspond to better functioning, primarily by lessening pain-related anxiety and patterns of avoidance and disability (Cho, Heiby, McCracken, Lee, & Moon, 2010; Schutze, Rees, Preece, & Schutze, 2010).

Another set of studies has investigated how experienced meditators react to experimentally induced pain. The evidence suggests that (1) experienced meditators report that they perceive painful stimuli as less unpleasant than inexperienced controls (Lutz, McFarlin, Perlman, Salomons, & Davidson, 2013), with the extent of meditation experience being inversely correlated to subjects' unpleasantness ratings (Brown & Jones, 2010); (2) experienced meditators report higher tendencies to observe and remain nonreactive to pain sensations than inexperienced controls (Grant & Rainville, 2009); (3) open monitoring (mindfulness per se) results in a significant reduction of pain unpleasantness among experienced meditators, but not novices (Perlman, Salomons, Davidson, & Lutz, 2010); and (4) experienced meditators, but not inexperienced controls, have significant decreases in anticipatory pain anxiety when in a mindful state (Gard et al., 2011). Interestingly, one study found that whereas concentration increased pain intensity for inexperienced controls, it did not do so for more experienced meditators—suggesting that the latter group was able to *be with* painful stimuli without having a strong aversive reaction to it (Grant & Rainville, 2009).

Although these studies suggest that extensive experience with meditation yields the greatest benefit in dealing with pain, there is evidence that training as little as 3 days of 20 minutes per day can significantly reduce pain intensity and pain-related anxiety in response to experimentally induced pain (Zeidan, Gordon, Merchant, & Goolkasian, 2010); that only six mindfulness training sessions can be sufficient to increase pain tolerance significantly (Kingston, Chadwick, Meron, & Skinner, 2007); and that a single 20-minute period of loving-kindness meditation can significantly reduce migraine pain (Tonelli & Wachholtz, 2012).

The central mechanism suggested by all of these studies closely parallels the Buddha's story about the two arrows. It appears that by accepting pain sensations, rather than resisting, fearing, or trying to avoid them, we are able to tolerate greater pain stimulation with less distress, whether the pain is caused by a medical condition or induced in the laboratory (Thompson & McCracken, 2011).

Another exciting line of research examines the brain regions that are activated when subjects adopt different meditative attitudes toward experimentally induced pain. The two components of mindfulness meditation, *focused attention* and *open monitoring* (Lutz, Slagter, Dunne,

& Davidson, 2008), correspond to concentration practice in which we repeatedly return attention to a single object, and mindfulness per se, in which we open and attend to whatever arises in awareness. In this research, open monitoring is understood to be a form of "cognitive disengagement" or letting go of control (Gard et al., 2012). Investigators have found that experienced meditators who were exposed to painful stimuli while practicing open monitoring had decreased activity in the lateral prefrontal cortex (lPFC), an area associated with executive control (Grant, Courtemanche, & Rainville, 2011). The meditators simultaneously had increased activation in the posterior insula (Gard et al., 2011; Grant et al., 2011), which is understood to be involved in interoceptive and sensory processing (Craig, 2009). These findings suggest that mindfulness practice decreases the experience of pain and pain-related anxiety through increased processing of the pain sensations themselves, coupled with cognitive disengagement that involves relinquishing attempts at control. Researchers seem to be observing how, on a neurobiological level, experienced meditators open to pain sensations while letting go of attempts to control them, and consequently experience less distress.

Interestingly, at least one study suggests that inexperienced meditators have different brain activation patterns than experienced meditators. When novice subjects attempted mindfulness meditation in the presence of a painful stimulus, they had an increase in activity in the lPFC, suggesting that they were trying to exert cognitive control over the pain. This strategy didn't work very well, however, and they did not experience the reduced pain unpleasantness or reduced anticipatory anxiety that occurred for experienced mediators (Gard et al., 2011).

OTHER PSYCHOPHYSIOLOGICAL DISORDERS

Processes quite similar to chronic back pain maintain a remarkable number of other psychophysiological disorders. Together, these account for a large percentage of all physician visits. Both mindfulness practice and its associated insights can be effective in treating these conditions.

Other Pain and Muscle Tension Disorders

The same factors that cause and perpetuate chronic back pain are often at work in other muscle and joint disorders. These include symptoms diagnosed as tendonitis, bursitis, bone spurs, plantar fasciitis, temporomandibular joint syndrome, repetitive strain injury, chronic headaches, and fibromyalgia. Although many of these pain syndromes can be caused by structural damage, injury, or disease processes, they are very often caused by muscle tension and/or anxious, vigilant attention to pain sensations (e.g., Bendtsen & Fernandez-de-la-Penas, 2011; Litt, Shafer, & Napolitano, 2004).

The process by which these conditions take root is parallel to the chronic back pain cycle. It may begin with either physical or psychological stress. Once the patient becomes concerned, he or she begins to focus on the painful area and often begins protecting it and abandoning normal activity. Worry and frustration set in, and a pain cycle becomes established.

Treatment for all of these conditions is similar. First a competent medical workup is needed to rule out other causes of the pain. This is followed by psychoeducation, which can be challenging, because patients and health care providers often assume that most of these pain syndromes, like chronic back pain, are caused by structural damage or disease. Next, patients are asked to list their abandoned activities. These are then reintroduced systematically, beginning with those that are pleasurable and minimally frightening. Mindfulness practice is then used to develop tolerance for the associated pain sensations, to increase awareness of disavowed affects, and to facilitate relinquishing the attempt to control symptoms.

Gastrointestinal and Dermatological Disorders

Like muscle tension disorders, these conditions are widely assumed to have a physical disease process at their root. Although some may be caused by infections, tumors, and other physiological processes, numerous cases of gastritis, irritable bowel syndrome, eczema, psoriasis, and related disorders are either caused or exacerbated by psychological stress (Gatchel & Blanchard, 1998). It is therefore not surprising that mindfulness practice has shown promise in their treatment (e.g., *gastrointestinal distress*: Gaylord et al., 2011; Kearney, McDermott, Martinez, & Simpson, 2011; *dermatological condition*: Kabat-Zinn et al., 1998).

All these disorders frequently follow a pattern similar to chronic back pain. The initial symptom may be caused by a physical event, such as an infection, but once patients become preoccupied with their symptoms, their worry causes activation of the fight-or-flight system, which in turn exacerbates or perpetuates the problem. The more diligently a patient pursues medical treatment, the more preoccupied he or she becomes with his or her symptom—and thereby trapped in a vicious cycle. When medical interventions fail to alleviate the problem, the same sorts of psychological interventions we've been discussing are often useful. Effective strategies include psychoeducation, self-monitoring of psychological reaction to symptoms, return to normal behavior, and guidance in working with negative, stress-causing emotions (R. Siegel, 2010).

As with the other disorders, mindfulness practice can be quite useful for developing an accepting, tolerant attitude toward the symptoms, as well as to increase emotional awareness and relax counterproductive attempts at control. Here is a typical example:

> Noah was a 45-year-old successful businessman who came into treatment complaining of a number of gastrointestinal symptoms. One week he would suffer from abdominal bloating and nausea, the next he would be plagued by constipation alternating with diarrhea. None of his numerous medical workups could identify a disease or structural cause for his suffering. He had taken many medications and tried restrictive diets. Each new intervention would appear to show promise, and then fail.
>
> Noah carefully monitored his eating, searching for correlations between what he ate and how he felt. He was always fearful that his symptoms would come at an inopportune moment, interrupting his work or causing embarrassment. Finding a cure for his condition had become the focus of his life.
>
> We started with an explanation of how preoccupation with alleviating symptoms can contribute to psychological stress, which itself can cause symptoms. This was followed by an introduction to mindfulness practice, for the purpose of observing anxious thoughts about his condition, as well as cultivating a nonrejecting attitude toward his symptoms. His catastrophic fears were examined, and he was encouraged to take an emotional inventory—observing which emotions were most difficult for him. He practiced using mindfulness to "be with" his symptoms, emotions, and thoughts without trying to fix them.
>
> Since he was generally action-oriented, this approach was difficult for him at first. Nonetheless, with continued support, Noah was able to see how fruitless his search for a cure had been, and how the search itself had kept him anxiously preoccupied with his gastrointestinal system. Over time he began to eat normally again, letting the symptoms come and go as they would. His discomfort began to abate, and he started to realize that in many areas of his life, an excessive zeal for control was the cause of his suffering.

Sexual Dysfunctions and Insomnia

These conditions also usually involve counterproductive attempts to control psychophysiological arousal. Although the disorders can be caused by a physical disease process or physiological condition, patients and health care providers more readily identify these as having a psychological component, and consequently they need less persuasion to try psychological interventions. A number of mindfulness-based empirically validated psychological treatments have been developed (e.g., *sexual dysfunction*: Brotto et al., 2008; Silverstein et al., 2011; *insomnia*: Gross et al., 2011; Ong et al., 2009; Yook et al., 2008).

Sexual Dysfunction

Initial efforts to treat sexual dysfunction involved psychoanalytic interventions designed to identify neurotic conflicts rooted in early psychosexual development. The field was advanced dramatically by the work of Masters and Johnson (1966; Masters, 1970) and their followers, who have focused on performance anxiety as a major factor (Singer-Kaplan, 1974).

Consider, for example, the treatment of erectile dysfunction. The most effective interventions, prior to the advent of Viagra, Cialis, and similar medications, involved helping patients to stop fighting their symptoms and focus on acceptance. After ruling out possible physical causes, therapists typically help men to understand that it is their very effort to control their erection that is creating the anxiety that interferes with a normal physical response. They then assign couples to engage in foreplay, but with instructions not to proceed to intercourse. "If an erection develops, so be it. If it doesn't, that's OK too." The goal is to attend to the sensations of foreplay in the present moment and relinquish concerns about getting or keeping an erection.

Mindfulness practice is well suited to such treatment—in fact we might view *sensate focus*, the technique pioneered by Masters and Johnson, as mindfulness practice using sensual touch as the object of awareness. By learning to watch mental and physical experiences come and go with acceptance in the present moment, patients learn the art of not controlling their experience. If this is first practiced in formal mindfulness practice, it can generalize nicely to sex therapy exercises.

Insomnia

Insomnia has received a great deal of attention by the medical community, mostly in the form of an ever-expanding offering of pharmaceuticals.

Most nonpharmacological treatments involve some combination of stimulus control therapy, sleep hygiene education, relaxation training, and sleep restriction therapy (Smith & Neubauer, 2003; Taylor & Roane, 2010). Stimulus control therapy, the central intervention of the sleep disorders field (Chessen et al., 1999), involves having the patient reserve the bed for only sleep or sex. This means that if the patient is still awake after 15–20 minutes, he or she is instructed to get out of bed and do something else until sufficiently sleepy to try again.

Most patients report that insomnia follows a pattern similar to sexual dysfunction. Anxiety about not sleeping leads to arousal, which prevents sleep. While some treatment regimens recognize this pattern and even employ paradoxical suggestions to "stay awake," (Shoham-Salomon & Rosenthal, 1987), most interventions focus on the goal of getting to sleep.

Mindfulness-based approaches offer an alternative that many patients find useful. First, medical and other psychiatric disorders are ruled out. Next the dynamics of insomnia are reviewed and the wisdom of giving up the fight against symptoms is explained. Patients are then taught mindfulness practice and invited to try it *instead* of sleeping.

People who practice mindfulness intensively in retreat settings notice an interesting phenomenon—they need less sleep. Mindfulness practice either produces some of the restorative benefits of sleep or makes sleep more efficient, reducing the time we need to be sleeping. Once this is explained to patients, mindfulness practice can be offered as an alternative, lessening concerns about falling asleep.

Patients are invited to practice mindfulness meditation both during the day and in bed at night. Worried thoughts about being tired the next day are allowed to come and go. If the practice brings relaxation that leads to sleep, the patient gets a good night's rest. If not, the practice can nonetheless provide a rejuvenating experience, with the patient feeling far more rested in the morning than if he or she had spent the night fretting. In either case, the struggle with insomnia is relinquished, which generally leads to a more normal sleep pattern.

It is interesting that this approach violates the cardinal rule of stimulus control therapy—reserving the bed only for sleep and sex. Nonetheless, by eliminating the central dynamic of the disorder, mindfulness practice can free many patients from chronic insomnia.

SILVER LININGS

Although few people say that they are glad to have had a psychophysiological disorder, it is not unusual for patients to appreciate the lessons they have learned through their recovery. In retrospect, many people come to understand their symptoms as wakeup calls, signals that their approach to life was in some way out of balance. A surprising number become drawn to regular mindfulness practice and to the philosophical understandings with which it has historically been associated.

As the disorder resolves, patients begin to notice that their suffering stems from trying to control things that are out of their control, and that they can gradually learn to let go. The reality of the impermanence of all things becomes clearer. They may develop an appreciation for experience in the present moment, realizing that this is where life is actually lived. They also gain confidence that they can learn to bear both emotional and physical pain and no longer need to rush to resolve it. Some are so taken by their recovery that they begin to investigate Buddhist or related teachings in depth. Their medical condition becomes a gateway to opening a spiritual dimension in their lives. And when adversity becomes an opportunity for learning and growth, life is enriched immeasurably.

11

Mindfulness, Insight, and Trauma Therapy

John Briere

We are healed of suffering only by experiencing it to the full.
—MARCEL PROUST (1925/2003)

*G*race was emotionally neglected and repeatedly sexually abused as a child. Later, in her 20s, she was involved with a man who also treated her very badly. When he was arrested for molesting a neighborhood girl, she attempted suicide and was briefly hospitalized. Many years of therapy have helped Grace a great deal. Now in her mid-30s, she reports few symptoms of posttraumatic stress, is not suicidal, and no longer takes antidepressant medication.

Referred by her therapist, Grace has been attending classes at a meditation center for about a year, and just finished a mindfulness-based cognitive therapy course. She states:

"Something is happening with the meditation. It's hard to explain, but sometimes when I get the usual hit of how little I've done with my life, or about my weight, I just go 'yeah, yeah . . . talk, talk, talk.' I just let the thoughts go. Maybe you don't always have to fix what's happening in your mind, sometimes you can just let it do what it does, but say 'Hello, mind. You're in the past, poor mind, but this isn't the past right now.' My problems aren't over, but I'm starting to think that maybe I'm not what happened to me, I'm not my thoughts. It's like, 'Hey mind, do whatever. But

I don't have to believe what you're saying, at least not all the time.' "

Over the last several decades, clinicians have developed a number of therapies for the treatment of posttraumatic stress disorder (PTSD) and other trauma-related difficulties. These interventions have considerable merit, and have improved the lives of many thousands of trauma survivors. However, the field is still evolving, and new, potentially even more helpful approaches will no doubt continue to emerge. After a brief introduction to trauma and trauma-related outcomes, this chapter describes a recent mindfulness-oriented approach in which the ideas and methods of Buddhist psychology are integrated with modern treatment models to assist those who seek help for trauma-related distress.

TRAUMA AND ITS EFFECTS

Trauma is usually defined as an event involving actual or threatened death, serious injury, or some other threat to physical integrity (American Psychiatric Association, 2013). Examples of such traumas include rapes, disasters, torture, physical assaults, and serious motor vehicle accidents. Memories of such traumatic events—as well as their associated emotions, cognitions, and sensations—can be quickly encoded in the brain and then triggered and relived at later points in time as symptoms of posttraumatic stress disorder (PTSD), in the form of flashbacks, intrusive thoughts, nightmares, and, indirectly, hyperarousal (Yehuda, 1998). These phenomena, in turn, can motivate cognitive, emotional, and behavioral avoidance responses that are themselves problematic.

In addition to PTSD, there are more complex effects of trauma, ranging from severe depression and anxiety to substance abuse, dissociation, relationship problems, suicidality, identity disturbance, and difficulties in regulating emotional states (Briere, 2004; Courtois & Ford, 2013). In addition, some trauma impacts are more obviously existential (Nader, 2006; Shay, 1995; Thompson & Walsh, 2010). A war veteran, torture victim, or sexual abuse survivor, for example, may emerge from successful treatment for PTSD and yet still suffer from a profound loss of meaning in life, fears about death, a sense of spiritual disconnection, alienation from others, or a worldview that no longer includes expectations of goodness, fairness, or justice.

This range of trauma responses, unfortunately, has not yet been met with an equivalent array of effective interventions. Although, for example, cognitive-behavioral therapy (CBT) has demonstrated efficacy in the treatment of PTSD (Cahill, Rothbaum, Resick, & Follette, 2009; Hembree & Foa, 2003), a substantial minority of clients do not experience significant improvement following treatment with this approach (Kar, 2011; Schottenbauer, Glass, Arnkoff, Tendick, & Gray, 2008). Similarly, more complex trauma effects can be resistant to traditional psychological interventions (Courtois & Ford, 2013), and the existential effects of adverse experience are rarely addressed by empirically informed treatments.

Fortunately, recent research and clinical practice indicate that there may be additional pathways to the resolution of psychological symptoms and distress, including those associated with trauma. One of the most studied of these is mindfulness. The possibility that a 2,500-year-old spiritual practice might assist in the treatment of present-day trauma survivors is intriguing, especially if this methodology does not just replicate the mode of action of existing treatments, but works in different ways and provides additional benefits. Before we can consider this approach, however, it is important to examine its antithesis—which turns out to be one of the most problematic aspects of posttraumatic disturbance.

AVOIDANCE AND THE PAIN PARADOX

When confronted with emotional pain, it is a common human response to avoid—to withdraw from the environment, numb or distract oneself, or suppress awareness, so that distress is not overwhelming. In fact, cognitive, behavioral, and emotional avoidance responses are hallmarks of PTSD (American Psychiatric Association, 2013). Yet, as it turns out, such activities may actually prolong, if not intensify, psychological distress. For example, trauma survivors who use drugs or alcohol, dissociate, externalize, or engage in denial or suppression of upsetting thoughts are more likely to develop intrusive and chronic posttraumatic problems and syndromes (e.g., Briere, Scott, & Weathers, 2005; Cioffi & Holloway 1993; Gold & Wegner, 1995; Morina, 2007; Pietrzak, Goldstein, Southwick, & Grant, 2011), seemingly because avoided material cannot be processed and resolved. As one Zen teacher and psychologist notes, more broadly, "What we cannot hold, we cannot process. What we cannot process, we cannot transform. What we cannot transform haunts us" (Bobrow, 2007, p. 16).

This tendency to inadvertently engage in pain-sustaining behaviors while trying to, in fact, avoid painful or upsetting internal states can be referred to as the *pain paradox* (Briere & Scott, 2012). In an effort to remediate distress and suffering, we may do things that specifically increase, not decrease, unwanted thoughts and feelings and even make them more chronic.

There are multiple reasons why people avoid unpleasant/painful stimuli. Some do so because they are overwhelmed by the intensity of the trauma they are experiencing, which may exceed their psychological or neurobiological tolerance for distress (Briere, 2002). In such situations, the trauma survivor is motivated to avoid posttraumatic thoughts or feelings in order to maintain internal equilibrium. For example, a homeless person or someone caught in prostitution may abuse alcohol or heroin or dissociate as a way to numb overwhelming emotional pain. Another person may use denial or thought suppression in an attempt to reduce the anxiety associated with awareness of fear-producing thoughts or memories.

Other aspects of avoidance are seemingly more cultural in etiology, reflecting socialization to deal with emotional pain and uncomfortable states through behaviors that distract, suppress, or numb. For example, people in North American society whose pain or suffering extends beyond some arbitrary period of time may be told by others to "just get over it," "put your past behind you," or "move on." Media advertisements often promote pain relievers or other medications to remedy simple discomfort, and encourage the acquisition of things as a way to feel better or address self-perceived inadequacies or dissatisfaction. Despite the conclusions of Western (and, as we will see, Buddhist) psychology, the social message is often that pain, distress, and dissatisfaction are bad things that should be removed, medicated, or otherwise avoided. The implication is that once one has done things to stop feeling bad, one will, by definition, feel good.

However, the opposite often proves true. In general, those who are able to more directly experience distress—whether through what we refer to as *mindfulness* or in response to psychotherapy, therapeutic exposure, or other ways of accessing and "sitting with" traumatic memory—are more likely to experience reduced distress over time (Foa, Huppert, & Cahill, 2006; Hayes, Strosahl, & Wilson, 2011; Kimbrough, Magyari, Langenberg, Chesney, & Berman, 2010; Thompson & Waltz, 2007). Various theoretical models suggest that direct engagement of psychological pain that is not overwhelming allows the psyche to desensitize and cognitively accommodate traumatic or upsetting material, until it no longer needs to intrude on consciousness (Briere, 2002; Horowitz, 1978; Rothbaum & Davis, 2003).

Thus, the pain paradox ultimately means that when in distress, to the extent possible, we should consider doing the exact opposite of what we or society may want us to do: Directly feel painful states and/or think painful thoughts, and avoid, in a sense, avoidance. As we will see, the Zen notion of "inviting your fear to tea" is critical to both Buddhist and some Western approaches to trauma treatment. To the degree that the trauma survivor can learn to apply full and focused attention to the products of consciousness, regardless of their emotional valence, he or she seemingly engages the polar opposite of psychological avoidance. In Buddhist psychology, this activity is referred to as *mindfulness*.

MINDFULNESS

Mindfulness can be defined as the learned capacity to maintain ongoing awareness of, and openness to, current experience, including internal mental phenomena and impinging aspects of the external world, without judgment and with acceptance (see Chapter 1). The ability to attend to the present moment and view oneself, one's internal experience, and others nonjudgmentally—as opposed to being preoccupied with negative aspects of the past or worry about the future—is thought to powerfully decrease psychological suffering (Kabat-Zinn, 2003).

A rapidly growing number of clinicians have integrated mindfulness into their therapies, both cognitive-behavioral (e.g., Hayes, Strosahl, et al., 2011; Segal et al., 2002) and psychodynamic (e.g., Bobrow, 2010; Epstein, 2008). In fact, even when mindfulness is not specifically employed, other aspects of Buddhist psychology or practice (e.g., compassion, metacognitive awareness, and appreciation of dependent origination, described later in this chapter) are likely to be helpful in work with traumatized people (Briere, 2012a; Germer & Siegel, 2012; Gilbert, 2009a).

Mindfulness Research

A number of different mindfulness-informed interventions have been developed over the last several decades. These include acceptance and commitment therapy (ACT; Hayes, Strosahl, et al., 2011), dialectical behavior therapy (DBT; Linehan, 1993a), mindfulness-based cognitive therapy (MBCT; Segal et al., 2002), mindfulness-based relapse prevention (MBRP; Bowen, Chawla, & Marlatt, 2011; Marlatt & Gordon, 1985), and mindfulness-based stress reduction (MBSR; Kabat-Zinn,

1982). One or more of these interventions have been shown to significantly reduce a wide variety of potentially trauma-related symptoms and disorders, including anxiety, panic, depression, substance abuse, eating disorders, suicidality, self-injurious behavior, low self-esteem, aggression, chronic pain, and borderline personality disorder (see reviews by Baer, 2003; Coelho, Canter, & Ernst, 2007; Grossman et al., 2004; Hofmann et al., 2010; Lynch, Trost, Salsman, & Linehan, 2007; and Chapter 1).

Surprisingly, there are relatively few empirical studies of mindfulness interventions for trauma survivors per se, nor much focus on PTSD, despite considerable theoretical discussion in the literature (e.g., Follette, Palm, & Hall, 2004; Follette & Vijay, 2009; Germer, 2005b; Orsillo & Batten, 2005; Vujanovic, Niles, Pietrefesa, Schmertz, & Potter, 2011; Wagner & Linehan, 2006; Walser & Westrup, 2007). This is beginning to change, however, as several mindfulness interventions have been developed for child abuse survivors (e.g., Kimbrough et al., 2010; Steil, Dyer, Priebe, Kleindienst, & Bohus, 2011), and meditation has been shown to reduce posttraumatic stress in combat veterans (Rosenthal, Grosswald, Ross, & Rosenthal, 2011). Apropos of this, the National Center for PTSD, of the U.S. Department of Veteran Affairs (2011) website notes that "research findings show that mindfulness can help with problems and symptoms often experienced by survivors. Mindfulness could be used by itself or together with standard treatments proven effective for PTSD" (*www.ptsd.va.gov/public/pages/mindful-ptsd.asp*).

INTERVENTION

By combining mindfulness research, Buddhist psychology, and modern perspectives on traumatic stress and avoidance, it may be possible to construct a hybrid of these perspectives and technologies that can be useful in the treatment of traumatized people. Both Buddhist and Western psychologies acknowledge that pain, illness, and death are unavoidable, but they also agree that (1) cognitive variables (e.g., excessive need for control, inaccurate expectations, or negative attributions) may increase trauma effects; (2) avoidance of distress may prolong and even intensify psychological suffering, whereas (3) greater awareness promotes processing and integration; and (4) greater insight into the basis for subjective/distorted reactions to adversity may decrease those reactions (Briere & Scott, 2012).

Most existing psychological treatments for trauma-related difficulties rely, to some extent, on the notion of disorder and treatment of disorder. However, there may be additional paths to well-being following adverse experience—those that not only provide relief from psychological pain, but also increase the survivor's awareness and acceptance of his or her experience and facilitate his or her understanding of certain realities of life and existence. To the extent that we can access such approaches, we may be able to do more than support "recovery" from traumatic events—that is, solely a return to one's general state before the trauma happened—with relatively little attention to contributory factors and dispositions that may already have been in place. A broader approach suggests, in addition, goals of growth, awareness, and capacity—moving, in some ways, beyond survival.

Mindfulness Training

Although the mindfulness-based interventions listed in this chapter have been shown to be helpful for symptoms and problems related to trauma, they have a serious limitation: with the exception of ACT and, to some extent, DBT, they are not conducted in the context of individual psychotherapy, which is a central modality in work with many seriously impacted trauma survivors (Pearlman & Courtois, 2005). Empirically based mindfulness interventions usually occur in group settings and tend to be nonclinically oriented, focusing more on the development of skills (e.g., mindfulness and the capacity to meditate) than on individual psychological symptoms, per se (Baer, 2003). This is entirely appropriate; skill development groups such as MBSR or MBCT can be very helpful adjuncts in work with traumatized persons.

At the same time, it is unlikely that a person suffering from some combination of the issues and problems described in this chapter would have the majority of his or her clinical needs addressed by a mindfulness-based group or a meditation practice alone. Perhaps most importantly, as indicated by the treatment outcome literature described later in this chapter, the therapeutic relationship—and the attuned, positive attention of the therapist toward the client—serve important functions in trauma therapy that cannot be replicated in a skills-oriented group intervention. Finally, because mindfulness is often best learned through meditation, which can be contraindicated for a minority of trauma survivors, the potential impacts of the client's trauma history should be taken into account and monitored on an individual basis so that the survivor is not adversely affected.

In this context, Catherine Scott and I (Briere & Scott, 2012) suggest a hybrid approach, outlined below.

- *Screen for the appropriateness of formal meditation training.* Experience suggests that some clients who are subject to intrusive thoughts, flashbacks, rumination, or easily triggered trauma memories are at greater risk of experiencing distress when meditating (Shapiro, 1992; Williams & Swales, 2004; see also Chapter 7), probably because meditation and mindfulness reduce experiential avoidance and provide greater exposure to internal experience, including memories and painful emotional states (Baer, 2003; Hayes, Strosahl, et al., 2011; Treanor, 2011). Furthermore, some trauma survivors suffer from reduced affect regulation/tolerance capacities (Briere, Hodges, & Godbout, 2010; van der Kolk et al., 1996), meaning that they may be more likely to be overwhelmed by the sensory and emotional material that can arise during meditation. More obviously, those experiencing psychosis, severe depression, a dissociative disorder, mania, substance addiction, suicidal thoughts, or proneness to relaxation-induced anxiety (Braith, McCullough, & Bush, 1988) generally should avoid meditation-based mindfulness training until these symptoms or conditions are resolved or improved.

Given these concerns, we recommend that those individuals considering formal meditation practice in the context of traumatic stress be assessed for contraindications beforehand. In most cases, there will not be any psychological impediment to undergoing meditation/mindfulness training, and multiple benefits may accrue. In the remaining instances, the issue may be less that the individual cannot ever attempt meditation, but rather that it is attempted only when he or she is more stable or less debilitated.

It is also possible—although not empirically evaluated to date—that some forms of contemplative activity are less activating for trauma survivors than formal mindfulness training; for example, loving-kindness meditation (Salzberg, 1995) or yoga (Yoga for Anxiety and Depression, 2009). For this reason, some trauma survivors may choose to begin with such practices before, or in lieu of, classic mindfulness training.

- *Refer those who have been screened to a mindfulness training group or a qualified meditation training center.* This recommendation might be questioned by some of those who are qualified both in psychotherapy and mindfulness training. However, extensive mindfulness training during psychotherapy sessions can be relatively inefficient in the average case; such skills development usually requires a significant investment of time, thereby reducing the availability of potentially more-needed trauma-focused interventions. Also, qualified meditation teachers typically have devoted years of training and experience to acquiring meditation and mindfulness skills, as well as knowledge of how to teach them to others—a background that may not be available to the average clinician, regardless of his or her own meditation practice.

In some circumstances, however, the clinician may be sufficiently experienced that he or she can teach mindfulness and conduct therapy simultaneously (e.g., see Brach [2012b]; Siegel [in press]). Even when this is true, the therapist should carefully consider what the traumatized client needs most at what specific point in treatment. For example, is meditation training the best option at a given moment in time, or does the client more immediately require additional affect regulation training, cognitive interventions, or titrated therapeutic exposure? This is not always an all-or-none scenario, of course. The trained clinician may introduce elementary meditation instruction or mindfulness exercises, but perhaps not spend an inordinate amount of time doing so, and/or may respond to client inquiries or interactions with a therapeutic style that is informed by a mindful perspective (see Chapter 1), while not necessarily teaching mindfulness directly.

Although the clinician may not be the client's primary meditation teacher, his or her personal experience with meditation and mindfulness nevertheless are important. When the client is simultaneously attending psychotherapy and mindfulness training, the meditation-experienced therapist can monitor and inform the process, helping the client to understand and integrate what he or she is learning and experiencing in both domains, while continuing to assess the appropriateness of formal or informal practice over time.

In general, candidates for mindfulness training should be provided with a description of this approach and information on its potential relevance to trauma-related problems or symptoms. A brief *Note to the Trauma Survivor* is included at the end of this chapter, which can be given to those clients for whom mindfulness training is appropriate.

• *As the client gains meditation and mindfulness skills, these capacities can be called upon during trauma-focused psychotherapy.* Minimally, this aspect of treatment may involve the following:

The use of settling skills learned in meditation. The client who is able to decrease his or her anxiety or hyperarousal through mindfulness practices—for example, by attending to his or her breath and engaging the here and now—can use these skills to downregulate distress when encountering painful memories or triggers of upsetting emotions. Similarly, mindfulness skills involving the ability to "let go" of intrusive or persistent mental content may be helpful for the client who is prone to repetitive or sustained negative cognitive–emotional states (Segal et al., 2002). As noted below for metacognitive awareness, settling skills represent a form of affect regulation and may be especially helpful for those easily overwhelmed by anxiety, depression, or anger (e.g., Linehan, 1993a).

Therapeutic exposure. Multiple writers (e.g., Baer, 2003; Germer, 2005b; Kabat-Zinn, 2003; Treanor, 2011) note that the decreased avoidance associated with mindfulness can expose the individual to emotionally laden memories in the context of a relatively settled state and a less-involved, nonjudgmental cognitive perspective—a process that is likely to desensitize and countercondition such material and decrease its power to produce distress (Briere, 2012a). In the therapy session, this process may be engaged by asking the client to recall traumatic events and to feel the attendant emotions, while intentionally engaging as mindful a perspective as possible (Briere & Scott, 2012).[1] To the extent that the client can experience traumatic memories with less judgment and more acceptance, their effects are less likely to be exacerbated or compounded by catastrophizing, shaming, or guilt-related cognitions, thereby decreasing their emotional impact. Less disturbing memories, in turn, require less avoidance and therefore increase exposure and psychological processing.

Metacognitive awareness. During therapy, the client may be invited to consider his or her trauma-related thoughts and perceptions from a metacognitive (Segal et al., 2002) perspective, viewing them as "just" memories or products of the mind that are not necessarily real in the current context. For example, the client may utilize a metacognitive perspective when undergoing flashbacks, or when in the grips of especially shaming cognitions, seeing them as merely transient trauma-related phenomena. This

---

[1] Although intentional processing of trauma and simultaneous maintenance of mindfulness may be somewhat contradictory endeavors (Semple, personal communication, November 3, 2011), induction of mindfulness-like states (including being a nonjudgmental participant–observer of one's own internal experiences) during memory processing is possible in many cases and appears to be helpful in decreasing the power of activated trauma-related emotions.

ability to observe one's thoughts—without necessarily identifying with them—increases the client's affect regulation capacity. For example, as he or she reinterprets intrusive cognitions as merely historic phenomena stored in memory, there may be less to be afraid of or angry about. And as the survivor comes to view triggered thoughts and memories as "old tapes" or "just trauma talking," avoidance strategies such as self-injury, substance abuse, or aggression may become less necessary (Briere & Lanktree, 2011).

Urge surfing is another form of metacognitive awareness found in MBRP (Bowen et al., 2011; Marlatt & Gordon, 1985). In this approach, the client learns to apply mindfulness skills to sudden, often trauma-related, cravings or urges to engage in substance abuse or tension-reduction activities. The survivor is encouraged to view the need to engage in such behaviors as similar to riding a wave: the need starts small, builds in size, peaks (often within minutes), and then falls away. If the client can experience triggered feelings as temporary intrusions of history that can be ridden like a surfboard—neither fought against nor acted upon—he or she may be able to avoid problematic behavior, whether taking a drink, using a drug, bingeing or purging, or engaging in self-mutilation.

FOSTERING EXISTENTIAL INSIGHT

It is not just the scientific literature on mindfulness that suggests a possible role for Buddhist psychology in modern trauma treatment. Also helpful may be what Buddhists call *wisdom* (Germer & Siegel, 2012), or, from a more secular perspective, *existential insight*. Existential perspectives are not always easily incorporated into a discussion meant for academically trained clinicians. For this reason, I ask the reader's permission to shift gears at this point: to consider what Buddhists refer to as the *dharma*, which is a more philosophical than empirical concept, at least from a Western perspective.

When the Buddha first described the "Four Noble Truths" (Anandajoti, 2010; see also the Appendix), he offered several organizing propositions. One was that life inevitably includes pain, loss, and trauma, because bad things happen, people we love die, and we are both fragile and mortal. These inevitable travails were especially apparent in Buddha's time, when disease was rampant, wars and violence were very common, poverty was a given for the vast majority—many of whom were oppressed by an inflexible caste system—and people, in general, did not live very long.

His second proposition was that pain and deprivation are not necessarily the primary reasons for lasting human distress; instead, suffering can arise when adverse events challenge one's investment in things that cannot last or never were true, and we respond with resistance when acceptance would be more helpful. The Buddha did not deny that the pain or loss hurts, but he contended that sustained states such as anxiety, depression, anger, frustration, obsession, or jealousy are often due to something more than pain. He maintained that suffering occurs when people's inaccurate expectations and emotional investments keep them from accepting the transient and ever-changing nature of things. For example, although a heart attack may involve great pain, it also may powerfully challenge false beliefs and expectations about personal immortality and—perhaps later, during recuperation—assumptions about autonomy, financial security, life trajectory, and the notion of life without pain or illness. These latter challenges, and struggles against them, may be at least as devastating as the pain and terror associated with a physically injured heart.

Thus, there typically are two sources of distress associated with any given traumatic experience: (1) the event itself and the pain it produces (including posttraumatic stress) and (2) the suffering associated with attempts to maintain previous models of self, others, and the basis for happiness in the face of intruding reality. In this regard, an early Buddhist teaching offers the parable of a person shot with two arrows in succession (Bhikkhu, 1997). The first arrow is the objective pain felt when encountering an adverse event or trauma. The second arrow is the extent to which the pain challenges long and tightly held expectations, needs, attachments, and worldviews, resulting in resistance and leading to more complex states that the Buddha called *suffering* (see also Chapters 10 and 14).

This distinction between immediate trauma-related pain and subsequent suffering has led some to suggest that whereas the first is inevitable, the second is optional. Although encouraging at one level, this notion can suggest that suffering is one's own responsibility—if one didn't "choose" to desire, love, need, or own and didn't resist subsequent loss, there would be no suffering following adverse events. However, it seems likely that all of us are, to some extent, afflicted by the second arrow—it is the human condition to value deeply our connections to others, care about our possessions and plans, and hope for sustained well-being for ourselves and loved ones. The story of the Buddha's second arrow may best counsel us that desires, needs, and expectations have a significant downside—they add to the effects of trauma and loss—not to mention suffering generally. And, yet, this may well be a reasonable tradeoff for most of us. For example, grief represents an interaction between an adverse event (e.g., the sudden death of a loved one) and a natural process (our intrinsic need and caring for certain people); in this context, love can produce great suffering but still may be worth it. Even so, Buddhist psychology can help the grieving individual process his or her loss by addressing second-arrow factors (e.g., guilt, preoccupation with control over uncontrollable events, a need to resist awareness of distress, or nonacceptance of mortality) in order to resolve the trauma of the loss more quickly and completely.

Thus, the wisdom teachings of Buddhist psychology offer significant opportunities for the client to address more directly the second-arrow issues associated with his or her trauma, including inaccurate beliefs and expectations regarding how the world actually works, and resistance to loss of the previous status quo. This process generally occurs as the client explores basic life assumptions in conversations with the clinician, as well as in meditation, during which the individual has a chance to "watch" his or her thoughts and feelings as they inevitably arise and fall away. Revision of unhelpful thoughts and beliefs is, of course, also possible through classic cognitive therapy. In the current instance, however, the material challenged and potentially updated is more existential in nature. Among the second-arrow aspects considered in this context are attachment, impermanence, and dependent origination.

In Buddhist psychology, *attachment* can be defined as the need to hang on to, rely upon, or overly invest in things and people that, ultimately, are impermanent. *Impermanence* refers to the fact that all things, animate and inanimate, are in a state of flux, and that no thing or event lasts forever, including our lives. As noted earlier, in Buddhism the need to hold on to things that do not last, or may not even exist, is thought to create human suffering. As a result, this perspective counsels against preoccupation with possessions or social status as well as rigid ideas, assumptions, or perceptions about oneself or others, since these things and ideas are inevitably unsustainable and unreliable, resulting in eventual crisis, loss, and unhappiness (Bodhi, 2005; see also Chapter 14).

To the extent that trauma therapy and mindfulness training can help the client access the reality of impermanence, two things may happen: (1) the client may initially feel distress associated with reduced belief in immortality or sustained happiness, and yet, eventually, (2) come to terms with such realities so that adverse events lose some of their associated qualities, such as feelings of abandonment, betrayal, crushing disappointment, or overwhelming loss. Although observers of Buddhist discourse often comment on the seeming dismal nature of a perspective that is so concerned with impermanence-related suffering, in actuality, the growing freedom from core false beliefs and other "accidents waiting to happen" can lead to greater emotional stability and acceptance of life as it is, as well as greater appreciation of things in the moment, whether they be the smell of fresh-brewed coffee, the smile of a child, or a rose. Importantly, in many cases the second-arrow suffering of the survivor of trauma has already occurred: He or she is currently experiencing chaos, loss, and crisis, and can gain from opening to existential insights that increase acceptance. In fact, in Buddhist psychology, adversity is often seen as a "good" thing, at least in part, because it provides the opportunity to challenge inaccurate beliefs and grow as a result of more complete awareness and understanding (Chödrön, 2002).

The third existential aspect, *dependent origination*, holds that all things arise from concrete conditions and sustaining causes, which, themselves, arise from other causes and conditions (Bodhi, 2005). In other words, all events occur because of previous events: No event occurs independently or in isolation. The concept of dependent origination suggests that attributions of inherent badness, inadequacy, or even pathology of self or others may be due to insufficient information: If we could know the logic of a given person's (or our own) problematic behavior or painful history, we would be less likely to judge or blame him, her, or ourselves (Briere, 2012b).

In the typical instance, the clinician might encourage the client to explore his or her thoughts, feelings, and reactions associated with a trauma, and provide nondirective opportunities for him or her to consider the "whats" surrounding the event: What did the client believe about life before the trauma? What, exactly, hurts the most now, after the trauma itself has passed? What is he or she resisting that is nevertheless true? What might happen if he or she didn't resist the feelings and thoughts that come and go? What was the first arrow? What is the second? When this process occurs without pressure from the clinician to decide on one version versus another, in the context of noncontingent acceptance and support, the client's detailed analysis may lead to a slow transition (1) from a view of self as weak or pathological to that of someone who is not "bad" because of what happened and whose responses (then and now) may be the logical effects of traumatization and violated expectations; and (2) in some cases of interpersonal victimization, from a view of the perpetrator as intrinsically evil to that of someone whose behavior arose from of his or her own predispositions and adverse history.

Importantly, this second notion does not mean that the client should immediately or necessarily ever "forgive" the perpetrator, especially to the extent that doing so implies that he or she is not entitled to negative feelings and thoughts (Briere, 2012b). In fact, as noted earlier, social or personal pressure to block or avoid unwanted internal states, including anger and desire for revenge, may inhibit the normal psychological processing necessary for recovery. Yet, it is also likely that sustained hatred and resentment are bad for people, whereas being less involved in such states can improve well-being (Dalai Lama & Goleman, 2003).

THE MINDFUL THERAPIST

Not only can it be helpful for the trauma client to increase his or her mindfulness and existential perspective, the clinician's capacities in these areas are also important. A therapist who is able to focus his or her attention on the client in an alert, accepting, and compassionate way will almost inevitably increase the quality of the therapeutic relationship (see Chapter 3; Siegel, 2007). A positive client–therapist relationship, in turn, appears to be the most helpful general component of treatment—often exceeding the effects of specific therapeutic interventions (Lambert & Barley, 2001; Lambert & Okishi, 1997; Martin, Garske, & Davis, 2000). This is certainly true for the trauma survivor in therapy, where a positive relationship can functions as both a minimal requirement and a powerful intervention (Cloitre, Stovall-McClough, Miranda, & Chemtob, 2004; Courtois & Ford, 2013).

Because mindfulness involves the capacity to pay close and nonjudgmental attention to internal and external phenomena, it can assist the clinician in maintaining a significant degree of attunement to the client (see Chapters 3 and 4; Shapiro & Carlson, 2009). In their discussion of the role of therapist mindfulness in the psychotherapeutic relationship, Bruce and colleagues (2010) note that "through mindfulness practice, a psychotherapist comes to increasingly know and befriend himself or herself, fostering his or her ability to know and befriend the patient" (p. 83). Not only does this *befriending* increase the capacity of the therapist to understand the client's ongoing experience, it may help the client to process negative interpersonal schema in the context of caring attention.

When attunement is continuously experienced by the client, especially if the clinician's compassion is also evident, the client may enter a form of relational activation, engaging psychological and neurobiological systems that encourage openness and connection, reduce expectations of interpersonal danger (and therefore defensiveness), and increase well-being (Gilbert, 2009a; Schore, 1994). These positive feelings, elicited in an interpersonal context that otherwise might trigger fear, tend to countercondition relational distress, producing an increased likelihood of trust and interpersonal connection (Briere, 2012a).

The therapist's mindfulness not only allows him or her to foster attunement and compassion toward the client, it also serves as a partial protection from his or her own reactivity during psychotherapy. By facilitating greater awareness of his or her internal processes, mindfulness helps the clinician to better understand the subjective and multidetermined nature of his or her own thoughts, feelings, memories, and reactions—a form of the metacognitive awareness described earlier. As he or she is more able to recognize specific emotional and cognitive responses to the client as potentially triggered phenomena—as opposed to arising solely from the client's actual clinical presentation—the clinician can place them in proper perspective before they result in significant countertransferential behaviors or, potentially, vicarious traumatization.

In this chapter we reviewed research indicating that mindfulness can be beneficial to people suffering from a variety of problems, symptoms, and disorders, many of which are associated with exposure to adverse events. Based on these findings, even in the absence of much equivalent research on PTSD, mindfulness training appears to be a helpful adjunct in the treatment of at least some people who have been traumatized. We also considered ways in which mindfulness may parallel or reflect processes that are well defined in modern trauma therapy. These include the notions that attention to painful internal states is a form of therapeutic exposure; that mindfulness-generated acceptance and metacognitive awareness can be considered forms of cognitive therapy; and that clinician mindfulness increases empathic attunement and compassion and protects against countertransference, much in the way that Rogers (1957), Freud (1912/1961b), and others described.

In other ways, however, mindfulness and other aspects of Buddhist psychology involve phenomena that are not well approximated by modern therapies. More than other approaches, mindfulness emphasizes the value of giving regular, ongoing attention to consciousness and the

products of consciousness, often attained through a methodology (meditation) that requires special training and self-observation skills. A side
effect of such regular practice may be the development of wisdom, or
existential insight, involving a clearer understanding of the transient and
interconnectedness nature of all things, people, and events. Although
sometimes disconcerting at first appraisal, this perspective can lead to
positive outcomes, including equanimity, emotional intelligence, and
compassion for oneself and others. In this way, applications of Buddhist
psychology to Western troubles represent more than psychotechnology;
they are also serve as encouragement to join a way of thinking and being
that is helpful to clients, therapists, and others willing to engage in this
process.

Note to the Trauma Client

Like many other people, if you are reading this, you have experienced
something in your life that hurt you in some major way. Whether it
was an accident, illness, a major loss, or done to you on purpose, this
kind of thing can bring with it a lot of suffering. Luckily, you sought out
therapy; not everyone does that.

You've probably heard of meditation. Maybe you've tried it.
Usually, it involves turning your attention inward, letting yourself watch
yourself without judgment. Sometimes a good way to do that is to
notice your breathing, and just stay with it, feeling yourself breathe in
and out, letting yourself slow down, allowing thoughts to come and go
without labeling them as good or bad. You can learn how to do this
in meditation classes, which are offered in cities throughout North
America and beyond.

Meditation can teach you to settle down, be less reactive,
and consider yourself more kindly. It also can help you to develop
mindfulness—the ability to stay more in the here and now, to be less
affected by your past, and to worry less about the future. A fair amount
of research and experience suggest that mindfulness skills can help
with the effects of trauma. You might ask your therapist about this, or
Google the phrase trauma and mindfulness to learn more.

12

Breaking the Addiction Loop

Judson A. Brewer

> Just as a tree, though cut down, can grow again
> and again if its roots are undamaged and strong, in
> the same way if the roots of craving are not wholly
> uprooted sorrows will come again and again.
> —BUDDHA (*Dhammapada*, in Bhikkhu, 2012d)

Addictions are among the most damaging of human conditions, significantly affecting the mental, physical, and economic health of individuals, families, and their communities. For example, cigarette smoking is the leading cause of preventable morbidity and mortality in the United States, and alcoholism can cost up to 6% of a country's gross domestic product (in the United States, this amounts to $2 every time anyone has a drink). But why are addictions so prevalent? Why can't individuals, who can often clearly see the harm that they are causing to themselves and others, stub out that cigarette or put down the bottle? What gets them and keeps them "hooked," and how can we as therapists help them unhook themselves from their addiction?

AN ADDICTION IS BORN

Before we can help our patients help themselves, both they and we must understand the fundamental underpinnings of the addictive process. Without this basic understanding, we may actually unknowingly

225

perpetuate it. How do addictions start? They often begin with a simple pairing of a drug or behavior with an affective state. For example, a girl goes to a party and has her first drink. When she drinks, she might notice that she feels that she "fits in," gets a "buzz" from the alcohol, and becomes less shy or awkward and more comfortable around others. She has just formed an associative memory, pairing her increased good feelings and decreased unpleasant feelings with drinking alcohol. The next time she's at a party, she will likely remember what happened last time: "Oh, last time I had a drink and felt much better." So she repeats the process by again having a drink, thus reinforcing the associative memory that she had laid down previously. This is positive and negative reinforcement in a nutshell. Basically, positive reinforcement is the addition of an appetitive stimulus to increase a certain behavior or response, and negative reinforcement is the removal of an aversive stimulus to increase a certain response (e.g., someone drinks when they are nervous, and the nervousness goes away). Importantly, the more often this associative learning process gets repeated and reinforced, the more automatic it becomes, until the girl heads straight for the booze at a party without thinking. Over time, she must consume more and more alcohol to get the desired effect because she develops a physical tolerance to alcohol. Eventually, she may consume so much alcohol that she starts blacking out, has debilitating hangovers, and so on. By now, in other challenging circumstances, she likely finds herself thinking, "I'm really stressed out—a beer or glass of wine sounds really good right now." Years later, she wonders how she became addicted to alcohol (see Figure 12.1).

This addictive loop is remarkable for several reasons. First, each link in the loop has been seen in both animal and human studies, suggesting that this process is primitive and therefore often resistant to cognitive manipulation (Nargeot & Simmers, 2011; Treat, Kruschke, Viken, & McFall, 2011). Second, it lines up remarkably well with Buddhist teachings, from which many mindfulness practices are derived, on the nature of stress and suffering and how to alleviate it.

WAS THE BUDDHA AN ADDICTION THERAPIST?

According to the ancient Buddhist teachings, on the night of his enlightenment, the Buddha, having spent countless hours in meditation, was sitting under a tree contemplating the causes of and conditions for the arising of suffering. He realized that suffering is caused by craving (or,

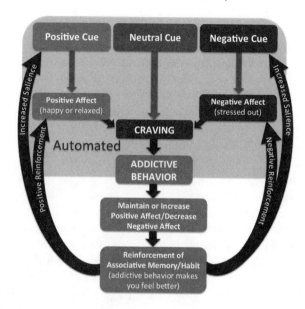

FIGURE 12.1. Associative learning addictive loop. Smoking, drinking, or drug use becomes associated with positive and negative affect through positive and negative reinforcement. Cues that trigger these states (gray arrows) lead to cue-induced craving, furthering this process, which becomes automated over time through repetition. Copyright 2011 by Judson A. Brewer. Reprinted by permission.

literally, *thirst—tanha*, in Pali), and that it was through the "relinquishment, release, and letting go of that very craving" that suffering is cured (Bhikkhu, 2011a, p. 76). These realizations became not only the foundational underpinnings for the teachings known as the Four Noble Truths (see the Appendix), but also the basis for understanding the causal nature of conditioned existence (i.e., that the perception of an experience may not be original to that experience but, instead, may initiate a preconditioned reaction that stems from a process made up of a series of mutually interdependent links that have been connected previously through cause and effect). This is the concept known as *dependent origination*. Simply put, when we come into contact with certain environmental cues (and thoughts are included here), depending on our previous experiences and memories of them, our brains interpret these cues as pleasant, unpleasant, or neutral. If it's pleasant, we want it to continue; if unpleasant, we want it to stop. Craving leads to clinging or attachment to the object, event, or behavior that perpetuates the pleasant state, giving rise to the "birth" of an identity around the object through the laying down of a memory. If the state cannot be sustained (i.e., "death" of the desired state), which is invariably the case, because all of conditioned existence is impermanent, stress and suffering may arise again. Stress feeds back into the cycle, leading to the next round of craving, attachment, and becoming. Not surprisingly, this loop of dependent origination is termed *endless wandering* (in Sanskrit, *samsara*), as there seems to be no clear way out once one is caught up in it (see Figure 12.2).

For example, if Jack smokes a few cigarettes with his friends because they say it is cool, he learns to associate smoking cigarettes with being cool. Over time, smoking just to be cool turns into a physical dependence on nicotine. Then, after several hours of not smoking, Joe's body goes into a withdrawal state and his brain interprets these bodily cues as unpleasant. He wants to feel better, smokes a cigarette, and when the unpleasantness passes, Joe develops a self-identity around smoking (e.g., "When I feel this unpleasantness, I should smoke and I will feel better"). His discomfort fuels the craving that then fuels the (smoking) behavior that further fuels the discomfort, and on and on. Each time he smokes with the intention of alleviating this suffering, he reinforces the cycle.

How to Put Out a Fire

Ancient mindfulness teachings on dependent origination often use the analogy of a burning fire to denote the process of birth and becoming. Interestingly, the Pali term *upadana,* often translated as *attachment,* has

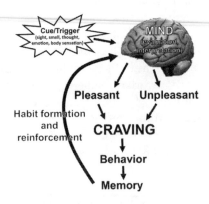

FIGURE 12.2. Early models of addiction: depenedent origination. From Brewer, Bowen, and Chawla (2010). Copyright 2011 by Judson A. Brewer. Adapted by permission.

an alternative translation that fits with the fire analogy: fuel or sustenance (DeGraff, 1993). So, in the case of addictive behaviors, the birth (associative pairing process) of the fire that becomes the addictive behavior is continuously fueled by the dependent origination loop. This point is important to note in relation to mainstay behavioral treatments for addictions, which have been only modestly successful success over the years. This unimpressive track record may be due in part to a failure to target core links in the addictive process, such as craving and clinging/sustenance. Typically these programs focus only on teaching participants to avoid triggering cues or to substitute other activities for smoking, drinking, or taking drugs. Avoidance and substitution likely treat "around" the core addictive loop rather than removing the fuel itself, thus leaving individuals vulnerable to relapse (see Figure 12.3).

So, with this understanding of how addictive processes start and are fueled, how does someone actually put out the fire? The Buddhist

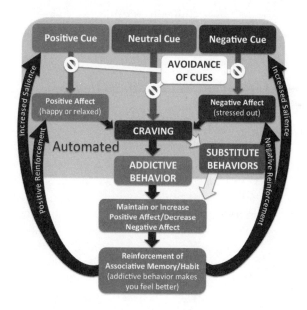

FIGURE 12.3. Limitation of current treatment paradigms in dismantling the addictive loop. Avoidance of cues (white circles) dampens input into the addictive loop (black arrows), whereas substitute behaviors (white arrows) circumvent the targeted addictive behavior. Strategies that teach avoidance of cues or substitute behaviors do not directly dismantle the core addictive loop (black arrows), leaving individuals vulnerable to relapse. Copyright 2011 by Judson A. Brewer. Reprinted by permission.

teachings are surprisingly simple and clear: By bringing mindful awareness to the core components of the addictive loop, an individual can
ride out the unpleasant feelings of craving instead of feeding the fire
by indulging in the addictive behavior. After some time and practice,
the fire burns out on its own, for lack of sustenance. Importantly, this
"bare" mindful awareness is, by definition, free from judgment, which
can often perpetuate an addiction rather than put it out (Bhikkhu,
2011c). For example, if someone uses willpower based on a critical judgment of him- or herself to not smoke (e.g., "I shouldn't do this, it's bad
for my health"), this judgment ("my smoking is *bad*") may work in the
short term, but it can create or foster other negative reinforcement loops,
such as detrimental self-judgments or judgments of others. Additionally,
when cognitive reserves are low, willpower may not prevail, and one
may tumble back into smoking, drinking, or using drugs. Alternatively,
mindfulness training specifically targets the critical links of affect and
craving in the addictive loop and, accordingly, works to extinguish the
associatively learned *process*, ideally putting the flames out for good
rather than just dancing around them (Bhikkhu, 2011a, 2011b; Gunaratana, 2002).

Does Mindfulness Training Really Help People with Their Addictions?

Mindfulness training has been incorporated into various treatments for
addictions. (See, e.g., acceptance and commitment therapy [ACT; Hayes,
Luoma, Bond, Masuda, & Lillis, 2006] and mindfulness-based relapse
prevention [MBRP; Bowen et al., 2009; Brewer et al., 2009].) It has also
been used as an "add-on" for other standard addiction treatments and
has shown preliminary success for treating various substance use disorders, including alcohol, cocaine, opioid, and others. However, up until
2009, only 1 of 22 published studies that included mindfulness training
was randomized, and none tested mindfulness training as a stand-alone
treatment. In the past couple of years, continuing work in this area is
showing promise. For example, an 8-week MBRP program has shown
preliminary efficacy as a next-step treatment for individuals who have
just completed an intensive inpatient or outpatient substance use disorder treatment program (Bowen et al., 2009). Additionally, MBRP has
also been adapted to make it more user-friendly in a standard outpatient
clinical setting. As it is important to "strike while the iron's hot" (bring
individuals into treatment as soon as they express readiness), MBRP has
been divided into two complementary 4-week modules, either of which
individuals can enter after an initial individual introductory session

(Brewer et al., 2009). This method not only cuts down on wait time for individuals wishing to start treatment (because they don't wait around for the beginning of another 8-week program as is standard for many mindfulness-based treatments), but also allows patients to learn from each other, as those who are just entering their first module of the program can learn from other patients who already have 4 weeks of training under their belts and are beginning their second module. This modality has shown preliminary efficacy for cocaine and alcohol dependence (Brewer et al., 2009). Interestingly, individuals who received mindfulness training in this setting showed adaptive physiological changes in their autonomic nervous system output when challenged with a personalized stressful story, suggesting that this training might help them when they need it most, as compared to a control group that received "gold-standard" cognitive-behavioral therapy (CBT) and did not show these adaptive changes.

A larger trial of mindfulness training as a stand-alone treatment for smoking cessation has also shown promising results (Brewer, Mallik, et al., 2011). Individuals who learned mindfulness (vs. the American Lung Association's Freedom from Smoking program—a gold-standard smoking cessation treatment), smoked fewer cigarettes at the end of this 4-week treatment and had significantly greater abstinence rates 4 months later (31 vs. 6%). Importantly, the more home practice the individuals in the mindfulness training group did, the better they fared. The control group also engaged in activities such as relaxation exercises at home as part of their treatment, but this type of practice didn't show any correlations with smoking cessation outcomes.

How do we know what mindfulness training was doing for these folks? Not only did individuals in the smoking study report that they were able to become much more aware of their automated, habitual smoking (one individual reported cutting down from 30 cigarettes/day to < 10 over just 3 days after noticing how habitually he smoked), but their relationship to craving seems to be affected as well. Why is this important? As craving is inherently unpleasant, it naturally drives individuals to act on it. People's brains tell them in a not-so-subtle manner, "This is uncomfortable, do something about it *now*," and the longer the craving goes unsatisfied, the more this unpleasant bodily sensation and the associated self-talk intensifies.

Mindfulness training teaches that instead of running away from unpleasantness by engaging in an addictive behavior, one can learn to accept what is happening right now and, paradoxically, move *into* it to explore what the craving actually feels like in their bodies, no matter how unpleasant it might be at the moment. Through this approach, individuals learn that cravings are inherently impermanent and that their heads don't actually explode if they don't act on them. They learn that indeed they can ride these out, and each time they do so, they gain greater insight, courage, and confidence in the mechanisms of dependent origination: Each time they feed a craving, it strengthens; each time they starve it, it weakens. It really is cause and effect in action. Especially at the beginning, cravings continue to arise (often with a vengeance), but literally sitting with these urges and pausing, instead of immediately reacting, disrupts both the automaticity and the strength of the associative learning loop. In fact, individuals who received mindfulness training for smoking cessation showed this exact pattern. Before treatment, they reported very strong correlations between cravings and the number of cigarettes they smoked, but these correlations had disappeared by the end of treatment, when many still reported cravings, but they were no longer coupled to smoking behavior.

So it seems that mindfulness training may actually work to help people break addictive cycles. And the clues that we have about how it might be acting seem to be directly in line with our modern theories of positive and negative reinforcement in addictions.

Does Mindfulness Training Actually Change Your Brain?

If we are looking to build our muscles, we might follow a regimen of weight training, such as doing a certain number of push-ups, pull-ups, and sit-ups each day. If we practice regularly, we will start to see the effects take hold, as our muscles tone and bulk up, and we are able to lift heavier objects. Our brains perform much the same way: The more we practice a mental task, the better we get at it, whether it is doing crossword puzzles or learning to read. Is this also true for meditation? Does mindfulness training actually change the brain?

A number of scientific studies have documented various different ways that mindfulness training improves our mental capacities, ranging from improved attentional focus, to decreased mind wandering, to improved emotion regulation. And with these findings, scientists have also shown that brain activity patterns, and even size, can change with meditation practice (for a good review on the subject, see Hölzel, Lazar, et al., 2011 and Chapter 15). For example, we compared brain activation patterns in experienced meditators (> 10,000 hours of reported meditation practice) to novices who had just learned how to meditate that morning (Brewer, Worhunsky, et al., 2011). Interestingly, we found that experienced meditators were much better at decreasing brain activity in the parts of the brain associated with mind wandering and self-referential processing during meditation (e.g.. worrying about how something will affect *me*). And it didn't matter what type of meditation they did—whether it was paying attention to their breath, wishing others well (loving-kindness), or just paying attention to whatever arose in their awareness—they still deactivated these regions. This result was nice to see, as it suggested that mindfulness training was doing what it set out to do: train the mind to pay attention to the present in a non-self-referential way. When we looked a little more deeply, we also found that the mind-wandering self-referential centers of the brain (which have been dubbed the *default mode* because we spend so much time activating them in regular daily life) were talking to different brain regions in experienced meditators, compared to novices. What were these other regions? Two prominent ones, called the dorsal anterior cingulate and the dorsolateral prefrontal cortex, have been implicated in self-monitoring and cognitive control, respectively. Putting all of this together, it is possible that experienced meditators may be constantly "on the lookout" for "self" (via the dorsal anterior cingulate), and when the self emerges (via mind wandering or thinking about oneself), their brains tell them to get back on task (via the dorsolateral prefrontal cortex), which is to pay attention to the present moment. This makes sense, as it is the intent of the training. Surprisingly, we found this pattern not only during meditation in experienced practitioners, but when they were just lying in the scanner, not doing anything in particular! The experienced meditators seem to have a different default mode! This finding suggests that after a bit of consistent practice, they had developed a new habit: paying attention and not being "sucked into" self-referential thinking.

How do the findings of this research relate to addiction and addiction treatment? Self-monitoring and cognitive control regions of the brain have been shown to be important in addictions, and in some cases, activity there can even predict how well people do in treatment (Brewer, Worhunsky, Carroll, Rounsaville, & Potenza, 2008). Mindfulness training may indeed build up the "mental muscle" in these brain regions in people who are trying to change addictive behaviors, so they are able to notice cravings and related self-referential thinking patterns, allowing them to "ride this wave" of experience rather than being sucked into it.

HOW IS MINDFULNESS TRAINING ACTUALLY TAUGHT TO INDIVIDUALS WITH ADDICTIONS?

A word of caution: For therapists who have an interest in, and may even have a daily practice of, mindfulness and meditation, this all may sound straightforward. It isn't. In our experience, individuals with addictions typically come into treatment having tried to quit on their own many times or having tried different treatments already (e.g., on average it takes someone five to seven attempts before he or she quits smoking), so they have little tolerance for treatments or therapists who aren't going to help them *now*. For example, in our smoking groups, new patients almost immediately ask if we (the therapists) have ever smoked (implied: quit smoking). It doesn't matter if you are a *jhana* (Pali: concentration practice) master and can hold unwavering concentration for hours, if you haven't practiced and applied these teachings in a very real way to the causes of suffering in your daily life, they won't trust you, and you likely won't be able to teach this approach to them. It is important to honestly consider your motivation and your own level of practice before proceeding. Otherwise patients will eat you up and spit you out, and nobody will benefit from these encounters. We would therefore strongly encourage therapists to get quite a bit of personal practice under their belts before proceeding.

At the Yale Therapeutic Neuroscience Clinic, where we have been implementing mindfulness training programs, we teach dependent origination in the very first class, using the diagram in Figure 12.2. Why? Here, we took yet another cue from the Buddha, who exclaimed, "I set out seeking the gratification in the world. Whatever gratification there is in the world, that I have found. I have clearly seen with wisdom just how far the gratification in the world extends" (Bodhi, 2005, p. 192). If individuals don't clearly see what they are actually getting each time they smoke or drink, there is much less hope that they will develop the resolve that is needed to ride out their (inherently unpleasant) cravings and urges as they attempt to quit. By walking them through the diagram step by step, using examples that are common to their lives, a seed is planted in their minds that yes, every time they smoke or use drugs, they are reinforcing these addictive habit patterns. We can also use analogies to illustrate this point, such as a screaming child in a grocery store.

The Screaming Child

Who has seen or parented a screaming kid at the grocery store? It certainly can be irritating if you are a couple of isles over, but imagine being the parent! Your kid screams because he wants something, and you desperately want him to shut up. So you fish around in your pocket or purse and find a lollipop. You immediately give it to him. He is happy for a few minutes. What just happened? You just created a habit, teaching your child to scream for lollipops. Now he's going to start screaming whenever he wants sweets, not just in grocery store. In a few years, he might be obese with rotted teeth from all the candy, not to mention poorly behaved.

Now imagine that your cravings for cigarettes or booze are the kid screaming, the drugs are the lollipops, and cancer, emphysema, or a lost job is the obesity. So what to do? Yell at your child? Gag him? Those approaches might work for a while, but the screaming will resume after the lollipop is gone, or only get worse if you gag him because you've just gagged him (which is painful) and haven't fixed whatever he is screaming about. Gagging in this analogy is you trying to resist the cravings. How about feeding him something else? That might be helpful for a while, but it too can cause other problems because you haven't addressed the craving (e.g., weight gain from substituting food for cigarettes).

What might you do instead? You might make sure his basic needs are met (his diaper doesn't need changing, he's not hungry or cold) and wait it out. Lovingly and patiently *hold* your child (your craving) until he stops screaming (your craving subsides). It might be unpleasant to get dirty looks from other people in the store at first, but eventually he will stop. And he will learn that he didn't get rewarded for his behavior, so the next time he screams, it will be less intense and shorter, and the next time even less intense and shorter still, until it dies off altogether. Now you have a well-trained child.

This analogy helps to illustrate the core components of mindfulness training: You can't ignore what's going on and expect it to magically disappear, and if you feed or push away your cravings, they only get more intense and more deeply ingrained.

After individuals have the opportunity to try this approach for a few days, we start giving them tools and techniques to help them ride out their cravings. In order to ride them out, they need to stay with them in their bodies from moment to moment, instead of acting on their fear through avoidance or running away.

To help guide patients, we have adapted a popular acronym— *RAIN*—to combine the recognition and acceptance components of mindfulness with moment-to-moment awareness techniques:

RAIN

We can learn to ride the waves of craving by surfing them. First, you Recognize that the wanting or craving is coming and Relax into it. Then, since you have no control over it coming, Allow or Accept this wave as it is; don't ignore it, distract yourself, or try to do something about it. This is your experience. Find a way that works for you, such as a word or phrase like, "I consent," "OK, here we go," "This is it," or perhaps a simple nod of the head. To catch the wave of craving, you have to study it carefully, Investigating it as it builds. Do this by asking, "What is the mind aware of now?" or "What's happening in my body right now?" Don't go looking. See what arises most prominently. Let it come to you. Finally, Note the experience in your body as you follow it. Keep it simple by using short phrases or single words, such as *restlessness in stomach, rising sensation, burning*, or *clenching*. When you get a better feel for wanting, you can simply note it too: *wanting getting stronger, rising in belly*, or *wanting, wanting, wanting*. Follow it until it completely subsides. If you get distracted, or the mind shifts to something else, simply return to the investigation by repeating the question: "What is the mind aware of now?" See if you can ride it until it is completely gone. Ride it to shore.

If you fall off the wave, or the wave feels unmanageable, you can start by returning your attention to a safe part of your body. The feet are usually a good spot to try. They are pretty neutral. So use "Feel your feet" as a backup, and just bring your attention there until the wanting/craving passes. This is like the surfer ducking under the wave and getting ready for the next one.

- Recognize/Relax into what is arising (e.g., craving).
- Allow/Accept this moment (use your phrase—"OK, here we go!"; "I consent").
- Investigate experience by asking, "What is happening in the body right now?"
- Note what is happening.

As part of this work, we teach individuals to wake up every morning and to set an aspiration to work with their cravings and drug use. We start by differentiating an aspiration from a desire, as a *desire* to quit can perpetuate the very fire an individual is wishing to put out. Simple analogies such as an *openhanded holding* of a wish to work with a craving (aspiration) versus *holding onto* something really tightly and wanting it to happen (desire) can help to illustrate simple, key differences between the two. Carefully chosen words can also be helpful here; using statements such as "May I work with my cravings" or "May I practice RAIN when I have a craving to smoke or drink" are usually more helpful than "I want to quit."

We also encourage individuals to learn and to use loving-kindness meditation throughout this process. Loving-kindness (*metta*) is a wonderful practice that can help individuals develop concentration as well as foster self-acceptance and acceptance of others. This attitude toward self is extremely important in treating a substance use disorder (and other behavioral addictions), as individuals often begin using drugs and alcohol to escape a psychologically traumatic past, and they suffer severe judgment from themselves and others due to their addictions. By learning to accept themselves as they are in this moment, loving-kindness can help individuals develop a stable and solid foundation from which to work with both negative affective states in their lives that trigger use, as well as cravings when they arise.

After a few weeks of learning to set daily aspirations, practicing the body scan and loving-kindness, and becoming familiar with using RAIN to ride out cravings, we then help individuals to integrate these approaches more seamlessly. We begin to point out (if they haven't already figured this out for themselves) how aspirations can align us with our goals of being happy, healthy, and harmonious with our surroundings (i.e., not suffer and not cause suffering for others). We help them see how urges and cravings to use derail us from reaching these goals. Here, traveling analogies can be helpful:

Staying on Track

Imagine that you are in Connecticut and want to go to California. You get in your car and head west on the highway. But soon this urge to stop at McDonald's pops up, so you stop for a bit to eat. Then you're back on the road and see a sign for Florida. You start thinking, "Hmmm, I've never been to Disney World. I'll stop off in Florida on my way. . . ." If you keep following every urge that pops up, you'll never get to your destination. And the longer you go without awakening to the situation (i.e., aren't mindful of your urges and resulting actions), the farther off track you get. But each time you notice your urges and note them ("Oh, there's that craving again") and ride out rather than act on each craving, you are able to stay on track and eventually get to your destination. The more you awaken to the situation and respond mindfully, the more momentum you build and the sooner you get there.

Bringing all of these points together, individuals can learn to (1) notice an urge, (2) use this as a mindfulness bell to remind themselves what their aspiration is, and (3) get back on track by using exercises such as RAIN or loving-kindness in the moment. In this sense, they notice when their car has veered off course (notice the craving), turn the steering wheel to get back on course (aspiration), and step on the gas (RAIN or loving-kindness practice). Once their momentum builds, they become unstoppable!

A benefit that we and our patients have seen from training individuals in mindfulness to help them with their addictions is that this practice naturally bleeds over into their daily lives. A burly auto mechanic sheepishly told me at the end of treatment that loving-kindness was his favorite practice, for in addition to helping him quit drinking, it helped him tremendously at work in dealing with his overbearing boss (his father). Another woman reported that she was able to accept extremely negative feelings surrounding the fact that she had discovered her dead brother, who had hanged himself in the closet. Not surprisingly, as rumination and other self-referential thought patterns are common to both addictions and other co-occurring conditions such as anxiety and depression, mindfulness training may be a useful as a dual-diagnosis treatment (Brewer, Bowen, Smith, Marlatt, & Potenza, 2010).

For centuries, we humans have been dealing with stress and suffering, both in our everyday lives and due to addictions. With its attention to the dynamics of craving and the process of dependent origination, mindfulness training aims to get at the core of this suffering, uprooting it or letting the fire burn out completely. Our modern views of the addictive process (backed up by research studies) are surprisingly similar to what the Buddha observed: that craving causes suffering, and by becoming disenchanted with and letting go of this very craving, we find relief from this condition. Mindfulness training is just beginning to be used by psychotherapists to help people with addictions step out of their addictive cycles. Preliminary work looks promising, though future studies are needed to confirm these initial successes and further link them with psychological and neurobiological mechanisms of change.

13

Working with Children

Trudy A. Goodman

> Try to be mindful, and let things take their natural
> course. Then your mind will become still in any
> surroundings, like a clear forest pool. All kinds of
> wonderful, rare animals will come to drink at the
> pool, and you will clearly see the nature of all things.
> You will see many strange and wonderful things
> come and go, but you will be still.
> —ACHANN CHAH (Chah, Kornfield, & Breiter, 1985)

*B*eginner's mind is a familiar expression in the Zen tradition for qualities of mindfulness: openness, receptiveness, and readiness to learn. Mindfulness practice cultivates the states of interest and relaxed spontaneity into which beginners in life—children—are born. Children live in a different country. As therapists we have to bridge a natural cultural divide to connect with them, and cultivating our own beginner's mind can help us do this. This chapter explores how mindfulness can help clinicians connect with children who come for psychotherapy, discusses its applicability in family therapy and parent guidance, and offers ways to teach mindfulness to kids.

RELATING MINDFULLY TO CHILDREN

What is unique about mindfulness-oriented child therapy? It is the intention and enhanced ability to return to the present moment, again and again, with openhearted, nonjudgmental attention, to stay with the experience of the child and one's own experience.

The Challenge of Working with Kids

Children do not communicate the way adults do. Many of their thoughts and feelings are expressed nonverbally, through play and body gestures. Mindfulness practice by the psychotherapist facilitates communicating with children, because mindfulness enhances nonverbal awareness. Moments of mindfulness are instantaneous, preverbal, preconceptual moments of clear seeing. The practice teaches us to open our senses, to be aware of what is happening in the moment, rather than engaging in discursive thinking or talking *about* experience.

Our operational definition of mindfulness—awareness of present experience with compassionate acceptance—provides a useful standpoint for relating to children. Children are more likely than adults to live in the present moment—in fact, they are notoriously confused by adult conceptions of time and sequence. I was reminded of this when treating a family with a 13-year-old daughter. When her mother told her a story about herself as a girl, the daughter responded, "Mom, I don't see how you can live in the past like that! Everything I think and do is now!" Mindfulness increases our capacity to relate empathically to a child's present-moment consciousness by helping us to experience life *ourselves* as a continuous series of present moments. It helps us be less caught up in concepts of time and to better attune to the way children experience life.

Because of the intensity of their attachments, and because adults are working continuously to socialize them, children are very sensitive to acceptance or disapproval by others. Therefore, *acceptance* is also critical to joining with children. The aspect of mindfulness that is non-judgmental and compassionate, accepting of what is—that understands without evaluating—creates a necessary atmosphere of emotional safety and trustworthiness in the therapy room.

Kids are also uniquely eager to return again and again to their chosen activities. The repetition of play that can be transformational and pleasurable for a child can be unnervingly tedious for the therapist. Mindfulness can help the therapist sustain enough interest to perceive subtle changes in otherwise boring, repetitive play sequences and stay emotionally connected with the child.

Mindfulness gives us the opportunity to know deeply, often in a nonverbal flash of insight, what is going on in the child. The child's world is different from our own; we can enter it with mindfulness by staying very present with what is happening in the moment. Our child patients can give us feedback when we become *un*mindful, perhaps through their misbehavior or withdrawal. Children, with their beginner's minds, teach us about the quality of our presence.

Psychotherapeutic Presence

Psychotherapeutic presence refers to more than being in the physical company of another person. It refers to a felt sense of being with another, of *mindfulness in relationship* (see Chapter 5). The opposite of therapeutic presence is absentmindedness or preoccupation. Children are especially sensitive to whether or not adults are emotionally engaged with them. The experience of being alone in the physical company of another can feel almost as abandoning as being left all alone.

> Cari, an 18-year-old patient, was upset after watching a video of her mother holding her when she was about 6 months old. In the video, Cari was on her mother's lap, being bounced on her mother's knee. Both Cari and her mother were facing her aunt, who held the camera. Her mother periodically bent over baby Cari and nuzzled, poked, and tickled her, then quickly returned to talking to her sister. Cari was strangely troubled by this seemingly benign scene. She felt that her mother had been oblivious to her as a baby as her mother talked and jiggled her in a mechanical way. Her mother's interactions felt intrusive, motivated by her mother's need to make contact and reassure herself.

Although physically present, Cari felt that her mother was emotionally absent. I taught Cari how to meditate; our shared experience of mindfulness created a compassionate field of attentive psychotherapeutic presence wherein Cari could discern a parallel between the feeling of being emotionally intruded upon by her mother and the patterns she observed in her meditation. Anxious thoughts would swoop into her consciousness when she was in a calm mental state, grab her attention, and pull her out of a state of peaceful presence, just as her mother did in the video.

Cari's experience illustrates two points. First, it shows how the therapist's kind attentiveness—his or her psychotherapeutic presence— can help children perceive their own experience in a new way. Cari took this insight a step further in seeing how the quality of a parent's attention can shape the way a child attends to his or her own experience (Bluth & Wahler, 2011). Second, we see how mindfulness practice may enhance social cognition in general; indeed, the neural circuits used for intrapersonal attunement may be the same as those used interpersonally (Siegel, 2007). Cari and I believed that her own mindfulness practice enabled her to perceive the legacy of her mother's mental states more accurately.

This enhanced mindful awareness also applies to the therapist doing psychotherapy. Awareness of the movements of his or her own mind during treatment can help the therapist learn a lot about a child's inner experience: warding off and being close, being present or being absent, feeling abandoned or abandoning.

Presence in Chaos

> When Carlos, age 9, arrived in my office, he asked, "Is this a place for kids who hate themselves?" He quickly confided that he, indeed, hated himself. Carlos was not able to wait to get to know me before becoming absorbed in wild dramatic play. The themes emerging were violent and explicitly sexual. Both his disregard for being in a room with an unfamiliar person and the uninhibited explicitness of his play were disconcerting.

At one point in the first session, we each had a puppet on one raised hand and were advancing across the floor on our bellies, slithering slowly along in Carlos's game. He suddenly looked over at me and asked incredulously, "Is this your job?" His sense of humor notwithstanding, I saw that, for Carlos, the line between real and pretend was unclear. His ability to move in and out of fantasy was dizzying, and I was beginning to feel flooded by all the emotional material surfacing in his play. Being with Carlos, I felt inner chaos and a swirl of overwhelming thoughts and feelings.

Mindfulness helped to focus my attention in the midst of the whirling impressions of the session. With three breaths in and out, I steadied my mind and recognized that my own chaotic state was a reflection of Carlos's. I felt his intense need to make sense of his world—which eventually became our clinical agenda.

I decided to introduce a mindfulness exercise to help us both. I suspected that Carlos might benefit from the same technique I used to disentangle from his emotional chaos. We developed a game called *three breaths* in which we would stop whatever we were doing, whenever he wanted, to explore how he was feeling, gently and slowly. Carlos liked the control this gave to our interaction and to his own experience in the moment. He also learned increasingly to use words for vulnerable and difficult feelings. In this way, Carlos began to benefit from mindful awareness of his tumultuous inner life, and I was able to remain more connected to him.

This quality of mind, which we might call *authentic presence, mindfulness in relationship*, or *therapeutic presence*, involves being aware of the fluctuations of our own attentiveness while we are emotionally engaged with a patient. Thomson (2000) suggests that "authentic presence . . . must sit somewhere between therapist and client" (p. 546). This means that we may be open and receptive to the patient's experience but simultaneously remain aware that the drama is a play of consciousness. Mindfulness enables the therapist to be compassionately engaged yet disentangled from the patient's experience. We can pop in and out of our own reactions and learn from what our body is sensing, from what our mind is doing, without losing connection with our patient. The process is subtler with children than with adults, because interactions with children are less verbal and structured; we must remain alert and receptive to visceral, preconceptual experience. It requires greater refinement of our attention.

Presence in Disconnection

Sustained awareness comes naturally as long as we are enjoying our experience and it remains interesting. However, unpleasant experiences also occur regularly in therapy, and our attention often begins to wander off in response. The cultivation of mindfulness helps us discern the patterns of connection and disconnection that occur in the office (Safran et al., 2011).

> Maria, a fifth grader, was referred for therapy by her school due to social withdrawal and emotional passivity. Although sweet and compliant, Maria was as emotionally disengaged in therapy as she was emotionally absent in the classroom. She was disinterested in most things, including her physical appearance, which is ordinarily a compelling concern at Maria's age. Her hair was unwashed, and she seemed generally neglected.

It was difficult to remain present in the room with Maria due to her emotional blandness and inability to engage in conversation. Despite my intention to be present with Maria in therapy, the temptation to space out, to plan or daydream, was almost irresistible. I sometimes found myself dreading our sessions. All my efforts to return, again and again, to presence and caring did not seem to enliven our connection. I often felt exhausted after our sessions.

After 6 long, lackluster therapy hours spent mindful of—and willing to explore—the perplexing sense of something missing in the relationship with Maria, I shared my puzzlement with her parents. A few weeks later, I received an early morning call at home from Maria's father. He told me that he had been sexually involved with his daughter. He described the emotional numbness and longing that had led him to seek that kind of comfort from her. He rationalized that his behavior might compensate for Maria's mother's neglect of the little girl, but her father had no apparent awareness of his own role in that neglect. I acknowledged his courage in telling me about what had happened.

Maria had checked out of being present to herself and to others. She was living in a dreamy, dissociated semblance of being a normal schoolgirl, going through the motions, without even knowing what was really wrong. My reactions—wanting to leave, to check out of being with her—reflected Maria's feelings with painful precision. I discovered later that Maria's mother was herself a victim of abuse, and my sense of disconnection reflected her mother's pervasive emotional disengagement as well. Mindfulness of connection and disconnection can sometimes be uncannily revealing if we are willing to linger with it and allow it to reveal its truths.

Our intention to return to the present moment with curiosity and caring, despite how it may feel, is an essential skill when working with patients who are bearing suffering without words. Children, especially, bring their struggles to therapy nonverbally. What is confusing or opaque to the therapist will eventually become interesting and clear if he or she has the open-minded intention to return to it again and again. Mindful awareness can go anywhere, exploring all corners, independent of our theoretical frame of reference. The question is, "What is happening here, now, in my experience and in my patient's experience?"

Beginner's Mind

In the beginner's mind there are many possibilities;
in the expert's mind there are few.
                              —SHUNRYU SUZUKI (1973)

Many teachers love to work with beginners because they are eager to learn, ask excellent questions, are curious, and are generally receptive to information and experience. What a delight! Our child patients are seeking the same receptiveness in their therapists. Can the therapist understand me, know me, be patient and kind enough to feel my struggle and recognize my strengths? Does the therapist like being with me? When the therapist can meet a child with beginner's mind, both are freed from preconceived notions rooted in the child's diagnosis or family history, and can meet with interest to see how it is simply to be together.

Leni, a 3-year-old girl with rosy cheeks and a ponytail, was referred to me by a well-known pediatrician who had raised the question of whether Leni had autism. Her frightened parents wanted a second opinion. When I first met Leni, her averted gaze, her silence, and her willingness to leave her mother without a backward glance all seemed to support the diagnosis. Leni was not ready to acknowledge me or respond to my words; in fact, she appeared to ignore me. When Leni came with me into the playroom and sat down, she painted a picture of a little girl sitting in the back of a big gray car being driven down a street all alone, surrounded by falling snow.

In other ways as well, Leni communicated what her world was like. Her play was repetitious, she perseverated verbally, and her behaviors were neither welcoming nor rejecting. Still, as I brought my attention fully into the moment and became mindful of all the sense impressions that were occurring in the field of my awareness, there was a felt sense of this little girl's presence and a slight connection. I sensed her presence in the form of her diligence, her energy, her anxiety, and her stubbornness. Leni evoked those same qualities inside of me. Her mother confirmed that those were some aspects of little Leni's personality.

It became evident over time that Leni did manifest elements of high-functioning autism, per DSM-5. Although the diagnosis was crucial for getting appropriate services during her school years, the focus of therapy was for Leni's parents and me to develop an empathic understanding of and connection to the little girl, buried behind her atypical neurology. Leni's needs could be flexibly addressed by this more attuned, mindful understanding.

As we search for the person behind the diagnosis, the willingness to *not know* is a precondition for discovery (see Chapter 3). Unlike true beginners, experienced therapists may move prematurely to conclusions due to overconfidence or anxious not knowing. As therapists, we need to restrain this tendency and learn to rest calmly in the midst of uncertainty, with patience and equanimity. I tried to hold my diagnostic understanding in suspension, so that it did not interfere with the task of making an authentic, warm connection with Leni's individuality and experience.

Mindfulness practice can be helpful in this regard; it trains the practitioner to suspend *cognitive construing*, to use Delmonte's (1986) term.

Child therapists in training often need to know that it is OK simply to be warmly receptive, to sit and be with a child, relaxed in what is yet to be revealed. Holding our concepts and theories lightly allows us to make a journey of co-discovery with the child. It is a collaboration in which our thoughts about treatment are deemphasized in favor of the *felt sense* (Gendlin, 1996) of the connection. The felt sense changes moment to moment, much like a child him- or herself. When the novice clinician asks for guidelines on how to think during the session, the answer is, "Not too much." If we feel the moment with the child, we trust that understanding will naturally occur to us when we need it.

Recent work in the emerging field of interpersonal neurobiology points to mechanisms by which one individual influences another (Iacoboni, 2008; Siegel, 2007). With this influence in mind, we understand something about how our beginner's mind is a gift to children. When we drop our preconceptions, they are free to come forward and inhabit our relaxed space of openness and receptivity. Our own peaceful state of being invites their calm and permits them to "come as they are," no part left out. All the scary, unacceptable, "strange and wonderful" creatures that live in the child's psyche are drawn to the "still forest pool" of our friendly receptivity (Chah et al., 1985, p. vi).

Preverbal Awareness

Difficult experiences occur for all children before they have the ability to speak. The traces of these experiences are buried in the body and feelings of the child. Even for adults, the results of traumatic experiences are often largely preverbal. Through compassionate, mindful awareness, clinicians can help to integrate preverbal experiences that have been exiled from awareness. Mindfulness, especially with the components of acceptance and self-compassion (Germer, 2009), may make it safe for difficult experience to come forth, like animals emerging silently and warily from the forest. With familiarity and comfort in the preverbal realm of experience, the therapist can remain quietly connected with the suffering child.

> Jason, a tousled 5-year-old with big brown eyes, had already been kicked out of every preschool program in which he was enrolled. He was entering a therapeutic school program when I met him. When limits to his behavior were set in the new school, Jason would scream, wail, flail his arms, and eventually collapse. Jason had often witnessed his mother being beaten by her live-in boyfriend

and naturally was unable to protect her. His mother compounded the problem by reacting to Jason's rages alternately with passive guilt and by verbally threatening to "tear [him] limb from limb." Both Jason and his mother felt helpless and out of control.

In his fantasy play in therapy, Jason could be a hero who saved people, a superman who could subdue any angry bad guy. Nonetheless, his small size and the vulnerability of a 5-year-old boy were keenly felt. The feeling of disempowerment caused by the limits set in his new school led to eruptions of fear and rage. I chose a new approach with Jason. What would it be like to hold him with steadiness and tender compassion, without anger or reactivity, in response to his storms? This approach had a profound effect. His anger exhausted itself and he sobbed softly, allowing himself to be rocked and comforted as felt his nearly unbearable sorrow.

As Jason learned to put his terror into words, he revealed that he was afraid his arms and legs would fall off. This fear echoed his mother's threats to tear him limb from limb. In the "country" where children live, words are swallowed literally. Jason was afraid I was going to pull off his arms and legs in retaliation for his anger. Little by little, Jason learned to tell the difference between his fears and reality. He learned that his arms and legs were securely attached to his body and that when his therapist stopped his rages, she would not hurt him. Jason's rages subsided.

The bulk of Jason's treatment was nonverbal. He was positively affected by my efforts to remain nonjudgmentally aware of his struggle and to stay lovingly connected throughout the course of his painful outbursts. Surprisingly, Jason later recognized himself in other little boys when *they* had temper tantrums, and he looked for opportunities to be kind and soothing.

Mindfulness in the presence of strong emotions takes practice—not years and years, but some period of regular practice with the intention to be receptive. As a reminder of my own intention to be mindful, I keep a quote on the wall of my therapy office:

> By being in alert attention, by observing oneself, with the intention to understand rather than to judge, in full acceptance of whatever may emerge, simply because it is there, we allow the deep to come to the surface and enrich our life and consciousness. . . . This is the great work of awareness. (Maharaj, 1997, p. 112)

Kids do not yet fully inhabit the verbal world, and adults sometimes cling to it too tightly. Adults have a tendency to foreclose a child's experience by offering verbal explanations or solutions. With mindfulness practice, this preverbal perceptual domain can become a safe and compassionate resting place for the psychotherapist, a bridge to helping a child with caring words.

The Present Moment

Therapeutic work always occurs in the here-and-now. Daniel Stern's (2003) reflections on the *now moment* in psychotherapy sound like a description of mindfulness practice.

> There is no remove in time. [The moment] is direct—not transmitted and reformulated by words. . . . Moments of meeting provide some of the most nodal experiences for change in psychotherapy. They are often the moments most remembered . . . that changed the course of therapy. (p. 57)

Although Stern suggests that we lack a theory of such moments, Buddhist psychology has elaborated in great detail the many nuances of the present moment and how to sustain compassionate moment-by-moment connection to both the contents of awareness and the process of change.

The present moment is exceptionally fleeting. When we conceptualize an experience of the moment, it is already gone. With mindfulness, we move closer and closer to the simple arising and passing of preverbal experience in the present moment. This sort of knowing, which is intuitive, is at the heart of our innate wisdom.

Clinical researchers have videotaped infant–parent interactions and have observed microcommunications flashing back and forth between the two individuals as quickly as 10 times a second (Beebe & Lachmann, 1998; Tronick, 1989). The baby glances, the mother responds; her response is echoed by the baby, who shapes the mother's next response, and so on. Mutual, reciprocal call and response happens so quickly that it cannot be followed by the conscious eye of an observer. Awareness of the present moment brings us closer to seeing this subtle, nonverbal process, and thereby makes it easier to enter and participate in the world of the child.

How does a therapist enter into a relationship of such subtlety? A therapist who is attuned emotionally to the child patient probably participates in these microcommunications with intuitive, participatory awareness rather than conceptual, objective knowledge. A sense of connection and understanding may be a result of a stream of reciprocal perceptions that is too fleeting to be tracked consciously. When this attunement is strong, the therapist is fully attentive to the patient and absorbed in the moment-to-moment "flow." Through emotional attunement and authentic presence, effective therapists are fully engaged in elusive, successive, fleeting present moments.

With some children, explicitly calling attention to the present moment facilitates treatment:

> Nine-year-old Maggie challenged me. She had previously seen two experienced clinicians without success. She was emotionally disconnected, frequently teased at school (where kids called her *poison-head*), and very sensitive to criticism. Maggie was battling with her parents about her refusal to do homework on a daily basis. It did not help that her younger brother was an excellent student and very popular in school. Her parents did not know how to help Maggie feel less victimized, angry, and lonesome.

A therapy veteran before the age of 9, Maggie was hyperalert to anything that smacked of psychology. Disdainful and distant, she would deflect every arrow in my therapeutic quiver by throwing a fit, followed by sullen silence.

Late one winter afternoon, Maggie and I sat facing each other on the floor of my office in a pool of lamplight. I wanted to connect but was frustrated in a way that was so familiar to Maggie herself. The silence was tense and uneasy. My thoughts wandered out the window. It was twilight, one of those hushed moments when the whole world turns deep blue. I felt the deep peace of meditation. I spontaneously turned to Maggie and said softly, "Look, it's all blue out there." She looked. I asked her if she had ever noticed this blue twilight world. She was curious, attentive in a new way. It was a moment of meeting, of presence and peace. For one brief "now" moment, we entered each other's world. As Stern (2003) writes, "As soon as a now moment arrives, all else is dropped and each partner stands with both feet in the present. Presentness fills the time and space" (p. 54).

A year later, I taught Maggie to practice mindfulness, sitting tall on an imaginary throne, focusing on the ebb and flow of the breath moving gently through the body. She learned to sit calmly, confident and absorbed, for 10 whole minutes, noticing her feelings and all the stories they tell, coming and going, appearing and disappearing, while she remained steadily there. She understood that she did not always have to believe her thoughts; she could choose to let them be, to let them go. She practiced in her room, sitting cross-legged on her bed, and found a haven in the present moment. To paraphrase Achaan Chah again, Maggie found the still forest pool, where all her wild things, scary things, unacceptable things, could come out and drink their fill. Children can learn that all their "strange and wonderful creatures" can coexist peacefully in the same young heart.

Play

Young children symbolically represent and express what they are thinking and feeling in their own language—the language of play. By cultivating mindfulness, therapists can become more skilled in attention and develop other qualities that are integral to successful play therapy (Landreth, 2002).

The space of play is intimate and immediate. In play, children explore, recreate, redo, and rework overwhelming life events and unbearable emotions into experiences they can assimilate. While playing, kids can be big and powerful, they can control their world, and they can design the game so they always win and never get left out or lose. Children can create healing distance from disturbing or traumatic events by having them happen to others, and by controlling their outcome.

> Six-year-old Hilary was hospitalized for surgery to correct a congenital heart defect. Well after recovering, Hilary still had nightmares and was wetting her bed. In play therapy, she organized a game of "hospital" in which a fleet of doctors roared up on motorcycles (Hilary was afraid of motorcycles) to stick needles in their little patients. "There, there, don't cry," Hilary comforted the patients. Hilary also made sure that all the patients fully recovered from the sticking and probing, just as she did.

In the safety and protection of play witnessed by her therapist, Hilary took charge of a situation in which she had formerly felt victimized and frightened. She regained her sense of competence and the bedwetting ceased.

For therapists to enter the arena of play, they must be willing to temporarily abandon their logical, linear, and verbal modes of thought and expression. Clinicians can develop comfort with the childlike emotional intimacy of play through intimate awareness of their own subjective experience.

Play is essential for all people. Adults differentiate between work and play, ordinarily calling work the activity that we do for an extrinsic goal (e.g., money) and play activity for its own sake. Work is *doing*, with an eye to the future, and play is *being*—spontaneous, wholehearted activity in the present moment. Absorption in play, like in meditation, generally increases energy: Attention is mindful, unified, and concentrated. (Perhaps this is why children have so much energy!)

When work, including clinical practice, becomes play, we find we have much more energy at the end of the day. Resting in the forgotten world of childhood—fresh, immediate, spontaneous, wide awake, immersed in the reality of here and now—can be a kind of mindfulness training for our adult minds. We can feel refreshed and renewed by working with, playing with, and being with our young patients. Children can become powerful teachers in the development of mindful presence.

FAMILY THERAPY

Many of the therapeutic skills discussed here are as relevant to family therapy as to individual child therapy. One goal of most family therapy is to enhance mutual understanding between children and their parents. Mindfulness practice can support this work by increasing the therapist's ability to relate to and understand children.

A great challenge of family therapy is remaining impartial toward family members, while remaining empathically attuned to each of them. This can be particularly difficult during moments of intense emotion or conflict. The ability to tolerate powerful affect, to remain present in the midst of chaos, and to be attentive to details of nonverbal communication, all help the family therapist navigate these tumultuous waters.

Beginner's mind is especially useful in family treatment. It is virtually impossible to plan family sessions effectively. Being in a room with several people, each with his or her own history and agenda, introduces so many variables that our only hope lies in trusting that we will be able to respond creatively and intelligently to whatever occurs. The comfort in being with new, changing, moment-to-moment phenomena that mindfulness practice brings is a real help to therapists in these circumstances.

As I discuss below, for family members who are open to it, actually practicing mindfulness together can also provide support to their growth and development.

PARENT GUIDANCE

It is no surprise that parents' degree of mindfulness should have a bearing on effective parenting. Parents' emotional attunement is essential to a child's growth and development. Several systematic studies have explored the impact of mindfulness practice on parenting (Bögels, Lehtonen, & Restifo, 2010; Coatsworth, Duncan, Greenberg, & Nix, 2009; Duncan, Coatsworth, & Greenberg, 2009; Goodman, Greenland, & Siegel, 2011; Singh et al., 2010; van der Oord, Bögels, & Pejnenburg, 2012), and there is mounting general interest in mindful parenting as evidenced by the rapid growth of popular publications (Kabat-Zinn & Kabat-Zinn, 1998; Kaiser Greenland, 2010; Kramer, 2004; Miller, 2006; Napthali, 2003; Placone, 2011; Rogers, 2005; Roy, 2007; Willard, 2010) and the proliferation of training programs for parents. How might we understand the influence of mindfulness on parenting?

Parenting is inherently challenging. Sometimes parents are angry with or alienated from their children, making it difficult to relate to them empathically. Other times, parents are hesitant to set necessary limits out of reluctance to tolerate the disconnection or tension that usually follows. Most parental guidance interventions focus on one of these difficulties, either increasing parents' ability to relate empathically to their children (e.g., Faber & Mazlish, 1999; Green, 2001) or enhancing their ability to establish clear, consistent consequences for behavior (e.g., Barkley & Benton, 1998; Patterson, 1977). Developmental psychologists generally agree that effective parenting involves finding an optimal balance between these strategies (i.e., skillfully providing both love and limits).

Parents who practice mindfulness often report that it helps strengthen both of these core dimensions of parenting. For the reasons discussed earlier in the context of child therapy, mindfulness allows for gentle presence, awareness of connection and disconnection, openness to a child's nonverbal communication, and ability to join a child in play—all of which help children to experience their parents' love and understanding more fully.

Equally important are the perspective and the patience cultivated by mindfulness. Many parents report that they have great difficulty responding wisely to their children's misbehavior, often reacting reflexively instead. The tired parent who is thwarted by a 2-year-old in the supermarket, or who is defeated in an argument with a teenager, may react with anger—even though he or she knows that this will be counterproductive. Even parents who would never come to the attention of the child protective services frequently commit these small "parenting crimes." Mindfulness practice can help parents deal with conflict and their own emotional reactivity, and set appropriate limits more skillfully.

To observe children grow is to be faced with evidence of constant change, of impermanence in childhood and in life itself. Being mindful of impermanence can enable parents to tolerate the loss of connection they face when setting a difficult limit, or their children's growing independence. This tolerance offers more ballast to parents, more courage to be with loss, frustration, or disappointment with wise understanding.

Teaching parents how to observe and communicate with their young children mindfully and empathically has been shown to increase secure attachment, cognitive development, and emotion regulation (Cohen et al., 1999; Cohen, Lojkasek, Muir, Muir, & Parker, 2002; Fonagy & Target, 1997; Grienenberger, Slade, & Kelly, 2005). Building on these findings, a number of explicit "mindful parenting" programs are being developed. For example, one mindful parenting program consists of weekly group meetings in which parents engage in a formal period of quiet observation, lasting from 20 to 30 minutes, and are encouraged to notice the details of their infant's behavior, as well as the quality of infant–adult interactions. Reynolds (2003) describes this approach: "Parents are encouraged to slow down inside to the pace of infant life, so they may notice the tiniest details of their baby's experience—and tease apart their own as well as their baby's emotional responses" (p. 364). Initial anecdotal reports suggest that the program increases parents' awareness and understanding of their baby's behavior.

Mindfulness practice helps people see that all of their experience is a series of changing moments, and that their thoughts and even their sense of self are contingent, influenced by myriad transitory conditions. This realization helps us take things less personally, a perspective that is absolutely essential for good parenting. Becoming more mindful allows parents to recognize the needs of their child rather than instinctually react out of personal injury or pride. A less personal perspective further reinforces the capacity to bear intense emotion as parents begin to see the universality of their predicament: "Oh, this is how it is to be a human reduced to despair by a 2-year-old," or "This is what it's like to be parents in the throes of frustration with their teenager." Compassionate awareness is the best way to *be with* intense affect.

It is easier for therapists to explain alternative parenting strategies than it is for parents to implement them. Habitual, automatic, emotionally charged parenting reactions tend to be quite tenacious and resistant to change. By bringing compassionate awareness to the present moment, mindfulness can help parents pause to see the steps that lead up to their responses. Parents can pause to observe their feelings in response to their children's behavior, observe their intention to react automatically with more self-compassion, and thereby respond to their children more wisely. This pause provides a vitally important moment in which to consider alternatives with kindness and clarity. The pause may not even involve stopping anything so much as a momentary redirection of attention from *inner mindfulness* (Analayo, 2003) toward what is happening externally. For example, Goodman and colleagues (2012) suggest:

> If we are mindfully slicing carrots and a child calls for our attention, our awareness can shift from inner personal carrot-focused experience to the external interpersonal environment (attending to the child), and our child's request simply becomes another expression of the way life is, endlessly changing its shape and appearance. (p. 299)

Mindfulness therefore has a valuable role to play in parent guidance by helping parents (1) to be more compassionate and loving with their children, (2) to see their own behavior more objectively, and (3) to set limits more skillfully. Parental mindfulness practice can take the simple form of asking parents to notice how emotions manifest in their bodies when they are with their children. When they find themselves becoming agitated in response to their child, parents can be shown how to follow their breath or to pay attention to their physical surroundings. For those receptive to the idea, mindfulness can be made into a family activity.

MINDFULNESS EXERCISES FOR CHILDREN

Mindful Magic

What's magic about mindfulness? We can move our attention up, down, sideways—anywhere we want! We can picture things (pretend they are real!) and play in our minds. And we can do this by ourselves or with friends. This is magic that we use for good things, like feeling safe, happy, peaceful, and free. When we feel safe and happy, we want everyone we love and care about—and everyone in the whole wide world, including all the plants and animals—to be peaceful and happy, too.

Magic Body

This exercise for the happiness and well-being of our bodies is easily adaptable for preschoolers by making it shorter and simplifying words. For older children it can be lengthened by adding more detail (neck, shoulders, arms, hands, fingers, right, left, etc.). Kids can practice this lying down when they wake up in the morning or before they go to sleep, or sitting comfortably anytime. You can close your eyes or leave them open, whichever way helps you feel most relaxed.

- Begin by belly-breathing in and out three times, feeling how each breath moves into your body, filling up your chest and belly, then feeling how the breath gently relaxes back out into the air around you.
- Then magically bring your attention to your wonderful head. How great it is to have a head! Notice all the things you can do with your head, nodding yes, shaking no, thinking and learning with your brain. Say quietly to yourself, "May my head be happy."
- With the magic of mindfulness, you can move your attention around to your face. Appreciate all the amazing things your face does, your eyes seeing, nose smelling, your mouth tasting, talking, singing, smiling, laughing, crying...now wish: "May my face be happy."
- Moving your mindful magic to your arms and hands, you can feel them relax. Arms and hands are truly magical, they can play all kinds of games, take care of dressing and feeding you. You can hug, hold hands, stretch, and wave. As a way of saying thank you, wish: "May my arms and hands be happy."
- Feel your in-breath fill your chest and tummy, feel your out-breath relax and let it all go. You can be mindful of how your heart beats and your breath breathes all day and night, healthy and strong. Your breath and your heartbeat keep you company every moment of your life, asleep or awake. "May my heart be happy."
- Magically move your attention to your legs and feet. You can say thank you to them for walking you everywhere you want to go, for running, jumping, sitting, riding, dancing, kicking, standing, lying down to rest. "May my legs and feet be happy."
- If your body is hurt or you're not feeling well, you can use the magic of mindfulness to take your attention to whatever needs some love. Remember your body knows how to get better—you truly have a magical body! You can wish: "May I be well and happy."

Magic Carpet

Mindfulness can help you find a safe place inside yourself, even when things outside are scary. Here is how to find this safe place using the magic carpet of mindfulness.

- Close your eyes and sit quietly for a moment. Imagine you are sitting on a magic carpet. Imagine that the magic carpet can float you way up into the clear, warm sunny sky. Even if it is cloudy or rainy, above the clouds the sun is shining brightly. Imagine yourself sitting on your carpet, floating above the clouds. Take your time. Feel how peaceful it is to look down at your world from high above it all. See how tiny it all looks from up here.
- Now ask your magic carpet to ride you back down to earth and land you in a safe place. This safe place might be in a corner of a room or under a tree, or a secret hideout, or any place where you feel protected, cozy, safe, sheltered, and warm. Imagine yourself landing softly there, what it looks like, how you want to be there. Feel how good it is to be safe and protected. Feel how your body can relax in this safe place, how your mind can be peaceful. You can always go to this safe place. You can imagine bringing your favorite toy or inviting a good friend to fly there on the magic carpet with you. For even more safety, you can imagine as many guardian lions or fairy godmothers or ninjas outside as you need to protect your space. Rest in this protected space for a while until you know you can be safe and strong.
- Now you are almost ready for the magic carpet to carry you back. As you get ready to go, imagine you are bringing this safe place with you. With mindfulness you can tuck this safe place anywhere, in your pocket, even somewhere inside your heart. Find the place inside you that can feel quiet, protected, safe, and cozy. Mindfulness helps you remember your own special safe place where you can feel OK even when hard things happen. And mindfulness is not afraid, even when things are scary; when you are scared, your mindfulness just knows and understands.
- Let the magic carpet fly you safely back. You can hop on anytime you remember, and ride to your safe place again. And now that you are back, mindfulness will help you remember; you carry the protection and safety of your special place inside you always.

Magic Happiness: How to Be Happy Right Here, Right Now

What Makes Me Happy?[1]

Materials: old magazines with pictures, scissors, glue, crayons, markers, colored chalk, paint, paper.

We can say that there are two kinds of happiness: eating-sweets happiness and peace-inside happiness. One comes from treats, like a new toy or a piece of cake. The other kind of happiness comes from a mind full of peace, like when you feel completely loved by your adults.

The first kind of happiness doesn't last . . . the second kind of happiness is more genuine, wider, and deeper, like an ocean.

Make a collage of the different things that make you happy, for example, eating an ice cream cone or hugging. If you can't find a picture, draw one instead. When you have finished, make two lists: short-term happiness and long-term happiness. In which list do each of your types of happiness belong? On a new sheet of paper, make a larger drawing of your favorite example of happiness.

Take three steps:

1. Enjoy things that make me happy.
2. Notice when I am sad.
3. Later, when I am not sad anymore, think about what made me sad and try to understand it and change it.

Magic Ball: Wishes for the World[2]

This is a variation of the loving-kindness meditation in which children are encouraged to offer their friendly wishes to other people. Children pretend that they are creating an enormous ball and filling it with their friendly wishes for other people and the world. When everyone has had a chance to add their wishes to the pretend ball, the group mimes tossing the ball up into the sky and then imagines that their ball will float around the world bringing friendly wishes to everyone, everywhere. Remember: Encouraging students to send friendly wishes isn't the same as encouraging students to change the way they feel about someone, or to like someone they don't like. It does offer

---

[1]This exercise is reprinted from *Planting Seeds: Practicing Mindfulness with Children* (2011) by Thich Nhat Hanh and the Plum Village Community with permission of Parallax Press, Berkeley, California. *www.parallax.org*.

[2]This exercise is reprinted with permission from Susan Kaiser Greenland, who pioneered Inner Kids and the Inner Kids Mindful Awareness Program for children, teens, and their families and is the author of *The Mindful Child* (2010).

students an opportunity to imagine a more loving, soothing, and safer world. Sending friendly wishes is one of several practices that offer students a direct experience of the mind/body connection. They'll notice that there's a difference between how their bodies feel when they are feeling warm-hearted and wishing others well compared to how their bodies feel when they are angry or upset.

- Squat down with hands out (in a circle, if with a group) as if holding one big ball. Imagine what the ball looks like, what color, etc.
- Ask each child to voice one friendly wish for someone or for the world, and mime putting it into the ball. One by one, wishes can be added. As the imaginary ball grows, mime holding a bigger and heavier ball.
- When all the wishes are in the ball, count to three and mime throwing the ball up into the sky and waving goodbye to it. Imagine the ball is bringing the wishes to everyone chosen and/or to everyone in the world.

Mindfulness practice and clinical work with children nourish each other. Both teach us to enter into a felt sense of the world of children, where we are free to hold our ideas more lightly, to disengage from familiar patterns of emotional reactivity, and to connect with our innate playfulness, creativity, and openness. By cultivating presence through practicing mindfulness, we can develop a more vivid, wholehearted attentiveness to the child's experience and our own. By setting the intention to be mindful, present, and open, therapists and parents can learn to meet the children where they live—in this precious, relational, transformational moment—which is the only moment we have.

Part IV

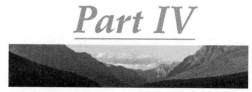

Past, Present, and Promise

*W*hile mindfulness practices can be enormously helpful in addressing a wide range of clinical conditions, this was not their original purpose. They were intended instead to bring about a radical transformation of human consciousness—liberation from the suffering inherent in the human condition. Chapter 14 reaches into the past to explore the central insights of Buddhist psychology and how mindfulness practices fit in this tradition's understanding of suffering and its alleviation. Chapter 15 fast-forwards to our modern scientific world and presents a review of our rapidly expanding knowledge of the neurobiology of mindfulness practices and our ability to functionally and structurally change the brain. Finally, Chapter 16 points us forward as it investigates parallels between positive psychology and Buddhist psychological insights into how we and our patients might live richer, more meaningful lives.

14

The Roots of Mindfulness

Andrew Olendzki

> Life, personhood, pleasure, and pain: This is all
> that's bound together in a single mental event, a
> moment that quickly takes place.
> —BUDDHA (*Maha Niddesa*, cited in Olendzki, 1998)

*E*mpirical studies are demonstrating the usefulness of mindfulness for alleviating psychological and physical problems, and modern researchers are beginning to identify the essential ingredients of mindfulness in clinical settings. It may seem entirely unnecessary to link mindfulness to its historical and philosophical roots, but the ancient understanding of mindfulness goes significantly beyond what is commonly considered in modern psychotherapy. Therefore, it may be helpful to look to the historical context of mindfulness and the system of thought underlying what we now call Buddhist psychology.

The practice of attending carefully to the details of one's present experience is probably as old as humankind itself. Doing so in a deliberate and structured way, however, seems to have particularly strong roots in the religious traditions of ancient India. It was in the forests and plains along the banks of the Indus and Ganges rivers that people began to explore the nuances of perceptual experience using methods a modern scientist might recognize as empirical, experimental, and repeatable—despite being entirely introspective. Carried out over the last four millennia, this program of self-study has yielded a descriptive science of the mind and body that is of growing interest to contemporary thinkers.

Ancient insights into the workings of human experience are preserved in the Hindu and Buddhist traditions, each leaving a rich legacy of sophisticated psychological material. Buddhist theoretical psychology, in particular, articulates a model of human consciousness that seems remarkably postmodern, based on a process view of noncentralized, interdependent systems for processing sense data and constructing identity. Its applied psychology is anchored in the practice of meditation, which can range from mindfulness, through various stages of concentration, to deeply transformative insights that can fundamentally restructure the organization of mind and body. The most basic and accessible form of the ancient Indian meditative arts, referred to in this volume as *mindfulness meditation*, is beginning to have a significant effect upon a wide range of contemporary scientific and therapeutic professions.

ANCIENT ORIGINS
A Unique View of the Human Condition

Each in its own way, the ancient Buddhist and Hindu schools of thought shared the view that human existence centers upon a node of conscious awareness, more or less identified as a soul, which is embedded in a sensory apparatus yielding both pleasant and painful experience. The nature of this existence is flawed by the fact that pain is inevitable, lasting pleasure is unobtainable, and humans have limited ability to see themselves or their world very clearly. Death provides no solution to this existential dilemma they called *dukkha* (loosely translated from Pali as *suffering*), for they believed that a person just flows on from one lifetime to another, without respite. Each time around, one will always encounter illness, injury, aging, and death. The religious agenda of ancient India was organized around liberating the soul from these rounds of rebirth and suffering, and, in the process, attaining a form of profound omniscience.

This is all very interesting to us today; because of the emphasis on awareness and direct experience, the problems posed by these ancient traditions, and the solutions offered to them, have a familiar psychological orientation. Unlike the dominant Western religions, which are grounded in a historical story line and come equipped with specific belief systems, Buddhism and its contemporaries were much more agnostic on matters of metaphysical revelation and focused instead on the practitioner's inner experience.

There is no particular religious explanation for why beings find themselves embedded in an unsatisfactory existence characterized by suffering, and there is nobody to call upon to bail them out. But through careful examination of the situation, they can begin to understand how their suffering is caused and can therefore learn how to work on undoing the conditions creating the discomfort. In these traditions, psychological and existential suffering are understood to have their origins in basic human drives and reflexes, which are for the most part unconscious and therefore apparently beyond one's control. But these can in fact be uncovered, behavioral responses can be modified, and it is possible to reprogram the mind and body substantially to avoid their instinctual shortcomings. What is required is a radical psychological transformation.

All the early schools shared the view that humans are actively participating in the endless turnings of this unsatisfying wheel of life through a combination of desire and ignorance. *Desire* is the deep compulsion to pursue pleasure and avoid pain, and *ignorance* points to the unconscious and unexamined nature of most of our attitudes and assumptions about the nature of things. Together, they condition how we construct our reality, lurching from one moment to another, trying, usually with only limited success, to satisfy an array of selfish and short-term needs.

The Importance of Experience

The Western intellectual tradition embraces rationality to govern unruly human nature. This rational bias can be seen in elegant and elaborated systems of law, social philosophy, and psychology. In the ancient Asian traditions, the rational and conceptual tools we value so highly in the West are seen as often being employed simply to rationalize and justify what we are driven to do, rather than offering much help in accurately understanding our predicament. So reasoning was not seen to offer much help. The revealed ancient truths, so highly valued by Western traditions, were also distrusted, because there was no assurance that the first in the file of blind men passing along the tradition had actually known or seen anything in his own direct experience. Another set of tools was needed to unravel the tangles of body and mind that held the soul in bondage to suffering, and this is where yoga, asceticism, and meditation became the crucial vehicles for self-exploration and self-transformation.

Yoga, in its original context, involved discipline, the yoking of body and mind, the binding of both to the will, and the fastening of human life to a higher purpose of discovery. It involved (and still may involve, depending on the practitioner) both asceticism and meditation, each of which works on loosening the bonds that tie the soul to suffering. Asceticism addresses desire by depriving the mind and body of what it desperately wants. In the practice of restraint, one can taste the flavor of desire, turn it over and examine its texture, and expose the hold it has upon the psychophysical organism. Meditation has more to do with learning to observe and to be keenly aware of what unfolds in the mind and body moment by moment. Honing an ever-sharpening experience of the present, the practice of meditation sheds light on processes that are otherwise invisible for their subtlety or overlooked for their ubiquity. All these techniques of experiential exploration were developed and cultivated over many centuries, and the lore they generated about the functioning of mind and body grew proportionally.

Meditation has much in common with the scientific enterprise of empirical observation. One simply regards the data of passing phenomenological experience as objectively as possible, using the apparatus of direct introspective awareness rather than the microscope or telescope. Until recently, meditation has not been amenable to outside measurement. However, it is by nature experimental insofar as one carefully notes the effect of various internal and external changes upon experience, and its techniques and findings are shown to be more or less replicated by whoever undertakes its rigors. This is why these practices are not so foreign and exotic to the modern psychological researcher, and why the ancient sciences of mind and body are being invited to contribute to the contemporary investigation of human consciousness and behavior.

THE CONSTRUCTION OF EXPERIENCE

The Emergence of Consciousness

The contemplative practices of ancient India gave rise to a very different way of viewing what we generally refer to as the *self* and the *world*. The sense of identity that every individual develops and the notion each has of the world in which he or she is embedded are regarded by the Buddhist tradition as an elaborate construction project. It is an edifice so complex and nuanced that it takes years of careful development and a tremendous amount of energy and attention to keep it in place. Ours is a universe of macro-construction, in which the continually arising data of the senses and of miscellaneous internal processing are channeled into structures and organized into schemas that support an entirely synthetic sphere of meaning—a virtual reality.

The mind is a world-building organ that pieces together a cosmos from the chaos of data streaming though the senses at breakneck speed. Beginning at the earliest possible age, human beings have to learn how to do this, and most of childhood development involves marching (in some reasonable order, one hopes) through various stages of growing complexity and, presumably, adaptation, during which the child learns to perceive the world as populated with stable objects that can be accurately known. It is a delicate process, and much can go wrong. Although the gradual building of identity that takes place over a lifetime is a well-studied subject in developmental psychology, the Buddhist tradition has considerably more to say about how world building can also be seen as occurring constantly, taking place each and every moment.

The process by which consciousness is constructed involves a number of components (see Figure 14.1). According to classical Buddhist analysis, the most elemental discernible unit of experience is a moment of *contact* between a sense organ, a sense object, and the awareness of that object. The coming together of these three factors, each itself the product of an entire process, sparks a synthetic incident of human cognition, an episode of sensory discernment, an event of "knowing" that forms the core around which human conscious existence is layered. *Consciousness* is thus an emergent, conditioned phenomenon, manifesting in

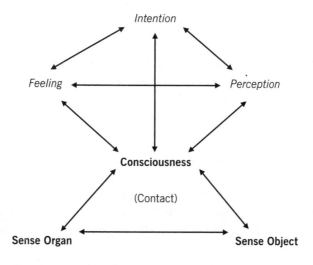

FIGURE 14.1. The interdependent construction of experience.

a series of momentary occurrences as simultaneously the agent, instrument, and activity of awareness (Bodhi, 2000).

The mode of the arising of conscious experience is codetermined by the nature of the organ and the object of its awareness with which it is interdependent. We call it *seeing* when the eye is used to discern a visible object, *hearing* when the ear is involved in noticing a sound, and depending on the other sensory supports, consciousness may manifest as *smelling*, *tasting*, *touching*, or *thinking*. This last is actually far more diverse than the term *thinking* usually covers and includes any mental event that is not already included in one of the other five sense modalities. According to Buddhist analysis, everything we are capable of experiencing arises in one of these six ways, and our entire world of experience is woven from the strands of such simple units of awareness.

Of considerable interest to the philosopher, if not the psychologist, is that in this view, none of the three elements of contact is ontologically primary; none possesses a privileged and enduring role. The material world presumably underlying the objects of the senses is irrelevant to the analysis of the human situation in an instant of awareness: The organs are not in the service of an entity that is "having" the experience, and consciousness is not something that can exist other than in the instant of its being enacted. Mind cannot be reduced to matter in this model, and neither is materiality merely a projection of mind. Rather, each is an equally important facet of a single psychophysical organism, which itself does not *exist* as much as it *occurs*. Early Buddhist thought has little interest in conceptual speculations about such matters, choosing instead to cleave to a rigorous empirical phenomenology. What one can actually see unfolding under scrutiny of the moment is considered to be of far more interest and use than theorizing from abstractions.

Perception and Feeling

The moment of contact between organs, objects, and consciousness is the seed around which a more complex manifestation of mind crystallizes. Also co-arising with these three are perception, feeling, and intention. In Buddhist psychology, these terms have unique and precise meanings.

Perception involves a host of associative functions that are learned gradually over time and are heavily conditioned by factors such as language and culture. It provides evaluative information about how the subject regards and construes the moment's experience; everything seen is *seen as* something; thus, every visual experience is automatically processed in light of previous understanding.

In this sense, perception is not the passive registration of the world received through the senses and represented accurately in awareness. In fact, it is a creative process of construction and categorization, drawing on past experience and the application of categories inherited from multiple sources. Consequently, it is not appropriate to say that we accurately perceive what is given; the act of perception often goes beyond the data present at the senses, potentially omitting details or filling in for missing information. Perception is also influenced by drive states; when we are hungry, we are more likely to notice restaurants than when we are not. This perspective is familiar to Western perceptual psychology.

This process offers a degree of efficiency, although, as the Buddhists would say, at the cost of considerable distortion and projection. The creative aspect of perception occurs without our conscious awareness that we bring more to the sense experience than is given (Bruner, 1973). The same is true of all the other senses, including the perception of all nonsensory cognitive experience, such as dreaming, planning, and imagining. The reflexive construction of perception is as ubiquitous to all mental activity as it is to every moment of sense experience.

Feeling is a word used in technical Buddhist vocabulary to refer to the affect tone associated with every object of sense or cognition. To the raw knowing that underlies every moment of experience is also added a hedonic tone, so that everything seen is *seen as* pleasant, unpleasant, or neutral. This feeling tone is also a natural and automatic part of the processing of every object known in any of the six modes of knowing (seeing, hearing, smelling, tasting, touching, or thinking) and becomes inextricably bound up with the way a moment is constructed.

In some cases, the clarity or strength of this charge is low, on which occasion the feeling tone is said to be neither pleasant nor unpleasant, but even when feelings are neutral, they play an important part in the texture of the moment. This process, too, ordinarily occurs outside of awareness, though it becomes an object of attention in meditation.

To summarize: Experience is so far seen to include five interdependent factors—an organ, an object, consciousness, perception, and feeling, all of which arise and fall together in the view of the attentive meditator.

The Role of Intention

One more psychologically important element—that of *intention*—is also added to this model of continuously arising factors. Intention involves the attitude taken toward what is happening in experience; it is the intentional stance one takes at any given moment. The word is used not in the sense of the goal to which action is directed, but rather of the *emotional quality of the mind* in the moment that action is initiated. Whereas the other factors are primarily contributing to our *knowing* what is going on internally or in the environment, intention is more a matter of what we are *doing* about it. Whereas objects appear to the organs of perception and are barely noticed by consciousness, and whereas perception and feeling have somewhat more to do with shaping the subjective significance of the object, intention is a more active and creative function that has a great impact on how the moment's experience is organized and presented by the mind.

Intention can have an active manifestation, for example, in a moment of attachment or aversion to present experience, an intentional stance of embracing or resisting what is happening. Put differently, intention is the factor that responds to the pleasant or unpleasant qualities of the arising experience by trying to hold on and perpetuate the experience, or to reject or terminate it. This is the pleasure principle, described by Freud (1920/1961d), in microscopic action.

Intention also manifests as action when activities of body, speech, and mind are initiated—either consciously or unconsciously—by the choice or decision to act one way or another. A *disposition to respond*, mentally or behaviorally, to circumstances in a characteristic or patterned way is an expression of a subtle, passive influence of intention. In Western psychological terms, dispositions resemble traits. Dispositions are learned from experience. We might also call these learned behaviors, conditioned responses, or personality characteristics.

According to Buddhist psychology, a person is continually shaped by his or her previous actions and their resulting dispositions. The personality is composed of bundles of such dispositions, laid down and regularly modified over one's entire lifetime, and it is from the background of these accumulated patterns that intentions, perceptions, and feelings in the next moment are shaped.

Every action is thus conditioned by all former actions, and every action also has an effect on all subsequent actions. In ancient India, the Sanskrit word for this process was *karma*. The great wheel of life, through which sentient beings "flow on" (as they conceived the mechanism of rebirth) from one lifetime to another, also functions on the microcosm: Beings flow on from one moment to another, continually being formed by previous selves and in turn continually forming and re-forming themselves and their world in each new moment. This is rebirth in psychological terms: Each moment is created anew from the conditions of previous events. Whether construed as occurring between lifetimes or between moments, the Buddhist notion of rebirth involves the perpetual *re-forming* of identity rather than the reemergence of a fixed entity suggested by the word *reincarnation*.

THE SELF

The Construction of Self

We can see from this basic overview of Buddhist psychology that a person is regarded as a process of continually unfolding dynamic systems, responding to a changing environment and perpetually reshaping itself as it constructs a meaningful order out of each moment's external and internal data. Mechanisms are in place to learn from experience and to retain information, and these structures stabilize over time such that each person acquires a unique set of characteristics. Some properties of this entire system change very rapidly, usually in response to some newly emerging stimuli, whereas other elements of character change very little or very gradually.

Although this process is fundamentally impersonal, as this system becomes sufficiently complex, the word *self* begins to be applied, bringing a whole new dimension to the model. As long as the psychophysical organism can be seen as a complex but impersonal process, one is able to maintain some intellectual and emotional detachment. But when self arises in experience as an existential entity—when the subsystems come to be misperceived as *belonging* to someone or as *owned* by a person—then the organism begins to respond in some very different ways.

According to classical Buddhist analysis, the application of the term *self* is a misunderstanding that causes considerable unnecessary difficulty. Much of this misunderstanding is rooted in the very way the mind has evolved to process information. It necessarily distorts reality in some important ways and on three different levels of scale: perception, thought, and view.

To begin with, the mind takes information from an uninterrupted flow of phenomena presenting at the sense doors. Perception consists of fixed bundles of data extracted from this background of perpetual flux, which amounts to constructing moments of apparent stability from an inherently unstable world. In Buddhist terminology, the mind is artificially creating moments of virtual permanence from an intrinsically impermanent universe. This is a distortion that is replicated at higher levels of processing. Thoughts, higher-level operations built upon such bundles of perception, also consist of staccato images and concepts, and views or beliefs are a further set of arbitrarily arrested attitudes and habits of mind.

The most important form of distortion fundamental to the way our minds operate involves creating the notion of self out of what is essentially an impersonal process. Selfhood is the expression of a particular kind of distorted view, a situation that develops gradually from basic misperceptions, to the casting of whole sets of misinformed thoughts, and eventually to a deeply rooted belief system that becomes imposed upon all further perception and thought. Here again we see a cyclical self-reinforcing pattern. Perceptions give rise to thoughts, which congeal into beliefs, and which then influence perception.

When the system operates optimally, it allows for growth, learning, and transformation. But when it is fundamentally misinformed, it can also give rise to a considerable amount of delusion. And this is what the Buddhists say is happening in the case of the ubiquitous belief in selfhood as a defining category of human psychology. They would not deny that stable patterns in this information-processing system provide a useful—perhaps even crucial—function in the organization of experience. But trouble arises when the constructed self becomes the main organizing principle, when it is unrealistically invested with qualities it does not innately possess, and, most importantly, when it becomes the node around which maladaptive behaviors coalesce. The self comes to be experienced as a central and dominant element of psychic life, mistaking what is a series of contingent patterns in constant flux for an enduring entity.

Self as a Cause of Suffering

Misunderstanding the nature of the self gives rise to suffering because it shapes our response to pleasurable and disagreeable experiences. Although pleasure and pain are a natural part of every moment's experience, the reflexive *desire* for pleasure to continue or for pain to cease introduces a different element not originally present in the barest elements of the experience. Desire is essentially the expression of a tension between what is happening and the person's intent to maximize gratification of the pleasure principle. It is the movement of mind that seeks for the next moment to be different from the present.

If I am adapted to an environmental temperature of 70 degrees, for example, and the temperature falls to 50 degrees, a *feeling* of discomfort might arise. This is my body's way of expressing its present state of disequilibrium. Now a desire might also emerge from this situation, manifest in my very much *wanting* to be warmer, to restore the feeling of pleasure that comes with being in balance with the environment.

Here is where my level of understanding makes a big difference. If my understanding is sufficiently developed to realize how all this is just the natural unfolding of cause and effect in a depersonalized psycho-physical system, the cold is merely cold; there is no expectation for it to be otherwise. Moreover, the presence of the cold is not a personal insult. Discomfort about the temperature may persist, but the desire for it to be different (i.e., the suffering) does not. This attentive but dispassionate quality is often described as *equanimity*, an attitude of mind capable of embracing both pleasure and pain, without being driven by them into the *action* of desire. Lacking equanimity and understanding, I might instead feel compelled to gratify my desire at any cost, an attitude the Buddhists refer to as *clinging* or *grasping*.

Much of our ordinary daily experience is colored by clinging, a process as dangerous as it is common, for a number of reasons. First there is the quality of compulsion, or being driven into action lacking in conscious choice. Without the mental ease to choose to act otherwise, we are in a cycle of conditioned responses, responding little differently than an animal or a machine might. We lose our humanity, our ability to act freely and with awareness.

Also, the pressing need to gratify the desire, whether in the pursuit of pleasure or the avoidance of pain, may lead us to overlook the needs and rights of others when they conflict with our own. Taking the former example to an extreme, we might hoard fuel and turn up the thermostat regardless of how much fuel is available for others, or we might even forcibly deprive a weaker person of clothing to keep ourselves warm.

Finally, clinging behavior reinforces the construct of selfhood. In the moment of grasping for something or pushing something away, the self as agent is created. This self experiences itself as the originator and beneficiary of this action. A sought-after object is labeled *mine* in the act of acquiring it, whereas a resisted or rejected object is defined in one's mind as *not mine*. In both instances, the world of experience becomes intensely personalized.

With this insight, the Buddhists are really offering a Copernican revolution to our understanding of selfhood and identity. It is not that a person *exists* (an assertion that so often goes unexamined) and then may identify with certain objects, ideas, and so on. Rather the person, conceived as an individual self with a particular identity, is *created* in a momentary act of identification. And with a *view* of selfhood underlying and shaping all experience, a person becomes motivated to create him- or herself moment after moment after moment. A sense of self is projected on to all experience. The solidity and coherence of the self is apparent, emerging from innumerable instants of self-building, just as the apparent reality of a movie emerges from the illusion of continuity generated by numerous individual frames of film.

The self is born and dies, rises and passes away, moment after moment, whenever one grasps after or clings to the gratification of desires. Yet each time one desire is satisfied, another will emerge, suggesting that no meaningful sense of peace or fulfillment can ever occur. This is the etiology of suffering in Buddhist psychology. The Buddhist word *dukkha*, mentioned earlier, is the term that denotes this suffering or unsatisfactoriness, a fundamental flaw in the mind–body operating system and thus in the human condition.

Identification with Self

Once we mistake the transient, constructed self for something enduring and central, we further reinforce it in our unexamined tendency to perceive that all experience is happening to "me." This is compounded by our use of the self as the yardstick of value; that is, an event is judged as good if I desire it and bad if I do not. Because of the way each moment carries a specific feeling tone, there is scarcely a moment that is not so judged. The world becomes divided into good *for me* and bad *for me*. So busy are we casting the world in light refracted through our desires, we miss the world as it is, intimate though impersonal.

The Buddhist analysis describes the self as a construct that arises with the requisite conditions and passes when those conditions are absent. It does not endure. However, once we come to mistake the self as somehow more real and enduring than it is, we have another problem on our hands. We spend much of our lives trying to fortify, defend, and aggrandize ourselves, fearing that failure to do so will result in our annihilation.

From this perspective the defenses, described so well in early psychoanalytic literature, are not enlisted so much against conscious knowledge of instinctual drives, but rather to buttress the illusion of self. Theorists as diverse as Alfred Adler (1927/2002), Ernest Becker (1973), and Erving Goffman (1971) have discussed how the drive to maintain self-esteem is a primary motive in psychological and social life. People often seek psychotherapy because of the elusive nature of achieving self-esteem. We calibrate our self-esteem by constant comparison with others, and we evaluate things and people based on whether they support or challenge our constructed identity. As a result, we can feel impoverished in the face of abundance. Others can become "part objects," judged by their value to our sense of self. When others become depersonalized in this manner, the way is paved for social cruelty.

Given the tremendous value placed on the self in Western culture, it is no surprise that disorders of the self are so prevalent. From a Buddhist perspective, these disorders are mere exaggerations of a fundamental misunderstanding about who we are.

MINDFULNESS AND THE HEALING OF SUFFERING

The Buddha characterized himself as a physician whose primary work was identifying the malady afflicting humankind, uncovering its causes, using that knowledge to see how it can be cured, and laying out a program through which each person can find well-being. He demonstrated all of these steps first himself. According to tradition, the prince Siddhartha became the Buddha one night when he finally saw clearly how the mind and body create their own suffering, and was able to so transform himself such that suffering entirely ended for him. Having cured himself, he then went on to help others.

Even the earliest path of development articulated in the classical Buddhist tradition is quite rich and diverse. It was understood that different people have different strengths and weaknesses, different capabilities, and find themselves in a wide range of worldly circumstances. The Buddha understood, as any physician would, that the healing process involves far more than just medicine. The understanding and cooperation of the patient, the level of care and support available from others, and environmental factors, such as nutrition, rest, and time, all play important roles in determining the success of the treatment. Therefore, although the naming of the illness, the identification of its root causes, and the core elements of its cure are all quite standard elements of the tradition, the number of ways to go about effecting that cure are tremendously variable. Each generation seems to develop a regimen that is best suited to its own unique environment. This is what has allowed Buddhism to adapt to so many different cultures over two and a half millennia.

The starting point for the program of healing prescribed by the Buddha is mindfulness meditation. It will not effect the cure entirely on its own, but no real progress toward well-being can occur without it. Because suffering is constructed each moment in reflexive and unexamined ways, it is first necessary to be able to illuminate something of the process. Whereas a healthy human being is working hard at creating and maintaining the conceptual edifice of personal identity most of the time, mindfulness meditation invites us to attend simply to the field of phenomena, to *that which arises* at the level of absolute sensory and cognitive immediacy. Phenomena will appear or arise at any of the five sense "doors" of the eye, ear, nose, tongue, and body, or they will arise as objects of awareness in the "mind door" itself. The capacity to be aware of these data *as phenomena,* rather than as the objects of our conceptually constructed world, takes a great deal of training and practice.

Our reflexes and instincts are entirely directed to overlooking the details of incoming experience in order to reinforce ongoing projects at the macro-level of construction. In simpler terms, we are so invested in the larger picture of goals, strategies, and the validation of assumptions and belief systems that we are in the habit of relating to sensory and cognitive detail as *means toward an end.* Mindfulness meditation gradually teaches us to regard this ongoing stream of textured experience as an *end in itself.* The aim is not to undermine completely the conventional world we construct, but rather to put it into its proper perspective. By learning to view this otherwise overlooked level of raw appearances, we begin to reveal the *process* of identity building and world construction itself, instead of remaining entirely focused on the *product* of this process.

Mindfulness practice helps to reverse our tendency to lean ahead into the next moment, to rush forward to the level of macro-construction. By bringing deliberate and sustained attention to the field of phenomena itself, we train the mind to inhabit the more open, unformed space of freshly arising experience. The mind will naturally incline into its various construction projects (thoughts, memories, plans, fantasies, etc.), but as it does so, we are able to see more clearly *that* it is doing so and *how* it is doing so. By observing the move from arising phenomena to thought creation, we begin to reveal the highly constructed nature of experience. From this starting point of heightened awareness of the mind's present-moment activity, a range of options for learning and growing becomes accessible. A detailed program of transformation was laid out in the early Buddhist literature (Nanamoli & Bodhi, 1995), and has been continually elaborated by centuries of tradition.

CLASSICAL MINDFULNESS TRAINING

Mindfulness of Body

In the classical tradition mindfulness is cultivated by applying it systematically to four general objects. The first is the body. Attending carefully to the physical sensations that arise in conjunction with breathing, for example, will yield an ever-present but continually changing set of phenomena to observe. The quality of attention brought to bear on these changing sensations gradually deepened as practice develops. The inbreath alone might at first seem to be accompanied by only a few discernible sensations at the nose, the abdomen, or as the clothing moves against the skin, but as skill increases, one will tend to notice more and more. Before long, a single inbreath might seem filled with a whole universe of nuanced physical phenomena, each, though exceedingly brief, with its own unique texture.

The same increasing acumen can be directed to the body as it assumes different positions: seated, standing, lying down, or walking. Each of these provides its own universe of unique sensations, an endless landscape for phenomenological exploration. Also centering on the body, mindfulness might be developed by observing physical objects of touch as one moves through the range of normal behaviors such as eating, drinking, falling asleep, or waking up. Or one might augment one's capacity to discern the raw physical manifestations of resistance, movement, and temperature, which the Buddhists identify as the basic components of all physical sensation.

Another exercise is to "sweep" the body with one's mindful awareness, from the tip of the head to the soles of the feet, identifying the sensation in each of the different components of the body. The aim in all these cases is to become and remain aware only of the physical sensations arising through one of the sense doors, the "body door," without reverting to seeing, hearing, thinking, or any of the other modes of experience.

Mindfulness of Feeling

Mindfulness can also be applied to feeling tones. Here the practitioner brings attention to the pleasant or unpleasant quality of every experience. It requires and develops the capacity to distinguish a bodily sensation, for example, from the feeling arising in conjunction with it. One becomes able to discriminate physical sensations arising in one's knee, for example, from the profound unpleasantness and even pain that is arising with it. The *touch* of the bodily sensation is one phenomenon; the *pain* of that touch is another. Classical mindfulness meditation seeks to nurture this level of precision.

The same is true even of mental objects arising in the mind. Each memory, thought, or image will be accompanied by a feeling tone that is *pleasant, unpleasant,* or *neutral.* Even when the feeling tone does not easily resolve itself under scrutiny as being particularly pleasant or unpleasant (as in the case of neutral feeling), it is still providing an ongoing, tangible sensation to all modes of experience that can be discerned by the practiced meditator. The temperature in the meditation room, for example, as experienced by the nerve receptors in the skin, may not seem too hot or too cold but may nevertheless yield a constant stream of feeling tones. Being able to unravel these two strands of experience—an object known through a sense door and the feeling tone accompanying that object—begins to reveal the restless movement of mind and contributes to a deeper understanding of its constructed nature.

Mindfulness of Mind

As the mind itself becomes the object of mindfulness meditation, the observer is invited to notice whether or not this particular moment of consciousness is accompanied by one of the three root causes of suffering, or afflictive intentional constructs: greed, hatred, or delusion. In any given moment, the mind is either caught up by one or more of these or it is not, and this is something of which one can learn to be aware. Greed and hatred are the two poles of desire, the intense *wanting* or *not wanting* of an object, whereas delusion is a strong form of the basic misunderstanding that gives desire its power over us.

For example, when discomfort is detected in the body because one remains unmoving in a seated position for some length of time, one can notice the growing resistance to the sensory information being received from the body. One can almost taste the building dissatisfaction, the "wanting the unpleasant physical sensations to go away" or to change into something else. At the next moment, one can experience the same situation in another light, the "wanting pleasant physical sensations to arise" in the body instead. It can be quite difficult to discern when the "not wanting unpleasant sensations" leaves off and the "wanting pleasant sensations" begins to arise and replace the former. Exploring the texture of this ambiguity, even though it may manifest as confusion, is what mindfulness of mind is all about, and it contributes to a growing phenomenological intelligence.

In yet another subsequent moment, the meditator may well experience the realization that both wanting and not wanting are just turnings of the mind's habitual response mechanisms, following from contact with certain physical sensations in the context of certain attitudes. Such a minor but significant insight might be followed by a return to awareness of the physical sensations, but recontextualized in a way that enables greater equanimity or less personal investment. Such a shift in attitude might be accompanied by a physical or mental sigh, a further attentive relaxing of the body, and a fresh resolve to look carefully but patiently at experience in whatever mode it is actually arising. Through the eye of equanimity, the quality of wanting or not wanting is temporarily absent from the mind, and the texture of this state, too, can be examined.

In this brief example, one has become aware of how the mind is at first afflicted with aversion, desire, and confusion, and then, following a moment of insight, how the mind manifests without these afflictions. By investigating the arising of these attitudes of mind in experience, mindfulness enters an evaluative stage that has the potential to transform. One might simply notice without judgment the variegated textures of physical sensations and even the alternating episodes of pleasure and pain; but as one sees a moment of aversive mind followed by a moment of nonaversive mind, or a moment of clear insight after innumerable moments of obscuration, one cannot help but notice the contrast.

It is not a matter of deciding conceptually that one is wholesome and the other unwholesome, for that is just the sort of *thinking about* experience that is counterproductive to the process. Rather, one develops an intuitive understanding, as a manifestation of insight or wisdom, about the relative effect of one mind state or another. We are still squarely in the realm of descriptive phenomenology rather than in higher level cognitive understanding.

Mindfulness of Mental Objects

A fourth foundation upon which mindfulness can become established is referred to as the *mindfulness of mental objects or mental phenomena*. Here one brings the same quality of nuanced awareness of that which arises to the actual content of mental experience. But since we are now at the culmination of the transformative path of mindfulness, it is not just a matter of being aware of whatever happens to arise and pass away in the mind. There is a detailed agenda, following the primary teachings of Buddhist psychology, of what to look for and how to work toward abandoning the factors that inhibit understanding, while cultivating the factors that augment it.

Five Hindrances

First, there are five *hindrances* or obstacles to clarity of mind that one can observe as present, absent, or arising in the mind when they had not been present. These are sense desire, aversion, indolence, restlessness, and doubt. One can also become aware of an attitude of nonattachment to such mental states that will cause them to pass away, and of an intentional stance toward such phenomena that will inhibit their re-arising in the future. Each of these five steps can be applied to each of the five hindrances. When one practices mindfulness in this particular way, these five qualities of mind will diminish and even cease, if only temporarily, and the mind will become considerably clearer as a result. Bringing focused awareness to the first hindrance of sense desire, for example, serves to uncover the innate reflex of the sensory apparatus to seek stimulation. Experientially, this presents as a subtle wanting that underlies all six of the human sense capabilities. Consciously working to set aside this stance of being primed for sensory stimulation, even temporarily, can bring open-mindedness to the moment that allows for a greater range of response.

Five Aggregates

Next in the classical scheme comes bringing awareness to the five *aggregates* of experience themselves, namely, materiality, feeling, perception, consciousness, and formations (referred to earlier as *intentions* and *dispositions*). Here the exercise is to simply be aware of each of these strands of compounded experience and to notice how each continually arises and passes away. This fivefold typology of experience is the Buddhist way of undermining the habitual tendency to reify personal identity. The tradition understands that people routinely assume the existence of a unified agent (the seer, feeler, thinker) underlying the flux of experience. Redirecting attention to each of these five categories gradually has the effect of emphasizing the flux of experience itself rather than the construction of a synthetic sense of unity. The phenomenological data merely reveal that seeing, feeling, and thinking occur; invoking the label of an agent noun (the *I* to whom it is happening) is unnecessary and unwarranted.

Six Sense Spheres

Following this focus, we have each of the six *sense spheres*, or sense doors, as objects of conscious awareness. In this case, the meditator observes, to take the first example, the eye or organ of perception and also the visual form or object of perception. These are referred to as the internal and the external manifestation of the sensory field. Moreover, the practitioner of mindfulness also notices phenomenologically how desire arises in conjunction with each of the sense spheres. Desire is not something general; in the momentary model of constructed experience, desire will always manifest for a specific mental or physical object.

Understanding the way any instance of desire is dependent upon and emergent from a particular sensory experience is an important insight yielded by these exercises in awareness. Having seen this, the practitioner is then in a position to notice, as with the hindrances, how abandoning one's attachment for this desire will facilitate its disappearance, and how attitudes can be expressed and repeated that will help effect its non-arising in the future.

Seven Factors of Awakening

Of great importance to the traditional form of mindfulness meditation is the awareness of seven positive factors in the growth toward wisdom. These are called the seven *factors of awakening*, and include mindfulness, the investigation of phenomena, energy, joy, tranquility, concentration, and equanimity (see Chapter 4 for a description of these qualities applied to psychotherapy). As before, one is guided simply to observe whether each of these is present or absent in any particular moment of consciousness, and when it is not present to see how it sometimes then arises. But unlike mindfulness of the hindrances, the object is not to abandon these mental factors, but to cultivate them. Again, there can be an intuitive understanding of the beneficial effect that each of these mental states has upon one's mind and body in the moment, and one can learn what sort of intentional stance will develop these factors.

Each of these particular states supports the others, so that guiding one's attention carefully through this list will gradually transform one's mind in the direction of greater wisdom and understanding. Again, mindfulness is the first step, and when the simple presence of mind upon currently arising phenomena matures, it will naturally lead to a deep interest in the coming and going of mental states. As each is investigated ever more closely, it will give rise to a natural energy and enthusiasm, which itself turns into a profound sense of joy that seems equally seated in the body and in the mind. The joy is effervescent, apparently bubbling up from deep springs, but this will gradually be tempered by tranquility. One does not replace the other, but what then ensues is the paradoxical state of tranquil energy. Here the mind is both peaceful and alert; it is calm, relaxed, and at ease, but acutely aware, without effort, of the rising and passing of phenomena. The tranquility brings greater *concentration*, defined as a focus or one-pointedness of mind that will naturally take one object of awareness at a time (see Chapter 1), but with such skill that it can mindfully process innumerable bits of data very quickly. Finally, as each of these factors fulfills and completes one another, a profound equanimity of mind, embracing all these qualities, becomes established. In this state, say the Buddhists, one is capable of overcoming, if only for a time, the obscuring and distorting effects of desire and misunderstanding upon the moment-to-moment construction of experience.

A TOOL FOR OUR TIMES

Such is a brief overview of how mindfulness may be understood and developed in the traditional context of classical Buddhist practice. The end toward which the practice is devoted is nothing less than the complete and radical transformation of the human psychophysical organism. This transformation may be modest at first, involving occasional moments of insight into one's motivations, of freedom from the hold of some conditioning, or of refuge from the constant onslaught of selfishness and desire. But these moments are cumulative and gradually gain momentum as more and more of the underlying patterns of our psychological process become revealed.

Mindfulness leads to insight, and insight leads to wisdom. The kind of insight referred to in this context is not the conceptual insight into one's personal narrative, but a more visceral and intuitive glimpse of the conditioned, constructed, changeable, and impersonal nature of our mental and physical life. It is an insight that loosens the bonds of attachment and opens the heart to a context wider than the merely self-referential. As unconscious patterns of behavior become exposed to the light of conscious awareness through the practice of mindfulness, they lose much of their power to deceive and compel us. The very way the data of the senses are organized each moment into the building of a personality and a view of the world begins to change. Eventually, recurring episodes of insight will contribute to more lasting alterations of the mind, a process the Buddhists refer to as the *deepening of wisdom*. This sort of insight changes us profoundly.

At its farthest point of culmination, the attainment of awakening (*nirvana* in Sanskrit), greed, hatred, and delusion are eliminated entirely. A person is still constructing experience moment to moment by means of sense organs and perception, and experiences both pleasure and pain. The difference is that the pleasure will not give rise to the desire for more pleasure, and the pain will not be met with aversion, resistance, or denial. Action is therefore no longer motivated by grasping after satisfaction, and identity as a node around which self-interested behavior is organized no longer gets constructed. A person moves through the world responding appropriately to events as they emerge, and his or her life becomes an expression of the more altruistic intentions of generosity (nongreed), kindness (nonhatred) and understanding (nondelusion).

We are left with a picture of a person who is content in any circumstance, free of involuntary conditioning, and in no way driven into action by compulsion. Such a person accepts the constant changeability of the world, no longer expects gratification beyond the meeting of certain contextual needs (e.g., eating or drinking when appropriate, but without attachment), exerts no claim of ownership over any object or element of experience, and perhaps most importantly, does not suffer under the narcissistic delusion of inflated personal identity. Such a view of human potential suggests the transformation of the human psychophysical organism to a higher stage of development.

Because mindfulness is being used as a psychotherapeutic intervention, we might predict that, in time, the way we understand the goals of therapy will be broadened to embrace a larger view of what is possible and the possibility of a deeper sort of contentment.

15

The Neurobiology of Mindfulness

Sara W. Lazar

Sow a thought, and you reap an act;
Sow an act, and you reap a habit;
Sow a habit, and you reap a character;
Sow a character, and you reap a destiny.
—19th-CENTURY ENGLISH PROVERB

*F*or over 2,000 years, it has been claimed that meditation can bring about a wide range of benefits to the body and mind. Only recently, however, has the scientific community begun to unveil the numerous changes that occur while one is meditating, such as decreases in stress hormones and increases in biological markers associated with physical relaxation.

Beyond the immediate effects of meditation, practitioners also report experiencing longer-lasting, trait-like changes. Although the sense of calm and clarity that arises during formal sitting meditation tends to diminish during the day, practitioners frequently report that morning meditation helps them cope more effectively with difficult situations, have more empathy and compassion, have better memory, and pay better attention. Scientists have begun to test these claims, and good research evidence now exists to support some of them, particularly increased ability to pay attention and more frequent experiences of compassion. However, it's still not clear exactly how the practice of meditation might lead to these widespread effects, and in particular, which neural mechanisms may underlie these beneficial changes. This chapter explores how meditation practice impacts the brain and how these brain changes may, in turn, lead to long-lasting benefits.

NEUROPLASTICITY

Before we dive into the structure and function of the brain, first we need to understand human behavior from a neural perspective. In this chapter, I use the word *behavior* to mean any action of the body or the mind. Under this umbrella, the aspects of human experience that meditators claim can be changed with practice, such as emotional responses, attention, or intention, are all defined as behaviors. And, from a neural perspective, all these behaviors are the product of brain *activity*, which is itself dependent on brain *structure* (see Figure 15.1).

Brain structure can be very loosely defined as anything related to the way in which neurons communicate with each other, ranging from the number of connections between neurons to the amount of neurotransmitter that is released between them. It is generally believed by neuroscientists that in order to have a long-lasting shift in behavior, there must be a corresponding change in brain structure. This possibility of change is called *neuroplasticity*. For example, as you read the words in this book, the neurons in your brain are processing the visual input into concepts and comprehending them in various ways. This is brain *activity*. In order to store the information for later use, somewhere in the brain neurons need to change something about how they communicate with each other (i.e., structure). We don't really understand this process yet, but we know that a series of events leads to changes that result in the formation of a memory. If you try to recall tomorrow what you have just read, those neurons will fire and produce a spurt of brain activity, and you will remember those ideas. When a behavior is repeated many times, such as bringing attention back to the present moment during meditation practice, the cascade of corresponding brain activity gradually changes and the pattern gets encoded differently than random behaviors. The structure of the brain has changed, and this new pattern now drives behavior. This is how habits form.

Neuroplasticity is also at the heart of the therapeutic process. For example, if a depressed patient goes to see a doctor, the doctor might prescribe antidepressant medication, which will alter the patient's brain structure (e.g., the receptors that reuptake serotonin). The medication will change the amount or type of communication between neurons, which will bring about changes in behavior, namely, a less depressed

Structure ⇌ Activity ⇌ Behavior

FIGURE 15.1. The interrelationship between brain structure, activity, and behavior.

mood. Similarly, a psychotherapist might challenge some of the patient's beliefs and self-doubts or encourage the patient to look at situations from a different perspective. When talk-therapy techniques are successful, there will be some change in brain structure that accompanies the change in perspective or attitude. Goldapple and colleagues (2004) provide an interesting example of this sort of change with patients suffering from major depression.

Now let's consider meditation. Using the framework described above, we can postulate that while engaged in meditation practice, the brain should display a specific pattern of brain activity that is different from normal brain activity. With repeated practice this activity should lead to changes in brain structure that are related to that practice. These alterations in structure should then support altered patterns of brain activity, even when the person is not meditating. Next, we consider the evidence that has been published to date to support each of these steps.

BRAIN ACTIVITY DURING MEDITATION

We begin with looking at what happens in the brain during meditation. From a cognitive neuroscience perspective, meditation is a highly heterogeneous and multifaceted task, involving both intense concentrative focus as well as an openness to sensory experiences, emotions, and thoughts. Furthermore, some meditation techniques, such as loving-kindness meditation (*metta*, in Pali), incorporate visualization and/or efforts to engender specific mind states. Consistent with this notion, researchers have begun to identify specific neural networks believed to underlie different forms of meditation. A drawback to these studies is that they have often varied significantly in their design and the type of meditation studied, making it difficult in some cases to compare results. However, several consistent findings have begun to emerge.

One of the most consistent findings is deactivation of a network of brain regions termed the *default mode network* (DMN; Bærensten et al., 2010; Brewer, Worhunsky, et al., 2011; Hasenkamp, Wilson-Mendenhall, Duncan, & Barsalou, 2012). Numerous studies have demonstrated the presence of certain networks of brain regions that are active during rest that carry out basic "housekeeping" tasks that are necessary to function normally. The most prominent of these is the DMN, which is thought to play a central role in creating and maintaining the *autobiographical self*, that is, supporting functions that create the sense of self and identity. This network is also hypothesized to generate spontaneous thoughts during mind wandering, and has been implicated in numerous psychiatric and neurological conditions, including Alzheimer's and autism. Deactivation of this network is consistent with meditation as a state of focused attention characterized by minimal mind wandering and self-referential activity.

These studies also revealed that brain regions important for attention, salience determination, and cognitive control were more active during meditation periods than during rest (Brewer, Worhunsky, et al., 2011; Hasenkamp et al., 2012; Tang et al., 2009). Brewer, Worhunsky, and colleagues (2011) further demonstrated that the DMN was more connected (i.e., more "in synch") with these cognitive control areas, consistent with the idea that during meditation there is more moment-to-moment monitoring and control of one's own mind state, which may help decrease the incidence of mind wandering. Hasenkamp and colleagues demonstrated that activity in one subregion of the DMN, the ventromedial prefrontal cortex (vmPFC), was inversely correlated with amount of meditation experience, suggesting that meditation experience may allow for a faster or more efficient disengagement of the cognitive processes subserved by this region.

Similarly, in a study with Tibetan monks, Brefczynski-Lewis, Lutz, Schaefer, Levinson, and Davidson (2007) demonstrated that the monks had considerably less activity in the anterior cingulate cortex (ACC) during meditation compared to controls who had been meditating for a week. The ACC is often associated with directing attention, so it might be expected that more experienced meditators would show greater activation than novice meditators. Alternatively, as more experienced meditators often report that they can sustain periods of uninterrupted attention longer than novice meditators, it may result in less need for ACC activity. When Hölzel and colleagues (2007) attempted to replicate these results using experienced lay insight meditation practitioners, they found that these participants showed *more* activity in the ACC as compared to nonmeditators. This discrepancy may result from the fact that Brefczynski-Lewis and colleagues tested highly trained monks, whereas Hölzel and colleagues tested lay practitioners, whose ability to sustain attention is undoubtedly less developed than the monks' ability.

An additional region activated during meditation in Tibetan monks is the anterior insula (Brefczynski-Lewis et al., 2007; Lutz, Greischar, Perlman, & Davidson, 2009). The insula is associated with interoception, which is the perception of visceral feelings such as hunger and thirst, as well as balance and detection of the heart and breathing rate. The insula has also been proposed as a key region involved in processing transient bodily sensations, thereby contributing to our experience of *selfness* (Craig, 2009). One hypothesis for the increased activation of the insula during meditation is that it reflects the mediator's careful attention to the arising and passing of internal sensations. The insula plays a key role in affective responses to pain (Casey, Minoshima, Morrow, & Koeppe, 1996) as well as in internally generated emotions (Rieman et al., 1997).

CHANGES IN BRAIN STRUCTURE THAT OCCUR AS A RESULT OF PRACTICE

We now consider brain structure. Magnetic resonance imaging (MRI) is like a giant camera, and there are two different types of images that can be taken: functional and structural. *Functional* MRI (fMRI) images capture changes in whichever part of the brain is active in real time. When someone is engaging in a particular task, we can observe on the scan which parts of the brain are active during that task, relative to rest or to other tasks. In contrast, *structural* MRI images reveal how much gray or white matter is present in different parts of the brain. This reveals information about how the brain is wired, and thus provides evidence that meditation practice can lead to long-lasting changes in how the brain works.

In 2005 we conducted a study that examined the brain structure of 20 lay practitioners of Theravada meditation and 15 control subjects who were matched with the meditators for gender, age, education and race, but had no experience practicing meditation (Lazar et al., 2005). We investigated brain structure by calculating the thickness of each person's gray matter. *Gray matter* refers to the parts of the brain where neurons talk to each other and where "thinking" and neural activity actually happen, whereas *white matter* refers to the parts of the brain that are comprised mostly of long-distance fibers carrying information from one part of the brain to another.

The core question we asked was: Does gray matter change as a result of meditation practice? We were led to this inquiry by several studies that compared specific groups of people and found differences in gray matter. One study looked at bilingual individuals and found that those who learn a second language as a young child have significantly more gray matter in brain regions associated with language when compared to those who learn a second language as a teenager, or individuals who speak only one language. Similarly, another study found professional musicians to have more gray matter than amateur musicians in areas of the brain related to musical ability, and that the amateurs had more gray matter than people with no musical training. In each of these studies, the amount of gray matter correlated with proficiency or experience (Gaser & Schlaug, 2003; Mechelli et al., 2004). The results of this research led us to hypothesize that there should also be differences in the brains of our subjects, who had all been practicing meditation for many years.

The long-term meditators had increased cortical thickness in the anterior insula and sensory cortex, regions involved in observing internal and external physical sensations, respectively. The insula was one of the regions found to be active during meditation that we discussed earlier (Brefczynski-Lewis et al., 2007). Given the emphasis on observing sensory stimuli that occurs during meditation, thickening in these regions is consistent with subjective reports of mindfulness practice. Interestingly, decreased volume in the anterior insula has been strongly implicated in several psychopathologies, including posttraumatic stress disorder (PTSD), social anxiety, specific phobias, and schizophrenia (Crespo-Facorro et al., 2000; Etkin & Wager, 2007; Phillips, Drevets, Rauch, & Lane, 2003; Wright et al., 2000). The insula has also been found to be active in monks when they are engaging in compassion practices (Lutz, Greischar, et al., 2009). Regions of the frontal cortex, an area devoted to decision making and cognitive processing, were also larger in meditators. It is well known that this part of the brain normally decreases in thickness as we age. Interestingly, when we plotted each person's cortical thickness in this region against his or her age, the graph suggested that meditation might help to slow down or even prevent this normal age-related decline in thickness.

Several additional studies have examined gray matter structure in long-term practitioners (Grant et al., 2011; Hölzel et al., 2008; Leung et al., 2012; Luders, Toga, Lepore, & Gaser, 2009; Luders et al., 2012; Pagnoni & Cekic, 2007; Vestergaard et al., 2009). Each study has reported different results, however, perhaps because each research group used subjects who practiced in different lineages of Buddhist meditation, had different criteria for how much the subjects needed to have practiced, or varied in the age of the subjects who were included. Each of these factors can influence results. Also, each study used slightly different methods for analyzing gray matter, and it is known that each method is sensitive to different aspects of gray matter structure. Therefore, it's difficult to directly compare the results.

Despite these differences, three brain regions have been identified in at least two studies, giving extra credence to the findings. These three regions are the right anterior insula, the left inferior temporal gyrus, and the hippocampus. The left inferior temporal lobe, which was identified in three studies (Hölzel et al., 2008; Leung et al., 2012; Luders et al., 2009), is involved in creating the sense of agency. The hippocampus plays a central role in memory, and has also been implicated in emotion regulation. The hippocampus is the only part of the brain that generates new neurons throughout our entire life. However, excessive cortisol levels, a steroid hormone that is released in response to stress, is toxic to these cells and can prevent new neurons from being generated. These neuroimaging studies with meditators suggest that meditation practice may hold the potential to prevent the detrimental effects of stress on the brain, which has important implications for numerous psychological conditions in which the structure and function of the hippocampus are important, such as depression and PTSD.

An important caveat to the structural findings discussed so far is that all the studies employed long-term meditation practitioners. Therefore, the observed differences could be due to other lifestyle differences between the groups, such as vegetarian diet, or the differences may have existed prior to the individuals' decision to start meditating. However, some of the studies (Hölzel et al., 2007; Lazar et al., 2005; Leung et al., 2012) have found correlations between amount of gray matter and amount of meditation practice, providing indirect evidence that these regions are the result of meditation and not a spurious finding.

To address these issues, we recently tested whether similar types of changes occur in novices who are just beginning to meditate (Hölzel et al., 2010; Hölzel, Carmody, et al., 2011). We recruited individuals from the Center for Mindfulness in Medicine in Worcester, Massachusetts, who were interested in undergoing the 8-week mindfulness-based stress reduction (MBSR) program. This highly structured program focuses on training participants in core mindfulness and meditative practices. We conducted MRI scans both before participants entered the course and after its completion and compared the imaging data collected from the participants to a wait-list control group. We found gray matter changes in four regions: the hippocampus, a region called the posterior cingulate cortex (PCC), a region called the temporal–parietal junction (TPJ), and part of the cerebellum. Gray matter in the insula was also increased, though the difference was not statistically significant when compared to the control group.

As discussed earlier, the hippocampus is integral to learning and memory, and it has been identified in numerous studies of both brain structure and function related to meditation. The PCC is part of the DMN and plays a central role in creating or understanding the context in which a stimulus or event occurs, and also determining the relevance of that stimulus to the self. As discussed above, activity in the PCC *decreases* during meditation (Brewer, Worhunsky, et al., 2011; Hasenkamp et al., 2012). Although finding increased amounts of gray matter in a region with decreased activity seems counterintuitive, this is not an uncommon finding, as the relationship between structure and function can be complex. Altered gray matter simply reflects a change in neural architecture in this area, which we presume supports altered functioning.

The third region with increased gray matter density was the TPJ, which plays a central role in empathy and compassion (Decety & Michalska, 2010). The TPJ also appears to play a central role in mediating the first-person perspective of bodily states (Arzy, Thut, Mohr, Michel, & Blanke, 2006; Blanke et al., 2005). TPJ deficits are associated with out-of-body experiences (Blanke & Arzy, 2005), suggesting that gray matter changes in this region might underlie increased sense of embodiment as a result of meditation training.

In addition to finding regions of increased gray matter, we also found a decrease in the gray matter density of the amygdala, which was correlated with a change in perceived stress levels (Hölzel et al., 2010; see Figure 15.2). The amygdala is well known to play a central role in emotional arousal and in mediating physiological responses to threats. The greater the decrease in a participant's stress levels following MBSR, the less dense the amygdala was. This finding has an important parallel with studies conducted on rats (Mitra, Jadhav, McEwen, Vyas, & Chattarji, 2005). In these animal experiments it was found that the amygdala of the rats had become *denser* after the animals were placed in a stressful living situation. The researchers then put the rats back in a nonstressful environment. Interestingly, even when they tested the rats again 3 weeks later, the amygdala remained denser and the animals behaved like they were still being stressed. Their environment returned to a peaceful state, but not their brains or their behavior. This was the opposite situation for our subjects. Following the 8-week mindfulness intervention, their lives were still the same; they still had the same stressful jobs and the same difficult people in their lives. Their environment had not changed,

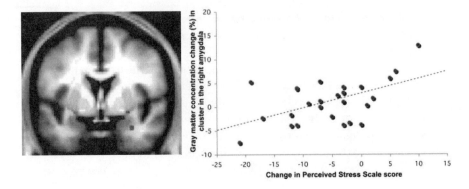

FIGURE 15.2. Change in stress is correlated with change in amygdala gray matter. From Hölzel et al. (2010). Copyright 2010 by Oxford University Press.

but their brains and *their relationship to their environment* had. The decreased size of the amygdala is a reflection of this internal shift.

Unfortunately, we do not know exactly what causes these changes in gray matter. In the hippocampus, it may be that more neurons are being created, as we know that neurons are formed in the hippocampus, though the magnitude of the observed change suggests that other factors are also contributing. For the other brain regions, the mechanism of change is uncertain. Increases in the number of connections between the neurons might be contributing to the changes.

The MRI can also be used to look at the white matter structure of the brain, which consists of the long fiber tracts between the two ends of a neuron. Recent experiments suggest that meditation practice promotes increases in white matter tracts in similar brain regions where gray matter changes are occurring (Kang et al., in press; Luders, Clark, Narr, & Toga, 2011; Tang et al., 2010, 2012). This increase in white matter tract density is consistent with the interpretation that changes in gray matter are due to changes in the number of connections between the neurons, as the fibers that connect neurons often stretch great distances. Studies with animals suggest that other mechanisms might also contribute to changes in gray matter, including increases in the number of small helper cells (called *astrocytes*) or increases in the diameter of blood vessels. A change in any of these neural components is consistent with neuroplasticity and the acquisition of new information or behaviors.

To summarize, structural changes have been found in brain regions that are important for emotion regulation, empathy, and self-referential processing. Furthermore, changes in stress levels brought about by mindfulness meditation correlated with changes in amygdala gray matter density. These data provide important information regarding how meditation works and lend considerable neural evidence to the claims of meditators that practice improves their mood, their emotion regulation capacity, and, in particular, their ability to handle stressful situations when not meditating. Regular meditation practice literally reshapes one's brain, leading to long-lasting changes in neural function.

CHANGES IN BRAIN ACTIVITY WHILE NOT MEDITATING

We now consider the evidence for this last part of the working model shown in Figure 15.1, namely, evidence that frequent meditation practice should lead to changes in brain activity throughout the day doing other tasks, not just while meditating. Over the last few years, a growing body of evidence has begun to demonstrate such changes. A commonly cited benefit of meditation practice is decreased reactivity to one's own emotional experiences. Several studies of healthy subjects have demonstrated that activity in the amygdala, the brain region most closely associated with emotional arousal, is often inversely correlated with activity in *executive control* regions of the prefrontal cortex (e.g., the ACC and dorsolateral prefrontal cortex), suggesting that these frontal regions play an important role in emotion regulation (Ochsner, Bunge, Gross, & Gabrieli, 2002).

Several studies have sought to explore this emotion regulation network in meditation practitioners. Studies that have explored longitudinal effects of short-term (1–8 weeks) meditation training in novices have found decreases in amygdala activity in response to a variety of affective stimuli, including emotionally evocative images (Desbordes et al., 2012; Taylor et al., 2011), facial expressions (Hölzel et al., 2013), and negative self-beliefs (Goldin & Gross, 2010). Interestingly, the only one of these studies that reported a concomitant increase in frontal executive regions utilized just 1 week of meditation training (Taylor et al., 2011). The other studies, which used 8-week mindfulness training programs, found no change in frontal executive regions, suggesting that meditation training provides a novel mechanism for regulating amygdala function. Indeed, one of the reports (Hölzel et al., 2013) found *increased* connectivity between the amygdala and a subregion of the dorsolateral prefrontal cortex that is thought to monitor (but not alter) amygdala activity, suggesting that the typical downregulation of emotional reactivity through the prefrontal cortex has been replaced with a less reactive neural response.

Intriguingly, studies with long-term meditation practitioners have found even more pronounced differences in neural responses to affective stimuli. Studies that employed affective images found that experienced Zen meditators perceived these images as less intense while being in a state of mindfulness than during rest, but that this occurred without *any* downregulation of the amygdala and without increased activity in modulatory prefrontal brain areas (Taylor et al., 2011). Other studies with experienced Zen practitioners have found that compared to controls, the meditators have less activity in brain regions responsible for conceptual reasoning during a lexical decision task, suggesting reduced elaboration and emotional reactivity to stimuli (Pagnoni, Cekic, & Guo, 2008).

Several studies have used experimentally induced mild pain or unpleasant sounds to explore how meditation practice can alter an individual's emotional response to these unpleasant stimuli. These studies have demonstrated that long-term meditators rate the intensity of the stimulus similarly to controls, but have significantly reduced self-reported ratings of unpleasantness to those stimuli (Gard et al., 2012; Grant et al., 2011; Lutz et al., 2013; Perlman et al., 2010). Importantly, these changes were accompanied by increased brain activation in sensory areas, including the insula, and decreased activation in executive control, evaluative, and emotion-related areas (prefrontal cortex, amygdala, and hippocampus). These data reflect a decrease in cognitive control rather than a decrease in the pain sensation per se. In one of the studies, the lower pain sensitivity in meditators was strongly predicted by decoupling between activity in the cognitive-evaluative prefrontal areas and sensory pain areas (Grant et al., 2011). This decoupling may correspond to the neural substrate of the meditators' capacity to view painful stimuli more neutrally. These altered neural findings are consistent with mindfulness training instructions to "just notice what is happening" and "let things be as they are." Farb and colleagues (2007) have also demonstrated increased activity in sensory regions, including the insula, during experiential processing of affective stimuli following mindfulness training. These findings have intriguing implications for using mindfulness practice to treat chronic pain (see Chapter 10).

In addition to demonstrating changes in brain activity during tasks, recent studies have also demonstrated altered brain activity associated with mindfulness training during simple rest. As discussed above, the

DMN is the primary set of brain regions that appears to be active during rest, is thought to play a central role in creating the sense of self and identity, and is understood to be more active during mind wandering. The PCC, which is deactivated during meditation (Brewer, Worhunsky, et al., 2011; Hasenkamp et al., 2012) and is one of the areas with altered gray matter density following MBSR (Hölzel, Carmody, et al., 2011), is a central hub of the DMN. Several studies have demonstrated that long-term meditation practitioners have increased connectivity between regions of the DMN (Brewer, Worhunsky, et al., 2011; Hasenkamp & Barsalou, 2012; Jang et al., 2011; Taylor et al., 2013). Changes in other resting state networks were identified in novices following MBSR participation (Kilpatrick et al., 2011). Several of the studies with experienced practitioners have also demonstrated that activity within the DMN is more tightly coupled to other networks during rest, in particular to networks associated with attention and executive control (Bærentsen et al., 2010; Brewer, Worhunsky, et al., 2011; Hasenkamp & Barsalou, 2012; Pagnoni et al., 2008), which has been suggested to reflect enhanced ability to maintain attention, disengage from distraction, and spend less time mind wandering, even when not meditating.

Interestingly, these findings are the opposite of what is seen in Alzheimer's or autism, in which decreased connectivity within the DMN has been reported (Brier et al., 2012). In these illnesses the differences in connectivity are related to clinical symptoms that are often profound. The fact that meditation experience is associated with changes of similar magnitude but of opposite direction has implications for the profound nature of changes that may be occurring with meditation practice.

This chapter has provided an overview of the recent neurobiological literature on mindfulness meditation and the evidence for mindfulness-based neuroplasticity. The data reported in this literature provide important insights about how meditation works and lend considerable evidence to the claims of meditators that practice improves their mood, their emotion regulation capacity, and, in particular, their ability to handle stressful situations. This review reflects only the tip of the iceberg, though, as there is still much to learn about how these brain changes lead to the myriad changes that meditators report. In particular, most of the neural research done to date has focused on MBSR and breath awareness meditation. There are myriad meditation techniques, and we need to better understand the similarities and differences, both neurologically and clinically, of different types of practices.

I am frequently asked, "Are these data telling us that people should meditate to make their brains bigger?" Or "I'm getting older—should I meditate to stop my brain from shrinking?" Although our data show that the brain does change with meditation practice, it is important to remember that learning *any* new task will lead to changes in your brain. The point of the data is to better understand how meditation may be working. However, I have heard from many meditation teachers that when people first come to classes, they are often a little skeptical. Students ask, "Is this really doing anything for me?" or "Do I need to practice for many years to get the positive benefits of meditation?" One use of the data is to help remove these doubts surrounding the efficacy of meditation and mindfulness, as opposed to presenting the brain changes as the primary goal of practice.

I will leave you with a Zen koan: "Intending to buy iron, they obtain gold." In my own case, I started practicing yoga as a form of physical therapy for knee pain. I didn't believe any of the health or cognitive claims that the teacher made, but after a few weeks I realized that there was much more to yoga practice than just a way to rehabilitate my knee. This is a common experience for those coming to yoga and meditation practices. They begin practice looking for stress reduction, or to increase their brain size, or to bring some other tangible benefit to their life—but they start to realize that these practices do much more: They enrich their lives in unanticipated directions and help them in ways that they didn't even know that they needed to be helped.

16

Positive Psychology and the Bodhisattva Path

Charles W. Styron

Enlightened means awakening to the basic goodness that is here, at the heart of our humanity. Society is the natural expression of that goodness. It manifests as a natural connection between beings that is experienced as kindness. Thus, an enlightened society is an awake and friendly association with others.

—SAKYONG JAMPAL TRINLEY DRADUL (2012)

Positive psychology is not new. Although it became a formal discipline in 1998 when Martin Seligman chose it as the theme of his year as president of the American Psychological Association, Abraham Maslow (1954) coined the term in the 1950s. He, too, was late to the party though—very late. As this chapter will show, the most important principles in positive psychology are really quite old. In some respects, positive psychology is serving ancient wine in new bottles, empirically supporting what has been known experientially for more than two millennia.

Everyone wants to be happy, and positive psychology takes the view that the cultivation of human well-being is as important as treating its maladies and pathologies. The Dalai Lama has even said that the very purpose of human life is to be happy (Dalai Lama & Cutler, 1998), and indeed mindfulness meditation has the attainment of well-being at its center. Positive psychology and mindfulness meditation, therefore, have very similar aspirations.

Since ancient times there have been many practices that facilitate the journey toward happiness. In early (*theravada*) Buddhist psychology, mindfulness meditation was conceived as a means of overcoming the inevitable pain of life. In later (*mahayana* and *vajrayana*) Buddhist psychology, realizing *buddha nature*—what Chogyam Trungpa (1984) more recently called "basic goodness" (see pp. 29–33)—became a focus. Glimpses of this state lead to the desire to bring it more fully into everyday experience through systematic and disciplined practice.

The integration of old and new is never easy, and in attempting it here, there is the risk of watering down ancient wisdom to appeal to modern understanding. On the other hand, there is also the contravening risk of accepting longstanding experiential claims on the basis of faith without objective evidence. Empiricism is the dominant paradigm for validating our understanding of the world at the present time, but as David Deutsch (2011) points out so eloquently, it is as much an intellectual construct as every other previous philosophical perspective has been. We need to work with the scientific tools available to us, but we need to do it with caution while honoring and respecting what our predecessors have passed on to us from their inner explorations.

THREE PILLARS OF POSITIVE PSYCHOLOGY

Seligman (2002) originally posited three principal avenues for the attainment of happiness: (1) the cultivation of positive emotions (including the experience of pleasure), (2) full engagement in one's activities, and (3) meaningful service to others. He more recently revised his formulation, adding the elements of (4) positive relationships and (5) achievement. He also changed his target objective from "happiness"—which he now characterizes as the narrow "entity of life satisfaction"—to the more inclusive and robust "construct of well-being" (2011, p. 15). *Well-being* is also the preferred expression in this chapter. As we examine the possibility of integrating positive psychology and mindfulness practice, furthermore, we will focus on Seligman's original three elements because of their broad acceptance in the field.

Cultivating Positive Emotions

Past

The first element for the attainment of well-being deals with positive emotion, and it is divided into three parts pertaining to the past, the future, and the present. In the quest for positive emotional experience of one's past, interpretation becomes enormously important. Although the past cannot be undone, reframing how we think about it can produce beneficial results. Practicing gratitude, for example, offers a strong return on investment. In a study at the University of Pennsylvania, Seligman (2003; Seligman, Steen, Park, & Petersen, 2005) found that writing a gratitude letter to an important person in one's past produced tangible improvements in the sense of well-being, and these effects persisted for up to 6 months. Lambert, Fincham, Stillman, and Dean (2009) also documented "that stronger feelings of gratitude are associated with lower materialism" (p. 32). Although considerably more challenging, writing forgiveness letters produces similar results.

Although gratitude is almost always appreciated and enhances the relationship in which it is expressed, the same cannot be said for forgiveness. Sometimes forgiveness is most effective as internal transformation, and mindfulness meditation can play an important role in reaching an inner state where it is possible. For example, meditation helps us to overcome the "availability heuristic" (Kahneman, 2011, p. 8), which is a strong, unconscious tendency to make *fast* intuitive judgments stemming from thoughts that are highly prevalent in our mind stream (e.g., revenge) rather than utilizing *slow*, more measured, reflective assessments of experience (e.g., forgiveness). Other ways that meditation may promote forgiveness are by (1) wearing down the sharp edge of the negative emotion through repetitive exposure; (2) gradually decentering us from the negative emotion and regarding our own pain more dispassionately; and (3) embracing our inherent interconnection with those who have wittingly or unwittingly caused us pain. Snyder, Lopez, and Pedrotti (2011) detail a similar path to forgiveness in their textbook on positive psychology. Patients tend to respond well to gratitude and forgiveness exercises because they give expression to important feelings that may never have been articulated before. These practices can even be beneficial when directed toward oneself (McCarthy, 2012; Snyder et al., 2011).

Future

Experiencing positive emotions regarding the future is as important as doing so for the past, though whenever future projections are entertained, anxiety is often close at hand. Mindfulness can help here as well. In meditation, we can witness the mind's nearly limitless capacity to churn out catastrophic thoughts. The meditative process of gently disengaging from such negative thinking can be quite beneficial, although it may take quite a bit of time on the cushion. Reframing catastrophic thoughts in realistic terms, using cognitive-behavioral tools, can provide further relief, but this step is much easier to take once we have begun to disengage from the thoughts. Meditation practice has no peer in facilitating this process, showing us that thoughts are thoughts, not facts. Joining mindfulness discipline with the positive psychology practice of cognitive disputation (Seligman, 2003), therefore, can powerfully reshape our feelings about the future.

Present

Finally, we come to the present and the role of pleasure. Pleasure is an important component of well-being, but personal set points limit the well-being attained by pleasure alone (Lucas, Clark, Georgellis, & Diener, 2003). According to Sonya Lyubomirsky (2007), for any given individual, about 50% of the potential for happiness is hereditary, 10% is due to external circumstances, and 40% can be affected directly by how we think and what we do. The experience of pleasure, therefore, is bounded by one's personal traits. Pleasure is also bounded by the phenomenon known as the *hedonic treadmill* (Ryan & Deci, 2001; Seligman, 2002). This refers to the tendency to habituate rapidly to significant changes in our lives. Unfortunately, habituation happens even more quickly in response to positive changes than to negative ones (Lyubomirsky, 2007). Research has shown that habituation to winning the lottery can take place within a year (Brickman, Coates, & Janoff-Bulman, 1978) and satiation with a sweet dessert occurs within minutes. Although pleasure is a limited and somewhat undependable partner in the pursuit of enduring well-being, it is still a very powerful motivator.

In the pursuit of pleasure, mindfulness meditation turns out to be a potent, unexpected ally. Meditation leads to *gratification*, which is satisfaction that accrues through conscious effort (Seligman, 2002), rather than through pleasure passively obtained. Meditation also contributes to the capacity to be *in* the present moment instead of wrapped up in thoughts about the past and the future. Being in the present, it turns out, is a key element of pleasure. Killingsworth and Gilbert (2010) employed a smartphone, experience-sampling, methodology that revealed participants' minds to be wandering 46.9% of the time—not thinking about what they were doing. It also turned out that a present-focused mind was a better predictor of the participants' happiness than the activity in which they were engaged. As anyone who has a regular mindfulness meditation practice will attest, life is tangibly more pleasurable when one is more present. Through cultivating a relaxed, gently focused mind, meditation enhances pleasure by allowing us to "savor" our pleasant experiences (Snyder et al., 2011). Savoring, however, is an unplanned byproduct of meditation rather than one of its articulated goals.

Dedicated, long-term meditators seem to have a remarkable capacity to enjoy the simplest things, displaying a joyful attitude toward every aspect of life. Contemporary neuroscientific research is corroborating this impression. For example, a positron emission tomography (PET) scan of a monk who had practiced meditation for many years showed left prefrontal cortex activation—an area associated with positive emotion— far more energetically than control subjects (Davidson & Harrington, 2001). Significantly less pronounced, but similar, effects were exhibited by subjects who had practiced as little as 8 weeks of mindfulness meditation (Davidson et al., 2003).

Positive emotional experiences of the past, future, and present remind us that life is good. Meditation practice takes this realization a step further. Time on the cushion almost always reminds us that life is good, and this is the case, paradoxically, *even when it isn't*. This is where we begin to taste the essence of what Buddhist traditions call *Buddha nature*—the undeniable, intangible, but utterly real experience of inherent goodness in all phenomena. It is not particularly logical, but it is there like bedrock. It is what keeps us going even when everything else seems to be falling apart. It is also probably what led Wittgenstein, the rather pessimistic positivist philosopher, to proclaim on his deathbed that it had all been "wonderful, absolutely wonderful" (Seligman, 2003).

Engagement and Service to Others

Let's turn now to the crux of positive psychology: full engagement in one's activities and meaningful service to others. Although considerable well-being can be experienced through practices that enhance positive emotions in the past, present, and future, there are limitations, and these limitations are nowhere more apparent than with the fleeting experience of pleasure. In contrast, the well-being attained through engagement and meaningful service is relatively unlimited. It is not bound by personal set points, satiation, or regret about the past and anxiety about the future. Engagement and meaningful service, therefore, assume a dominant role in the overall positive psychology enterprise, and they are intimately linked with the exercise of what Peterson and Seligman (2004) call *signature strengths*. To emphasize this point, Snyder and colleagues (2011) entitled their excellent textbook *Positive Psychology: The Scientific and Practical Explorations of Human Strengths.*

Signature strengths are skill sets that are inherently strong and familiar for a given individual, and Peterson and Seligman argue that engagement and meaning materialize fully in one's life only when employing them quite liberally. The full array of strengths that Peterson and Seligman identify covers the gamut of human activity and includes assets such as courage, love, humanity, and temperance—24 of them in all. Although all familiar, each individual will find several signature strengths to be frequent, close companions whereas others will remain more distant and challenging. Signature strengths are defined as those that are typically the most prevalent, productive, and effortless contributors to the successful conduct of one's activities. They are the modes of expression or action in which a given person performs best—*best* as compared to all of the other ways that that same individual could perform, not best as compared to others. Therefore, *everyone* has a collection of signature strengths. Conveniently, there is a web-based tool that helps to identity one's signature strengths via a forced-choice assessment. It is called the Virtues in Action (VIA) Survey of Character Strengths, and it can be found at *www.authentichappiness.sas.upenn.edu/default. aspx* (Seligman, 2004).

Engagement, the second element for the attainment of well-being, occurs when several components come together for an individual: signature strengths, an activity or project suited to the exercise of those strengths, an aspect of challenge, an absence of excessive time pressure, and a degree of passion or interest. It is important for the level of skill in the identified strength to be well matched to the level of difficulty associated with the activity. Excessive skill will lead to boredom, whereas excessive challenge will lead to anxiety or worry (Snyder et al., 2011), so some challenge is necessary to keep things interesting. In fact, the well-known Zen teacher Ezra Bayda (2010) says, "We can't be truly happy *until* our life is difficult" (p. 85).

When we're engaged in an activity that is demanding and we're also skilled at doing it, a measure of absorption takes place. Mihaly Csikszentmihaly (1991) identified this absorption as an optimal experience called *flow*. Flow is the hallmark of peak engagement—we lose awareness of time, work effortlessly, remain focused with ease, and perform unselfconsciously.

Although unfettered flow marks the zenith of engagement, flow isn't required for significant satisfaction. Flow occurs on a continuum, and entering into it even modestly is always preferable to the alternative.

The real prerequisite for life satisfaction is the exercise of one's signature strengths. There are no time limits for the expression of our signature strengths—we can be engaged for hours, days, weeks, or even years. It also doesn't matter what the particular strength happens to be, although some (e.g., curiosity) can be more readily put into action than others (e.g., bravery).

As originally defined by Seligman (2002), *engagement* is distinguished from meaningful service to others primarily by intention. Engagement arises in the pursuit of personal goals, whereas meaning finds expression when one is "using [one's] signature strengths in the service of something larger than [oneself]" (p. 249). But since strengths and virtues have to do with our interactions with other people so much of the time, the boundary between engagement and meaningful service frequently blurs.

Virtue

The field of positive psychology originally focused on the individual achievement of well-being. Reference to *interpersonal* relationships was often implied by Seligman (2002, 2004) and others in the early literature, but the emphasis remained on the attainment of happiness through individual effort. Although happiness per se is still ultimately experienced and measured empirically at the individual level, much of the relatively recent literature in positive psychology has been considerably more social in nature. Although there are many explanations for this new interpersonal emphasis in positive psychology, the primary reason is the important role of virtue.

As noted above, Peterson and Seligman (2004) identified 24 character strengths in their seminal work *Character Strengths and Virtues*. These were distilled from an exhaustive examination of the world's principal spiritual, ethnic, and cultural traditions. (This is a work in progress, by the authors' own admission.) The 24 strengths are grouped together under six overarching virtues: wisdom, courage, humanity, justice, temperance, and transcendence. All of world's great traditions, they argue, have found well-being to be a product of the practice of these six specific virtues (or virtues very similar to them). This collection of virtues, furthermore, attempts to cover the full domain of positive human expression. The idea that the practice of virtue leads to well-being, of course, is not a surprise for most of us (see Chapter 6). We may have studied it in a philosophy class on Aristotle, heard about it in any of many religious traditions, or had it inspired in us by our parents and teachers. The pursuit of virtue is so familiar, in fact, that we may have become somewhat inured to it.

By making the practice of virtue central to positive psychology, Peterson and Seligman bring us back to familiar ground. Although we may have been holding out for something more novel, exciting, and less demanding, we realize with this practice that we do not have to start over from scratch. We can continue our journeys in many instances without even skipping stride if we have heart. Fortunately, empirical evidence supporting the practice of virtue has begun to accumulate, and such evidence may inspire us further (Frederickson, 2003, 2009; Frederickson & Branigan, 2005). In our skeptical culture, this is no small matter, and in clinical work, framing what a patient is doing in terms of inherent virtue or aspiration is hard to surpass.

In light of the fundamentals of positive psychology discussed so far, the centrality of practicing virtue to attain well-being and the recent prosocial trend in the positive psychology literature make a lot of sense (see also Chapter 6). Virtue, it turns out, is both socially determined and socially constructed, and so are many of the strengths that give it particular expression. It appears in relationship to other living beings. It is not surprising, therefore, that a great deal of the recent literature has a relational perspective, and Seligman has even identified the domain of positive relationships as a new element in his reformulation of positive psychology. In his 8-week teleclasses, Peterson (2007, 2008) devoted almost half of the class time to overtly social topics. To drive the interpersonal point home, Peterson and Park (2007) sum up the thrust of positive psychology with the phrase, "Other people matter" (p. 172). Peterson (2007b) adds, along similar lines, "If you're going to do something, do it with somebody else." Other people not only matter, as they say; they matter a lot, and we would do well to include them as often as possible in our activities. Expanding on these two expressions, finally, we could add a third: "If you're going to do something, do it *for* somebody else." We'll return to this perspective and its logic shortly.

The Mahayana Path

The Buddhist mahayana (Sanskrit: *maha* = great, *yana* = path) tradition emphasizes working for the benefit of others. Operationally, this boils down to the practice of the six *paramitas*, or the six perfections. *Paramita* is a Sanskrit term that means "that which has gone beyond" or "that which is most excellent." *Param* means "other side" or "other side of the river," whereas *ita* means "arrived." *Paramita*, therefore, means "arriving on the other side," and it refers to the transcendent action of going beyond one's own personal, egoistic concerns.

The *paramitas* are *metavirtues* that transcend ordinary conceptions of virtue because they are practiced without ego attachment, with some realization of emptiness and no-self as they were described in Chapters 2 and 14. Naturally, this is a very tall order for most people and works best when entertained as an aspiration rather than as a reality. The *paramitas* are actually practiced simultaneously most of the time, but they are usually presented in a certain order. They are (with their Sanskrit names):

1. Generosity (*dana*)—giving without expectation of recognition, without attachment.
2. Discipline (*sila*)—practicing ethical behavior; restraint from causing harm.
3. Patience (*ksanti*)—unconditional forbearance; waiting without a goal in mind.
4. Exertion (*virya*)—joyful, effortless, wholesome activity for its own sake.
5. Meditation (*samadhi*)—pervasive mental balance, arising from a mind at peace.
6. Wisdom (*prajna*)—innate, discriminating awareness, arising from within.

Notice that the *paramitas* have an uncanny resemblance to the overarching virtues catalogued in Peterson and Seligman's *Character Strengths and Virtues*. A pairing of the six *paramitas* and the six virtues is shown below with assessments of their comparability shown in parentheses.

PARAMITA	POSITIVE PSYCHOLOGY	VIRTUE
Generosity	(generally equivalent)	Humanity
Discipline	(generally equivalent)	Temperance
Exertion	(moderately comparable)	Courage
Patience	(mildly comparable)	Justice
Meditation	(virtually equivalent)	Transcendence
Wisdom	(virtually identical)	Wisdom

The absence of a perfect fit here doesn't really matter—my point is to show the striking consonance between the *paramitas* and the positive psychology virtues. This compatibility makes good sense, of course, because the virtues were identified by their recurring prominence in a large number of traditions. One of these, undoubtedly, was the Mahayana Buddhist tradition.

Generally speaking, mahayana practice can be described as working consistently for the benefit of others, and to a certain extent, this is a discipline that many of us practice in our daily lives. The operative words here are *to a certain extent*, however, because mahayana practice is quite ambitious. When officially embarking on this path, a meditation practitioner typically takes the *Bodhisattva Vow* in the presence of his or her teacher. The vow is quite poetic and it derives from a lengthy presentation by Shantideva, an eighth-century Buddhist scholar, called the *Bodhicaryavatara* (1979, pp. 685–763). It reads in part:

> As earth and the other elements, together with space,
> Eternally provide sustenance in many ways for the
>   countless sentient beings,
> So may I become sustenance in every way for sentient
>   beings
> To the limits of space, until all have attained nirvana.
> —Morning Liturgy for Mahayana Students
>   (Nalanda Translation Committee, 2004, pp. 6–7)

This vow is wildly ambitious, so it remains an aspiration—*traveling the bodhisattva path*. *Bodhi* (in Sanskrit) means "awake," and *sattva* means "being," so *bodhisattva path* means the "awake being path." This is what one does, supposedly, if one is truly awake, truly aware of one's place in the world. It is an interesting declaration, to be sure, but why has it been made in the first place?

The answer seems paradoxical, at least initially. Mindfulness practitioners have discovered over the last 2,500 years that working for the benefit of others is actually a far more felicitous and effective path to well-being than pursuing one's own interests alone. Remember, though, the issue here is *well-being*. The bodhisattva path leads to well-being; it may or may not lead to pleasure or praise or wealth or fame. Contemporary research has shown, furthermore, that conventionally valued, worldly attainments like those just mentioned have little, if any, correlation with enduring happiness (Lyubomirsky, 2007). The bodhisattva impulse is quite promising, therefore, because it presents us with a challenge about how to conduct our lives. The challenge is a difficult one, and in a complex world, it may require a finely tuned compromise between goals and practicalities.

Many Western practitioners find the bodhisattva ideal to be somewhat stifling, and a cautionary note is essential for those who choose to practice it. In Buddhist thinking, the context and intention associated with one's actions are extremely important, so traveling this path needs to be as free of expectations as possible. Serving others under duress because one is expected to do so is dramatically different from doing so by choice, and it often leads to powerful, understandable resentments. Embarking on this path prematurely or with excessive zeal can also backfire. It's like running a marathon—it takes abundant training, pacing, endurance, and above all, a desire to do it. Angela Duckworth has researched self-discipline extensively in children and adolescents, and Seligman cites her work at length in his discussion of the element of achievement in developing well-being. She would undoubtedly conclude that the bodhisattva path requires considerable character strength and "grit" (Duckworth, 2007, lecture, March 29, 2012; Seligman, 2011).

Meaningful service to others entails the use of signature strengths for purposes larger than one's personal concerns. Erik Erikson (1950) referred to this activity as the life-stage practice of *generativity*. He posited that without it, we cannot arrive at the end of our lives with a feeling of *integrity*—his final stage. The mahayanists go even further; they say that without the pervasive practice of unselfishness, it is impossible to be fully alive and awake.

Prosocial actions can be contagious: They are likely to engender similar behaviors in those who are observing them. This is known as *elevation* in positive psychology (Algoe & Haidt, 2009; Cox, 2010; Landis et al., 2009; Steger, Kashdan, & Oishi, 2008; Vianello, Galliani, & Haidt, 2010). Elevation has been studied alongside admiration and gratitude. Algoe and Haidt (2009) found that "elevation (a response to moral excellence) motivates prosocial and affiliative behavior, gratitude motivates improved relationships with benefactors, and admiration motivates self-improvement" (p. 105). Elevation arises when we witness virtuous action, and it motivates others to take up arms and join the campaign for a stronger, more humane social fabric. These are activities that social entrepreneurs such as those in Ashoka Innovators for the Public (*www.ashoka.org*) explicitly target in developing countries around the world as they seek to engage others in pursuing innovative approaches to seemingly intractable problems. Such activity has to be kindled, however—there must always be a spark. And the spark is a person acting unselfishly, acting for a purpose larger than him- or herself, employing signature strengths for the benefit of others.

The clinical setting, finally, offers unparalleled possibilities for practicing and modeling meaningful service—it can be a doorway to unselfish connection. When we fall short, we can point out our failure, apologize for it, and even laugh a little at it with our patient if the mood in the room permits. The slightly bad news in all of this is that it's very challenging to practice meaningful service consistently—to travel the bodhisattva path. The unmitigated good news is that we have countless opportunities to do it.

Building an Enlightened Society

In his remarkably insightful book about the war in Afghanistan, Sebastian Junger (who was an embedded reporter) points out that untrained soldiers in the presence of modest danger are far more likely to break down than well-trained soldiers in situations of extremity (Junger, 2010). Training is essential for combat against external adversaries, which we know intuitively as well from experience, but it's actually no less important in the daily communication that we conduct with our own minds. This is something that we *do not* generally recognize. Without some training in a meditative discipline, for example, the reflective, slow part of our minds will lose the moment-to-moment battle that we wage internally throughout the day against our instinctual reactivity (Kahneman, 2011). Most of the time, furthermore, we won't even know it because this struggle takes place largely outside of normal awareness. It is through meditative discipline that we are able to resolve these conflicts consciously and turn our minds into allies (Sakyong, 2003). We are then able to share our best intentions wholeheartedly with the global community instead of doubting them and keeping them largely to ourselves.

According to the Tibetan Buddhist teacher Sakyong Jampal Thinley Dradul (2012), an *enlightened society* places kindness at its center and regards inherent goodness in all individuals as its first principle, its primary signature strength. This aspiration is at once lofty and quite ordinary, and it resonates with the sensibility of Janet Surrey (see Chapter 5) and others who call for a more relational model of mindfulness. Most importantly, though, an enlightened society is one in which individuals are fundamentally unashamed of who they are and instinctively unhesitating in their appreciation of others. It is a social order that aspires to realize its ultimate potential. Because it is comprised of individuals who acknowledge their fundamental goodness, it is also inherently good itself, unconditionally good in spite of any confusion that may episodically beset it. Finally, an enlightened society is one in which individuals practice meaningful service when they are able to do so; they *do* things for each other. Here's an exercise along these lines that anyone can try.

A Bodhisattva To-Do List

- Choose a week in your regular schedule—all 7 days.
- Start the week on Monday.
- Make a to-do list of things that you are going to do for someone on each day.
  - You may do things for many people or for only a few—your call.
  - If it's not something *for* someone else, leave it off the list.
  - Small things that you routinely do for someone else are OK.
  - Do them consciously. Make the entries count—no throwaways.
- Do not leave any days vacant.
- Aim for two or three items per day.
- Do not have more than one day with only one item on the list.
- Spread the items around, putting them at different times of the day.
- Treat Saturday and Sunday like you might treat any other weekend—do something more ambitious or time-consuming.
- Check things off the list as you would check them off of any other to-do list.
- Before bed, reflect for a few minutes on your activities of the day.
- Jot down what worked best.
- Forgive yourself for whatever you didn't do.
- In the coming weeks, gradually integrate bodhisattva items into your ordinary to-do lists.

Every society finds a way to strike a balance between personal needs and service to others. An enlightened society simply tilts the scale a bit toward *meaningful service*, recognizing that well-being is more likely to arise when the strengths of its citizens are actively engaged. Although ambitious in scope, such a society evolves one citizen at a time. It is one in which being awake to the spontaneous play of one's mind is both valued and cultivated, and it is one where individuals are somewhat less likely to be kidnapped by habitual patterns. Well-being is abundant as the fortuitous side-effect of living with awareness that other people's happiness is essential for one's own. It is one where kindness is common and not particularly newsworthy, and where actual enlightenment, although highly valued, is neither required nor expected. It is, finally, a vision of community where the cultivation of positive attitudes and mindfulness can grow together—a community that's within our reach if we simply have the courage to reach for it.

If you want to be happy today, make someone else happy;
If you want to be happy tomorrow, make someone else happy today;
If you want to be happy indefinitely, accept a modicum
of difficulty in your life with equanimity, and put others first.

Appendix

Glossary of Terms in Buddhist Psychology

Andrew Olendzki

THE TWO TYPES OF MEDITATION

Many different forms of meditation are practiced in the Buddhist and non-Buddhist traditions of Asia. The two practices most prevalent in the earliest teachings of the Buddha are:

1. *Concentration* (calming, *samatha* in Pali; focused attention). Focusing the mind on a single object to the exclusion of other objects fosters concentration, or a *one-pointed* mode of mental function. As distracting thoughts or sensations arise, one abandons giving attention to those objects and gently returns awareness to the primary object of experience (e.g., the breath, a word or phrase). As the mind steadies on one particular aspect of the phenomenal field, it gains tranquility, stability, and power.

2. *Mindfulness* (insight, *vipassana* in Pali; open monitoring). In mindfulness meditation, one allows awareness to move from one object to another as stimuli present themselves in experience. When this practice is done in a sustained manner, it leads to insight into the subjective construction of experience and into the three characteristics of existence.

THE THREE CHARACTERISTICS OF EXISTENCE

Construed as three fundamental attributes of the human condition, the three characteristics of existence are normally obscured from view by distortions of perception, thought, and view, and are revealed through careful and disciplined investigation of experience. Insight into these characteristics contributes to wisdom.

   1. *Impermanence* (*anicca* in Pali). The stream of consciousness that makes up the subjective flow of human awareness—and hence the world constructed by the mind—is actually composed of very brief episodes of cognitive activity that arise and pass away with great rapidity. More generally, it refers to the observation that all conditioned phenomena are transitory.
   2. *Suffering* (*dukkha* in Pali). This word is used in a very broad and existential manner in the Buddhist tradition. It refers not only to the inevitability of physical pain, injury, illness, aging, and death, but also to the subtler psychological distress resulting from the fundamental insatiability of desire. Not getting what one wants, having to cope with what one does not want, and confusion about conflicting desires are all encompassed by the word *suffering.*
   3. *Non-self* (*anatta* in Pali). Ever a source of perplexity to Westerners, the Buddhist insight of non-self does not deny that there are unique and more or less stable patterns of personality that develop throughout a person's lifetime. Rather it points out that these patterns are *just* patterns of conditioning and learned behaviors, and that they lack any essence or numinous core. The reflexive assumption of *ownership* of thoughts, feelings, sensations, etc. (these are *mine*, this is *me*) is unwarranted, maladaptive, and the source of a host of psychological difficulties.

THE THREE UNWHOLESOME ROOTS

These are the three underlying tendencies of human behavior from which all the other afflictive emotions are derived. They might be thought of as three primary colors that can mix in many different ways to form the full spectrum of unhealthy emotions. The terms *wholesome* and *unwholesome* can refer to active *states* of mind; to *behaviors* of body, speech, and mind; or to character *traits* that lie dormant in the unconscious mind.

1. *Greed.* Also known as *craving, wanting,* or *attachment,* greed is the impulse to reach for or hold on to something that is desirable. It is a reflexive response to the feeling tone of pleasure.

2. *Hatred.* Also referred to as *aversion* or *ill will,* hatred involves pushing away, denying, or attacking something that is experienced as undesirable. It is usually generated as a response to pain or displeasure. Greed and hatred are the bipolar expressions of desire.

3. *Delusion.* Also referred to as *ignorance* or *confusion,* delusion is used in a technical way in Buddhist thought to denote blindness to certain facets of reality, such as the three characteristics and the construction of experience.

THE THREE WHOLESOME ROOTS

1. *Non-greed.* This quality of mind is the opposite of greed and usually manifests as generosity or renunciation. Both involve some degree of nonattachment and a temporary suspension of selfishness and the need for gratification.

2. *Non-hatred.* The opposite of hatred is non-hatred, a word that covers both loving-kindness, which is a stance of friendliness or goodwill (see below), and compassion, which involves caring deeply for the well-being of another.

3. *Non-delusion.* Other words for non-delusion include *insight, understanding,* or *wisdom.* It is wisdom that is ultimately transformative in Buddhist psychology; it involves the ability to see things clearly, as they really are.

THE THREE KINDS OF FEELING

The word *feeling* in Buddhist thought refers to a hedonic tone rather than to the more complex emotions the word denotes in English. One of the three feeling tones is always present in every moment, accompanying both physical and mental experience.

1. *Pleasant feeling.* Arising from contact between a sense object and a sense organ, a feeling of pleasure may arise. It is always a very brief and very specific event, conditioned by the particular sense and one's underlying attitude toward the particular object.

2. *Unpleasant feeling.* Also arising from contact between a particular sense object and organ, a feeling of displeasure or pain may arise. Both pleasure and pain give rise to a response of wanting or not wanting the sensation to continue. This feeling is distinguishable from the ensuing response.

3. *Neither-pleasant-nor-unpleasant feeling.* Sometimes careful attention will reveal a sensation as pleasant or unpleasant, whereas other times one can be aware of feeling tone that is neutral—neither pleasant nor unpleasant.

THE FOUR NOBLE TRUTHS

A basic organizing principle of Buddhist doctrine, the four truths taught by the Buddha are considered noble because they help raise one's understanding above the level of automatic response into the realm of transformation through wisdom. Based on an ancient medical lore, the truths may be taken as analogous to a physician's diagnosis, etiology, prognosis, and treatment plan for a patient afflicted with a disease.

1. *Suffering.* The term *suffering* is used in a broad sense to point out a fundamental unsatisfactoriness of the human condition (see the above section on the three characteristics of existence), ranging from simple discomfort to the existential challenges of sickness, aging, and inevitable death. Much of our effort works to obscure these truths, but as with all healing, an important first step is to face the nature of the affliction with honesty and courage.

2. *The origination of suffering.* All human suffering has a simple and consistent cause: desire. Whenever there is a disequilibrium between what is arising in experience and what one *wants* to have happen, suffering is inevitable.

3. *The cessation of suffering.* Understanding the causal interdependence of these two, suffering can be brought to cessation simply by the elimination of desire. Unpleasant thoughts and sensations may still exist, and are in fact inevitably part of all experience, but by changing one's attitude of resistance to what is unpleasant, suffering can be reduced and even eliminated.

4. *The path leading to the cessation of suffering.* Many different strategies and programs for bringing suffering to an end have been developed over Buddhism's 2,500 years. Traditionally, the healing program is articulated as the *Noble Eightfold Path.*

THE NOBLE EIGHTFOLD PATH

These eight guidelines for living one's life and holding oneself in the present moment constitute a broad ethical context for development in the Buddhist tradition. The word *right* is used before each one not to impose a rigid normative mold, but more in the sense of *appropriate* or *well-tuned*. These eight dimensions are practiced in parallel, and each supports and reinforces the others.

1. *Right view.* This is the first element in the series but also culminates the list. At the near end of the progression, one needs a certain amount of confidence in the teachings to put them into practice, and one needs to be pointing in the right direction for any journey to be effective. At the far end of the path, right view can be taken to refer to awakening fully to "seeing things as they really are."

2. *Right intention.* In Buddhist psychology, *intention* is the principle tool of transformation. When intention is skillfully crafted in each moment, it guides the mind wisely to its state in the next moment, and thus, like the rudder of a ship, can be used to navigate through the changes of arising and passing experience. It is also sometimes known as *right aim*.

3. *Right speech.* Since speech molds and reflects the quality of thoughts, it becomes quite important that one's habits of speech are truthful, helpful, kind, and free of selfish and manipulative motives. It is speech used for healing and education, and never for harmful or divisive purposes.

4. *Right action.* Traditionally, right action is expressed in terms of living by five ethical precepts: not killing, not stealing, not lying, not misbehaving sexually, and not indulging in intoxicants. Each of these precepts is open to more or less strict interpretation, depending on one's level of commitment (e.g., for a monastic vs. a layperson).

5. *Right livelihood.* This is also construed traditionally as a series of ethical constraints upon a layperson's mode of livelihood and culminates in the monastic code of living for monks and nuns. Laypeople should avoid professions that involve killing, for example, and mendicants should keep their intentions pure as they wander for alms.

6. *Right effort.* Right effort primarily involves the mindful cultivation of wholesome states both before and after they arise in experience, and the deliberate abandoning of unwholesome states, also both before and after they occur. It describes a level of mental hygiene that is quite

scrupulous, and requires considerable ongoing attentiveness to the quality of the inner life.

7. *Right mindfulness.* When mindfulness is well developed following the guidelines of the foundations of mindfulness (see the next section), it is said to be *right mindfulness*, which means applying attention carefully and evenly to phenomena as they appear.

8. *Right concentration.* This calls for the steady application of one-pointed awareness from time to time, outside of everyday activities, and is particularly encouraged as a tool for development in Buddhist psychology. Regular meditation is a foundational aspect of the eightfold path.

THE FOUR FOUNDATIONS OF MINDFULNESS

Basic instructions for the cultivation of mindfulness are given in this classical form. Each category is considered a *foundation* in the sense of providing a basis for practicing those techniques of mind training that involve being fully aware, in the present moment, of one sensory or thought object at a time, and of thereby understanding the changeable and ultimately selfless nature of phenomenological experience.

1. *Mindfulness of body.* Beginning with sitting in a quiet place with legs crossed and back straight, mindfulness practice commences with deliberate awareness of breathing, of the tranquilization of body and mind, and with attention to the bodily sensations arising in conjunction with bodily postures, movements, and activities.

2. *Mindfulness of feelings.* The practice progresses by focusing present moment, nonconceptual awareness upon the feeling tone running through all arising and passing experience. Whether each moment is accompanied by a pleasant, unpleasant, or a neutral feeling, the practitioner seeks to know, with great precision, the feeling tone of the experience.

3. *Mindfulness of mind.* Shifting attention from bodily sensations and feelings to the purely mental sphere, the meditator is invited to bring awareness to the quality of mind as it arises and passes away moment by moment. This is done by noticing if any of the three unwholesome roots (greed, hatred, and delusion) are present or absent.

4. *Mindfulness of mental objects.* An even more detailed and nuanced investigation of mental events involves noticing the presence, absence, and changing dynamic of a number of other factors outlined in Buddhist psychology: hindrances, aggregates, sense spheres, factors of awakening, and noble truths. It is not a discursive analysis of these factors, but rather an experiential and intuitive exploration of the texture of the phenomenal landscape.

THE FOUR LIMITLESS QUALITIES OF HEART
(*Brahma Viharas* in Pali)

There are four qualities of heart that are particularly healing and can be developed using a form of concentration meditation on each of the four unique mental states. These meditations are also called *divine abidings* in a figurative sense, insofar as they involve elevating the mind to very subtle and sublime states. They are classically presented by analogy to a mother's feelings toward her child:

1. *Loving-kindness* (*metta*). As a mother would feel boundless loving-kindness for her newborn baby, wishing deeply for his or her health and well-being, a person deliberately cultivates and develops the same quality of universal and selfless love toward all beings, by focusing the mind unswervingly on such intentions as "May they be happy," "May they be well."

2. *Compassion* (*karuna*). As a mother would respond to a child who is sick or injured, so also a meditator can intentionally develop an attitude of compassion that meets the experience of suffering with the wish for all beings to be safe, secure, and healed of their afflictions. Compassion is a particular state of mind that can be singled out and cultivated by concentration and absorption.

3. *Sympathetic joy* (*mudita*). The quality of mind that responds to the good fortune of others with happiness and goodwill rather than with jealousy or envy is called *sympathetic joy*. This state, too, can be deliberately strengthened by practice and is similar to a mother's response to her grown son or daughter leaving home to marry or pursue his or her profession. An unselfish perspective is a key ingredient of this absorption.

4. *Equanimity* (*upekkha*). As a mother might listen to her grown son or daughter recount his or her various business decisions, neither being attracted to nor repelled by any particular outcome as long as he or she is healthy and happy, so the tradition describes the state of mind called *equanimity*. It is not a detachment due to distancing from phenomena, nor a desensitized neutrality of feeling, but is rather an advanced state of being able to embrace both pleasant and unpleasant experience without the responses usually conditioned by desire.

THE SEVEN FACTORS OF AWAKENING

These seven states of mind or attitudes are particularly helpful in gaining the sort of insight into experience that Buddhist psychology encourages; each factor therefore contributes greatly to the development of wisdom. In some formulations of the teaching, each one of these factors provides the basis for the natural unfolding of the next in an organic process of development.

1. *Mindfulness.* This is the practice of being fully aware in the present moment, without self-judgment or other forms of linguistic and conceptual overlay, of the arising and passing away of phenomena in the field of direct experience.

2. *Investigation.* This is willingness and ability to bring interest, enthusiasm, and an attitude of detailed exploration to experience. The states investigated are the arising and passing of the awareness of sensory objects, mental objects, and whatever else may be unfolding in the moment.

3. *Energy.* When mental effort is brought to a situation, there is the application of energy. It is not the counterproductive striving or straining to attain a goal, but involves the diligent and consistent application of effort to the present moment.

4. *Joy.* Often the mind and body can become exuberant and appear to bubble over with happiness, contentment, or thrill. Though many people are more familiar with this experience when it is induced in unwholesome ways, the positive and transformative value of wholesome joy is an important quality of mind in Buddhist psychology and is to be cultivated.

5. *Tranquility.* Of equal value is the deep serenity that can emerge in the mind and body when there is an absence of conflict, distress, or suffering. This tranquility is not the opposite of joy, for the two can easily coexist. Rather than a tranquility that reduces energy, it is described more as a quality of mental luminescence that emerges as the mind becomes unified, stable, and focused.

6. *Concentration.* As described earlier, concentration involves a one-pointed attentiveness over time to a particular sensation or object to the exclusion of others.

7. *Equanimity.* Also described earlier, equanimity is the quality of mental equipoise in which the mind is neither attracted to a pleasant object nor averse to an unpleasant object.

References

Abramowitz, J. S., Deacon, B. J., & Whiteside, S. P. (2011). *Exposure therapy for anxiety: Principles and practice*. New York: Guilford Press.

Adler, A. (2002). *The collected clinical works of Alfred Adler: Vol 1. The neurotic character* (H. Stein, Ed., & C. Koen, Trans.). San Francisco, CA: Alfred Adler Institutes of San Francisco & Northwestern Washington. (Original work published 1927)

Aggs, C., & Bambling, M. (2010). Teaching mindfulness to psychotherapists in clinical practice: The mindful therapy programme. *Counselling and Psychotherapy Research, 10*(4), 278–286.

Aitken, R. (1984). *The mind of clover: Essays in Buddhist ethics*. New York: North Point Press.

Alexander, F. (1931). Buddhist training as an artificial catatonia. *Psychoanalytic Review, 18*, 129–145.

Algoe, S. B., & Haidt, J. (2009). Witnessing excellence in action: The "other-praising" emotions of elevation, gratitude, and admiration. *Journal of Positive Psychology, 4*(2), 105–127.

American Psychiatric Association. (2013). *Diagnostic and statistical manual of mental disorders* (5th ed.). Washington, DC: Author.

Analayo. (2003). *Satipatthana: The direct path to realization*. Birmingham, UK: Windhorse.

Anandajoti, B. (2010). *The earliest recorded discourses of the Buddha (from Lalitavistara, Mahākhandhaka & Mahāvastu)*. Kuala Lumpur, Malaysia: Sukhi Hotu.

Arch, J. J., Eifert, G. H., Davies, C., Plumb Vilardaga, J. C., Rose, R. D., & Craske, M. G. (2012). Randomized clinical trial of cognitive behavioral therapy (CBT) versus acceptance and commitment therapy (ACT) for mixed anxiety disorders. *Journal of Consulting and Clinical Psychology, 80*(5), 750–765.

Aronson, H. B. (2004). *Buddhist practice on Western ground: Reconciling Eastern ideals and Western psychology*. Boston: Shambhala.

Arzy, S., Thut, G., Mohr, C., Michel, C. M., & Blanke, O. (2006). Neural basis of embodiment: Distinct contributions of temporoparietal junction and extrastriate body area. *Journal of Neuroscience, 26*(31), 8074–8081.

Asmundson, G. J., Coons, M. J., Taylor, S., & Katz, J. (2002). PTSD and the experience of pain: Research and clinical implications of shared vulnerability and mutual maintenance models. *Revue Canadienne De Psychiatrie, 47*(10), 930–937.

Auerbach, H., & Johnson, M. (1977). Research on the therapist's level of experience. In A. Gurman & A. Razin (Eds.), *Effective psychotherapy: A handbook of research* (pp. 84–102). New York: Pergamon.

Baer, R. A. (2003). Mindfulness training as a clinical intervention: A conceptual and empirical review. *Clinical Psychology: Science and Practice, 10*, 125–143.

Baer, R. A. (2010). Self-compassion as a mechanism of change in mindfulness and acceptance-based treatments In R. Baer (Ed.), *Assessing mindfulness and acceptance processes in clients: Illuminating the theory and practice of change* (pp. 135–153). Oakland, CA: Context Press/New Harbinger.

Baer, R. A., & Krietemeyer, J. (2006). Overview of mindfulness- and acceptance-based treatment approaches. In R. A. Baer (Ed.), *Mindfulness-based treatment approaches: Clinician's guide to evidence base and applications* (pp. 3–27). London, UK: Academic Press.

Bærentsen, K., Stødkilde-Jørgensen, H., Sommerlund, B., Hartmann,T., Damsgaard-Madsen, J., Fosnæs, M., et al. (2010). An investigation of brain processes supporting meditation. *Cognitive Process, 11*(1), 57–84.

Bandura, A. (1986). *Social foundations of thought and action: A social cognitive theory.* Englewood Cliffs, NJ: Prentice Hall.

Banks, A. (2010). *The neurobiology of connecting* (Work in Progress). Wellesley, MA: Stone Center Working Paper Series.

Barkley, R. A., & Benton, C. M. (1998). *Your defiant child: Eight steps to better behavior.* New York: Guilford Press.

Barlow, D. (2004). *Anxiety and its disorders: The nature and treatment of anxiety and panic* (2nd ed.). New York: Guilford Press.

Barnard, L., & Curry, J. (2011). Self-compassion: Conceptualizations, correlates, and interventions. *Review of General Psychology, 15*(4), 289–303.

Barnouw, V. (1973). *Culture and personality* (rev. ed.). Homewood, IL: Dorsey Press.

Batchelor, S. (1997). *Buddhism without beliefs.* New York: Riverhead Books.

Bayda, E. (with Bartok, J.). (2005). *Saying yes to life (even the hard parts).* Boston: Wisdom.

Bayda, E. (2010). *Beyond happiness: The Zen way to true contentment.* Boston: Shambhala.

Bechara, A., & Naqvi, N. (2004). Listening to your heart: Interoceptive awareness as a gateway to feeling. *Nature Neuroscience, 7*, 102–103.

Beck, A. T. (1972). *Depression: Causes and treatment.* Philadelphia: University of Pennsylvania Press.

Beck, A. T. (1976). *Cognitive therapy and the emotional disorders.* New York: International Universities Press.

Becker, E. (1973). *The denial of death.* New York: Free Press.

Beckham, J. C., Crawford, A. L., Feldman, M. E., Kirby, A. C., Hertzberg, M. A., Davidson, J. R., et al. (1997). Chronic posttraumatic stress disorder and chronic pain in Vietnam combat veterans. *Journal of Psychosomatic Research, 43*(3), 379–389.

Beebe, B., & Lachmann, F. (1998). Co-constructing inner and relational processes: Self and mutual regulation in infant research and adult treatment. *Psychoanalytic Psychology, 15*(4), 480–516.

Beecher, H. K. (1946). Pain in men wounded in battle. *Annals of Surgery, 123*(1), 96–105.

Bell, D. C. (2001). Evolution of care giving behavior. *Personality and Social Psychology Review, 5,* 216–229.

Bendtsen, L., & Fernandez-de-la-Penas, C. (2011). The role of muscles in tension-type headache. *Current Pain and Headache Reports, 15*(6), 451–458.

Benson, H. (1975). *The relaxation response.* New York: Morrow.

Bhikkhu, T. (Trans.). (1997). Sallatha Sutta: The Arrow (SN 36.6). Retrieved December 27, 2011, from *www.accesstoinsight.org/tipitaka/sn/sn36/sn36.006.than.html.*

Bhikkhu, T. (2011a). Dhammacakkappavattana sutta: Setting in motion the wheel of truth (SN 56.11) (T. Bhikkhu, Trans.). Retrieved October 7, 2011, from *www.accesstoinsight.org/ tipitaka/sn/sn56/sn56.011.than.html.*

Bhikkhu, T. (2011b). Paticca-samuppada-vibhanga sutta: Analysis of dependent co-arising (SN 12.2) (T. Bhikkhu, Trans.). Retrieved June 17, 2011, from *www.accesstoinsight.org/tipitaka/sn/sn12/sn12.002.than.html.*

Bhikkhu, T. (2011c). Satipatthana sutta: Frames of reference (MN 10) (T. Bhikkhu, Trans.). Retrieved June 14, 2011, from *www.accesstoinsight. org/tipitaka/mn/mn.010.than.html.* Archived at *www.webcitation. org/5sOcjl76K.*

Bhikkhu, T. (Ed.). (2012a). Anguttara Nikaya, 10:108. In *Beyond coping: A study guide on aging, illness, death, and separation.* Valley Center, CA: Metta Forest Monastery. Retrieved March 4, 2012, from *www.accessto-insight.org/lib/study/beyondcoping/index.html.*

Bhikkhu, T. (2012b). Dhammapada: Tanhavagga [Craving] (338) (SN 56.11) (T. Bhikkhu, Trans.). Retrieved October 17, 2012, from *www.accesstoinsight. org/tipitaka/kn/dhp/dhp.24.than.html.*

Bhikkhu, T. (2012c). Sallatha Sutta [The Arrow] (T. Bhikku, Trans.). In *Samyutta Nikaya XXXVI6* (chap.). Retrieved January 18, 2012, from *www.accesstoinsight.org/canon/sutta/samyutta/sn36-006.html#shot.*

Bhikkhu, T. (Trans.). (2012d). Upaddha Sutta: Half (of the Holy Life). Retrieved November 2, 2012, from *www.accesstoinsight.org/tipitaka/sn/sn45/sn45.002.than.html.*

Bickman, L. (1999). Practice makes perfect and other myths about mental health services. *American Psychologist, 54*(11), 965–979.

Biegel, G. M., Brown, K. W., Shapiro, S. L., & Schubert, C. M. (2009).

Mindfulness-based stress reduction for the treatment of adolescent psychiatric outpatients: A randomized clinical trial. *Journal of Consulting and Clinical Psychology, 77*(5), 855–866.

Bien, T. (2006). *Mindful therapy: A guide for therapists and helping professionals.* Boston: Wisdom.

Bigos, S. J., Battie, M. C., Spengler, D. M., Fisher, L. D., Fordyce, W. E., Hansson, T. H., et al. (1991). A prospective study of work perceptions and psychosocial factors affecting the report of back injury. *Spine, 16*(1), 1–6.

Bigos, S. J., Bowyer, O. R., Braen G. R., Brown, K., Deyo, R., Haldeman, S., et al. (1994). *Acute low back problems in adults. Clinical practice guideline no. 14* (AHCPR publication no. 95-0642). Rockville, MD: U.S. Department of Health and Human Services, Public Health Service, Agency for Health Care Policy and Research.

Bion, W. (1967). Notes on memory and desire. *Psychoanalytic Forum, 2,* 271–280.

Birne, K., Speca, M., & Carlson, L. (2010). Exploring self-compassion and empathy in the context of mindfulness-based stress reduction (MBSR). *Stress and Health, 26,* 359–371.

Bishop, S. R., Lau, M., Shapiro, S., Carlson, L., Anderson, N. D., Carmody, J., et al. (2004). Mindfulness: A proposed operational definition. *Clinical Psychology: Science and Practice, 11*(3), 230–241.

Blanke, O., & Arzy, S. (2005). The out-of-body experience: Disturbed self processing at the temporo-parietal junction. *The Neuroscientist, 11*(1), 16–24.

Blanke, O., Mohr, C., Michel, C. M., Pascual-Leone, A., Brugger, P., Seeck, M., et al. (2005). Linking out-of-body experience and self processing to mental own-body imagery at the temporoparietal junction. *Journal of Neuroscience, 25*(3), 550–557.

Bluth, K., & Wahler, R.G. (2011). Does effort matter in mindful parenting? *Mindfulness, 2,* 175–178.

Bobrow, J. (2007). Tending, attending, and healing. *Psychologist–Psychoanalyst, 27,* 16–18.

Bobrow, J. (2010). *Zen and psychotherapy: Partners in liberation.* New York: Norton.

Boccio, F. (2004). *Mindfulness yoga.* Somerville, MA: Wisdom.

Bodhi, B. (Ed.). (2000). *A comprehensive manual of Abhidhamma.* Seattle, WA: BPS Pariyatti Editions.

Bodhi, B. (2005). *In the Buddha's words: An anthology of discourses from the Pali Canon.* Boston: Wisdom.

Boellinghaus, I., Jones, F., & Hutton, J. (in press). The role of mindfulness and loving-kindness meditation in cultivating self-compassion and other-focused concern in health care professionals. *Mindfulness.*

Bögels, S., Lehtonen, A., & Restifo, K. (2010). Mindful parenting in mental health care. *Mindfulness, 1*(1), 107–120.

Bohart, A., Elliot, R., Greenberg, L., & Watson, J. (2002). Empathy. In J. C. Norcross (Ed.), *Psychotherapy relationships that work: Therapist contributions and responsiveness to patients* (pp. 89–108). Oxford, UK: Oxford University Press.

Bohlmeijer, E., Prenger, R., Taal, E., & Culjpers, P. (2010). The effects of mindfulness-based stress reduction therapy on mental health of adults with a chronic medical disease: A meta-analysis. *Journal of Psychosomatic Medicine, 68*(6), 539–544.

Bond, T. (2000). *Standards and ethics for counseling in action*. London, UK: Sage Publishing.

Boorstein, S. (1994). Insight: Some considerations regarding its potential and limitations. *Journal of Transpersonal Psychology, 26*(2), 95–105.

Boorstein, S. (2012, Fall). Medicine for the brain, dharma for the mind: An interview with Sylvia Boorstein. *Inquiring Mind*. Retrieved from *www.inquiringmind.com/Articles/MedicineForTheBrain.html*.

Borkovec, T. D., Alcaine, O. M., & Behar, E. (2004). Avoidance theory of worry and generalized anxiety disorder. In D. S. Mennin, R. G. Heimberg, & C. L. Turk (Eds.), *Generalized anxiety disorder: Advances in research and practice* (pp. 77–108). New York: Guilford Press.

Borkovec, T. D., & Sharpless, B. (2004). Generalized anxiety disorder: Bringing cognitive-behavioral therapy into the valued present. In S. C. Hayes, V. M. Follette, & M. M. Linehan (Eds.), *Mindfulness and acceptance: Expanding the cognitive-behavioral tradition* (pp. 209–242). New York: Guilford Press.

Bowen, S., Chawla, N., Collins, S. E., Witkiewitz, K., Hsu, S., Grow, J., et al. (2009). Mindfulness-based relapse prevention for substance use disorders: A pilot efficacy trial. *Substance Abuse, 30*(4), 295–305.

Bowen, S., Chawla, N., & Marlatt, G.A. (2011). *Mindfulness-based relapse prevention for addictive behaviors: A clinician's guide*. New York: Guilford Press.

Brach, T. (2003). *Radical acceptance: Embracing your life with the heart of a Buddha*. New York: Bantam Dell.

Brach, T. (2012a). Mindful presence: A foundation for compassion and wisdom. In C. K. Germer & R. D. Siegel (Eds.), *Wisdom and compassion in psychotherapy: Deepening mindfulness in clinical practice* (pp. 35–47). New York: Guilford Press.

Brach, T. (2012b). *True refuge: Finding peace and freedom in your own awakened heart*. New York: Bantam Books.

Brach, T. (2013). *True refuge: Three gateways to a fearless heart*. New York: Bantam.

Braehler, C., Gumley, A., Harper, J., Wallace, S., Norrie, J., & Gilbert, P. (in press). Exploring change processes in compassion-focused therapy in psychosis: Results of a feasibility randomized controlled trial. *British Journal of Clinical Psychology*

Braith, J. A., McCullough, J. P., & Bush, J. P. (1988). Relaxation-induced anxiety in a subclinical sample of chronically anxious subjects. *Journal of Behavior Therapy and Experimental Psychiatry, 3*, 193–198.

Brefczynski-Lewis, J. A., Lutz, A., Schaefer, H. S., Levinson, D. B., & Davidson, R. J. (2007). Neural correlates of attentional expertise in long-term meditation practitioners. *Proceedings of the National Academy of Sciences of the United States of America, 104*(27), 11483–11488.

Breines, J. G., & Chen, S. (2012). Self-compassion increases self-improvement motivation. *Personality and Social Psychology Bulletin, 38*, 1133–1143.

Brewer, J. A., Bowen, S., & Chawla, N. (2010). *Mindfulness training for addictions*. Unpublished manuscript.

Brewer, J. A., Bowen, S., Smith, J. T., Marlatt, G. A., & Potenza, M. N. (2010). Mindfulness-based treatments for co-occurring depression and substance use disorders: What can we learn from the brain? *Addiction, 105*(10), 1698–1706.

Brewer, J. A., Mallik, S., Babuscio, T. A., Nich, C., Johnson, H. E., Deleone, C. M., et al. (2011). Mindfulness training for smoking cessation: Results from a randomized controlled trial. *Drug and Alcohol Dependence, 119*(1–2), 72–80.

Brewer, J. A., Sinha, R., Chen, J. A., Michalsen, R. N., Babuscio, T. A., Nich, C., et al. (2009). Mindfulness training and stress reactivity in substance abuse: Results from a randomized, controlled stage I pilot study. *Substance Abuse, 30*(4), 306–317.

Brewer, J. A., Worhunsky, P. D., Carroll, K. M., Rounsaville, B. J., & Potenza, M. N. (2008). Pretreatment brain activation during Stroop task is associated with outcomes in cocaine-dependent patients. *Biological Psychiatry, 64*(11), 998–1004.

Brewer, J. A., Worhunsky, P. D., Gray, J. R., Tang, Y. Y., Weber, J., & Kober, H. (2011). Meditation experience is associated with differences in default mode network activity and connectivity. *Proceedings of the National Academy of Sciences of the United States of America, 108*(50), 20254–20259.

Brickman, P., Coates, D., & Janoff-Bulman, R. (1978). Lottery winners and accident victims: Is happiness relative? *Journal of Personality and Social Psychology, 36*(8), 917–927.

Brier, M. R., Thomas, J. B., Snyder, A. Z., Benzinger, T. L., Zhang, D., Raichle, M. E., et al. (2012). Loss of intranetwork and internetwork resting state functional connections with Alzheimer's disease progression. *Journal of Neuroscience, 32*(26), 8890–8899.

Briere, J. (2002). Treating adult survivors of severe childhood abuse and neglect: Further development of an integrative model. In J. E. Myers et al. (Eds.), *The APSAC handbook on child maltreatment* (2nd ed., pp. 175–202). Newbury Park, CA: Sage.

Briere, J. (2004). *Psychological assessment of adult posttraumatic states: Phenomenology, diagnosis, and measurement* (2nd ed.). Washington, DC: American Psychological Association.

Briere, J. (2012a). When people do bad things: Evil, suffering, and dependent origination. In A. Bohart, E. Mendelowitz, B. Held, & Kirk Schneider (Eds.), *Humanity's dark side: Explorations in psychotherapy and beyond* (pp. 141–156). Washington, DC: American Psychological Association.

Briere, J. (2012b). Working with trauma: Mindfulness and compassion. In C. K. Germer & R. D. Siegel (Eds.), *Wisdom and compassion in psychotherapy* (pp. 265–279). New York: Guilford Press.

Briere, J., Hodges, M., & Godbout, N. (2010). Traumatic stress, affect dysregulation, and dysfunctional avoidance: A structural equation model. *Journal of Traumatic Stress, 23,* 767–774.

Briere, J., & Lanktree, C. B. (2011). *Treating complex trauma in adolescents and young adults.* Thousand Oaks, CA: Sage.

Briere, J., & Scott, C. (2012). *Principles of trauma therapy: A guide to symptoms, evaluation, and treatment* (2nd ed.). Thousand Oaks, CA: Sage.

Briere, J., Scott, C., & Weathers, F. W. (2005). Peritraumatic and persistent dissociation in the presumed etiology of PTSD. *American Journal of Psychiatry, 162,* 2295–2301.

Brotto, L. A., Basson, R., & Luria, M. (2008). A mindfulness-based group psychoeducational intervention targeting sexual arousal disorder in women. *Journal of Sexual Medicine, 5*(7), 1646–1659.

Brown, C. A., & Jones, A. K. (2010). Meditation experience predicts less negative appraisal of pain: Electrophysiological evidence for the involvement of anticipatory neural responses. *Pain, 150*(3), 428–438.

Brown, C. A., & Jones, A. K. (in press). Psychobiological correlates of improved mental health in patients with musculoskeletal pain after a mindfulness-based pain management program. *Clinical Journal of Pain.*

Brown, K., & Ryan, R. (2003). The benefits of being present: Mindfulness and its role in psychological well-being. *Journal of Personality and Social Psychology, 84*(4), 822–848.

Broyd, S., Demanuele, C., Debener, S., Helps, S., James, C., & Sonuga-Barke, E. (2009). Default-mode brain dysfunction in mental disorders: A systematic review. *Neuroscience and Biobehavior Reviews, 33*(3), 279–296.

Bruce, A., Young, L., Turner, L., Vander Wal, R., & Linden, W. (2002). Meditation-based stress reduction: Holistic practice in nursing education. In L. Young & V. Hayes (Eds.), *Transforming health promotion practice: Concepts, issues, and applications* (pp. 241–252). Victoria, BC, Canada: Davis.

Bruce, N., Manber, R., Shapiro, S., & Constantino, M. J. (2010). Psychotherapist mindfulness and the psychotherapy process. *Psychotherapy Theory, Research, Practice, Training, 47*(1), 83–97.

Bruner, J. (1973). *Beyond the information given: Studies in the psychology of knowing.* New York: Norton.

Buber, M. (1970). *I and thou* (W. Kaufmann, Trans.). New York: Charles Scribner's Sons.

Buhr, K., & Dugas, M. J. (2006). Investigating the construct validity of intolerance of uncertainty and its unique relationship with worry. *Journal of Anxiety Disorders, 20,* 222–236.

Burgmer, M., Petzke, F., Giesecke, T., Gaubitz, M., Heuft, G., & Pfleiderer, B. (2011). Cerebral activation and catastrophizing during pain anticipation in patients with fibromyalgia. *Psychosomatic Medicine, 73*(9), 751–759.

Burns, D. (1999). *The feeling good handbook.* New York: Penguin Putnam.

Burns, J. W. (2000). Repression predicts outcome following multidisciplinary treatment of chronic pain. *Health Psychology: Official Journal of the*

Division of Health Psychology, American Psychological Association, 19(1), 75–84.

Burns, J. W., Quartana, P. J., Gilliam, W., Matsuura, J., Nappi, C., & Wolfe, B. (2012). Suppression of anger and subsequent pain intensity and behavior among chronic low back pain patients: The role of symptom-specific physiological reactivity. *Journal of Behavioral Medicine, 35*(1), 103–114.

Buser, T., Buser, J., Peterson, C., & Serydarian, D. (2012). Influence of mindfulness practice on counseling skills development. *Journal of Counselor Preparation and Supervision, 4*(1), 20–45.

Cahill, S. P., Rothbaum, B. O., Resick, P. A., & Follette, V. M. (2009). Cognitive behavioral therapy for adults. In E. B. Foa, T. M. Keane, M. J. Friedman, & J. A. Cohen (Eds.), *Effective treatments for PTSD: Practice guidelines from the International Society for Traumatic Stress Studies* (pp. 139–222). New York: Guilford Press.

Campbell, J. (1995). *Reflections on the art of living: A Joseph Campbell companion.* New York: Harper Perennial.

Carmody, J. (2009). Evolving conceptions of mindfulness in clinical settings. *Journal of Cognitive Psychotherapy, 23*(3), 270–280.

Carmody, J., Baer, R., Lykins, E., & Olendzki, N. (2009). An empirical study of the mechanisms of mindfulness in a mindfulness-based stress reduction program. *Journal of Clinical Psychology, 65,* 613–626.

Carmody, J., Crawford, S., Salmoirago-Blotcher, E., Leung, K., Churchill, L., & Olendzki, N. (2011). Mindfulness training for coping with hot flashes: Results of a randomized trial. *Menopause, 18*(6), 611–620.

Carr, L., Iacoboni, M., Dubeau, M.C., Mazziotta, J. C., & Lenzi, G. L. (2003). Neural mechanisms of empathy in humans: A relay from neural systems for imitation to limbic areas. *Proceedings of the National Academy of Sciences of the United States of America, 100*(9), 5497–5502.

Carson, J. W., Carson, K. M., Gil, K. M., & Baucom, D. H. (2004). Mindfulness-based relationship enhancement. *Behavior Therapy, 35*(3), 471–494.

Carter, C. (1998). Neuroendocrine perspectives on social attachment and love. *Psychoneuroendocrinology, 23,* 779–818.

Casey, K. L., Minoshima, S., Morrow, T. J., & Koeppe, R. A. (1996). Comparison of human cerebral activation pattern during cutaneous warmth, heat pain, and deep cold pain. *Journal of Neurophysiology, 76*(1), 571–581.

Cassidy, E. L., Atherton, R. J., Robertson, N., Walsh, D. A., & Gillett, R. (2012). Mindfulness, functioning, and catastrophizing after multidisciplinary pain management for chronic low back pain. *Pain, 153*(3), 644–650.

Center for Mindfulness in Medicine, Health Care, and Society. (2012). Dear Friend of the Center. Retrieved September 23, 2012, from *www.umassmed. edu/cfm/appeal/index.aspx.*

Chah, A., Kornfield, J., & Breiter, P. (1985). *A still forest pool: The insight meditation of Achaan Chah.* Wheaton, IL: Theosophical Publishing House.

Chen, K., Berger, C., Manheimer, E., Forde, D., Magidson, J., Dachman, L., et al. (2012). Meditative therapies for reducing anxiety: A systematic review and meta-analysis of randomized controlled trials. *Depression and Anxiety, 29, 545–562.*

Chessen, A. L., Anderson, W. M., Littner, M., Davila, D., Hartse, K., Johnson, S., et al. (1999). Practice parameters for the nonpharmacologic treatment of chronic insomnia. *Sleep, 22, 1128–1133.*

Chiesa, A., Calati, R., & Serretti, A. (2011). Does mindfulness training improve cognitive abilities?: A systematic review of neuropsychological findings. *Clinical Psychology Review, 31, 449–464.*

Childs, D. (2007). Mindfulness and the psychology of presence. *Psychology and Psychotherapy: Theory, Research, and Practice, 80*(3), 367–376.

Cho, S., Heiby, E. M., McCracken, L. M., Lee, S. M., & Moon, D. E. (2010). Pain-related anxiety as a mediator of the effects of mindfulness on physical and psychosocial functioning in chronic pain patients in Korea. *Journal of Pain, 11*(8), 789–797.

Chödrön, P. (2001). *Tonglen.* Halifax, NS, Canada: Vajradhatu.

Chödrön, P. (2002). *The places that scare you: A guide to fearlessness in difficult times.* Boston: Shambhala.

Chödrön, P. (2007). *Practicing peace in times of war.* Boston: Shambhala.

Chou, R., Qaseem, A., Snow, V., Casey, D., Cross, J. T., Shekelle, P., et al. (2007). Diagnosis and treatment of low back pain: A joint clinical practice guideline from the American College of Physicians and the American Pain Society. *Annals of Internal Medicine, 147*(7), 478–491.

Christensen, A., & Jacobson, N. (2000). *Reconcilable differences.* New York: Guilford Press.

Christopher, J., Chrisman, J., Trotter-Mathison, M., Schure, M., Dahlen, P., & Christopher, S. (2011). Perceptions of the long-term influence of mindfulness training on counselors and psycotherapists: A qualitative inquiry. *Journal of Humanistic Psychology, 51*(3), 318–349.

Christopher, J., & Maris, J. (2010). Integrating mindfulness as self-care into counseling and psychotherapy training. *Counseling and Psychotherapy Research, 10*(2), 114–125

Chung, C. Y. (1990). Psychotherapist and expansion of awareness. *Psychotherapy and Psychosomatics, 53*(1–4), 28–32.

Cigolla, F., & Brown, D. (2011). A way of being: Bringing mindfulness into individual therapy. *Psychotherapy Research, 21*(6), 709–721.

Cioffi, D., & Holloway, J. (1993). Delayed costs of suppressed pain. *Journal of Personality and Social Psychology, 64, 274–282.*

Cisler, J. M., & Koster, E. H. (2010). Mechanisms of attentional biases towards threat in anxiety disorders: An integrative review. *Clinical Psychology Review, 30, 203–216.*

Clark, D., Fairburn, C., & Wessely, S. (2008). Psychological treatment outcomes in routine NHS services: A commentary on Stiles et al. (2007). *Psychological Medicine, 38, 629–634.*

Cloitre, M., Stovall-McClough, K. C., Miranda, R., & Chemtob, C. M. (2004). Therapeutic alliance, negative mood regulation, and treatment outcome in child abuse-related posttraumatic stress disorder. *Journal of Consulting and Clinical Psychology, 72,* 411– 416.

Coatsworth, J.D., Duncan, L. G., Greenberg, M. T., & Nix R. (2009). Changing parents' mindfulness, child management skills, and relationship quality with their youth: Results From a randomized pilot intervention trial. *Journal of Child and Family Studies, 19*(2), 203–217.

Cocoran, K., Farb, N., Anderson, A., & Segal, Z. (2010). Mindfulness and emotion regulation: Outcomes and possible mediating mechanisms. In A. Kring & D. Sloan (Eds.), *Emotion regulation and psychopathology: A transdiagnostic approach to etiology and treatment* (pp. 339–355). New York: Guilford Press.

Coelho, H. F., Canter, P. H., & Ernst, E. (2007). Mindfulness-based cognitive therapy: Evaluating current evidence and informing future research. *Journal of Consulting and Clinical Psychology, 75,* 1000–1005.

Cohen, N., Lojkasek, M., Muir, E., Muir, R., & Parker, C. (2002). Six-month follow-up of two mother–infant psychotherapies: Convergence of therapeutic outcomes. *Infant Mental Health Journal, 23*(4), 361–380.

Cohen, N., Muir, E., Lojkasek, M., Muir, R., Parker, C., Barwick, M., et al. (1999). Watch, wait, and wonder: Testing the effectiveness of a new approach to mother–infant psychotherapy. *Infant Mental Health Journal, 20*(4), 429–451.

Cohen-Katz, J., Wiley, S., Capuano, T., Baker, D., Kimmel, S., & Shapiro, S. (2005). The effects of mindfulness-based stress reduction on nurse stress and burnout, Part II: A quantitative and qualitative study. *Holistic Nursing Practice, 19,* 26–35.

Collum, E., & Gehart, D. (2010). Using mindfulness meditation to teach beginning therapists therapeutic presence: A qualitative study. *Journal of Marital and Family Therapy, 36*(3), 347–360.

Cosley, B., McCoy, S., Saslow, L., & Epel, E. (2010). Is compassion of others stress buffering?: Consequences of compassion and social support for physiological reactivity. *Journal of Experimental Social Psychology, 46,* 816–823.

Courtois, C. A., & Ford, J. D. (2013). *Treatment of complex trauma: A sequenced, relationshp-based approach guide.* New York: Guilford Press.

Cox, K. S. (2010). Elevation predicts domain-specific volunteerism 3 months later. *Journal of Positive Psychology, 5*(5), 333–341.

Cozolino, N. (2010). *The neuroscience of psychotherapy: Healing the social brain.* New York: Norton.

Craig, A. D. (2009). How do you feel—now?: The anterior insula and human awareness. *Nature Reviews Neuroscience, 10*(1), 59–70.

Craig, C., & Sprang, G. (2010). Compassion satisfaction, compassion fatigue, and burnout in a national sample of trauma treatment specialists. *Anxiety, Stress, and Coping, 23*(3), 31–339.

Craigie, M. A., Rees, C. S., & Marsh, A. (2008). Mindfulness-based cognitive therapy for generalized anxiety disorder: A preliminary evaluation. *Behavioural and Cognitive Psychotherapy, 36,* 553–568.

Cramer, H., Haller, H., Lauche, R., & Dobos, G. (2012). Mindfulness-based stress reduction for low back pain: A systematic review. *BioMed Central: Complementary and Alternative Medicine, 12*, 162.

Craske, M. G., & Barlow, D. H. (2008). Panic disorder and agoraphobia. In D. H. Barlow (Ed.), *Clinical handbook of psychological disorders: A step-by-step treatment manual* (4th ed., pp. 1–64). New York: Guilford Press.

Cree, M. (2010). Compassion focused therapy with perinatal and mother–infant distress. *International Journal of Cognitive Therapy, 3*(2), 159–171.

Crespo-Facorro, B., Kim, J., Andreasen, N. C., O'Leary, D. S., Bockholt, H. J., & Magnotta, V. (2000). Insular cortex abnormalities in schizophrenia: A structural magnetic resonance imaging study of first-episode patients. *Schizophrenia Research, 46*(1), 35–43.

Crits-Chrisopth, P., & Gibbons, M. B. (2003). Research developments on the therapeutic alliance in psychodynamic psychotherapy. *Psychoanalytic Inquiry, 23*(2) 332–349.

Crits-Christoph, P., Gibbons, M., & Hearon, B. (2006). Does the alliance cause good outcome?: Recommendations for future research on the alliance. *Psychotherapy: Theory, Research, Practice, Training, 43*(3), 280–285.

Crocker, J., & Canevello, A. (2008). Creating and undermining social support in communal relationships: The role of compassionate and self-image goals. *Journal of Personality and Social Psychology, 95*, 555–575.

Crombez, G., Vlaeyen, J. W., Heuts, P. H., & Lysens, R. (1999). Painrelated fear is more disabling than pain itself: Evidence on the role of pain-related fear in chronic back pain disability. *Pain, 80*(1–2), 329–339.

Csikszentmihalyi, M. (1991). *Flow: The psychology of optimal experience.* New York: HarperCollins.

Dahlsgaard, K., Peterson, C., & Seligman, M. (2005). Shared virtue: The convergence of valued human strengths across culture and history. *Review of General Psychology, 9*(3), 203–213.

Dalai Lama, XIV. (1999). *Ethics for the new millennium.* New York: Riverhead Books.

Dalai Lama, XIV. (2000). *Transforming the mind.* New York: Thorsons/Element. Retrieved February 19, 2011, from *www.dalailama.com/teachings/training-the-mind/verse-7.*

Dalai Lama, XIV. (2003). *Lighting the path: The Dalai Lama teaches on wisdom and compassion.* South Melbourne, Australia: Thomas C. Lothian.

Dalai Lama, XIV. (2005a, November 12). Op-Ed: Our faith in science. *New York Times.* Retrieved from *www.nytimes.com/2005/11/12/opinion/12dalai.html?pagewanted=all&_r=1&.*

Dalai Lama, XIV. (2005b, November 12). *Science at the crossroads.* Presentation at the annual meeting of the Society for Neuroscience, Washington, DC. Retrieved February 5, 2011, from *www.dalailama.com/messages/buddhism/science-at-the-crossroads.*

Dalai Lama, XIV. (2010, May 25). Many faiths, one truth. *New York Times,* Op-Ed., p. A27.

Dalai Lama, XIV, & Cutler, H. C. (1998). *The art of happiness*. New York: Riverhead Books.

Dalai Lama, XIV, & Goleman, D. (2003). *Destructive emotions: How can we overcome them? A scientific dialogue with the Dalai Lama*. New York: Bantam Books.

Dalrymple, K. L., & Herbert, J. D. (2007). Acceptance and commitment therapy for generalized social anxiety disorder: A pilot study. *Behavior Modification, 31*, 543–568.

Darwin, C. (2010). *The works of Charles Darwin, Vol. 21: The descent of man, and selection in relation to sex (part one)*. New York: New York University Press. (Original work published 1871)

Dass, R. (1971). *Be here now*. New York: Crown.

Daubenmier, J., Kristeller, J., Hecht, F., Maninger, N., Kuwata, M., Jhaveri, K., et al. (2011). Mindfulness intervention for stress eating to reduce cortisol and abdominal fat among overweight and obese women: An exploratory randomized controlled study. *Journal of Obesity, 2011*, 651936.

Davidson, R. J. (2004). Well-being and affective style: Neural substrates and biobehavioural correlates. *Philosophical Transactions of the Royal Society, 359*, 1395–1411.

Davidson, R. J. (2009, May 1). *Neuroscientific studies of meditation*. Paper presented at the Harvard Medical School's conference Meditation and Psychotherapy: Cultivating Compassion and Wisdom, Boston, MA.

Davidson, R. J. (2012). The neurobiology of compassion. In C. K. Germer & R. D. Siegel (Eds.), *Wisdom and compassion in psychotherapy: Deepening mindfulness in clinical practice* (pp. 111–118). New York: Guilford Press.

Davidson, R. J., & Harrington, A. (2001). *Visions of compassion: Western scientists and Tibetan Buddhists examine human nature*. Oxford, UK: Oxford University Press.

Davidson, R. J., Kabat-Zinn, J., Schumacher, J., Rosenkranz, M., Muller, D., Santorelli, S. F., et al. (2003). Alterations in brain and immune function produced by mindfulness meditation. *Psychosomatic Medicine, 65*(4), 564–570.

Davis, D. M., & Hayes, J. A. (2011). What are the benefits of mindfulness?: A practice review of psychotherapy-related research. *Psychotherapy, 48*(2), 198–208.

Davis, J. H. (2011, November). What feels right about right action? *Insight Journal*. Barre Center for Buddhist Studies, Barre, MA.

Decety, J. (2006). Human empathy through the lens of social neuroscience. *Scientific World Journal, 6*, 1146–1163.

Decety, J. (2011). The neuroevolution of empathy. *Annals of the New York Academy of Sciences, 1231*, 35–45.

Decety, J., & Cacioppo, J. (2011). *The Oxford handbook of social neuroscience*. New York: Oxford University Press.

Decety, J., & Jackson, P. (2004). The functional architecture of human empathy. *Behavioral and Cognitive Neuroscience Reviews, 3*, 71–100.

Decety, J., & Meyer, M. (2008). From emotion resonance to empathic understanding: A social developmental neuroscience account. *Development and Psychopathology, 20,* 1053–1080.

Decety, J., Michalska, K. J. (2010). Neurodevelopmental changes in the circuits underlying empathy and sympathy from childhood to adulthood. *Developmental Science, 13*(6), 886–899.

DeGraff, G. (1993). *Mind like fire unbound: An image in the early buddist discourses* (4th ed.). Valley Center, CA: Metta Forest Monastery.

Deikman, A. (2001). *Spirituality expands a therapist's horizons.* Retrieved July 6, 2004, from *www.buddhanet.net/psyspir3.htm.*

Delmonte, M. (1986). Meditation as a clinical intervention strategy: A brief review. *International Journal of Psychosomatics, 33*(3), 9–12.

Depue, R. A., & Morrone-Strupinsky, J. V. (2005). A neurobehavioral model of affiliative bonding. *Behavioral and Brain Sciences, 28,* 313–395.

Desbordes, G., Negi, L., Pace, T., Wallace, A., Raison, C., & Schwartz, E. (2012). Effects of mindful-attention and compassion meditation training on amygdala response to emotional stimuli in an ordinary, non-meditative state. *Frontiers in Human Neuroscience, 6,* 292.

Deutsch, D. (2011). *The beginning of infinity: Explanations that transform the world.* New York: Viking Press.

Devettere, R. J. (1993). Clinical ethics and happiness. *Journal of Medical Philosophy, 18,* 71–89.

Deyo, R. A, Rainville, J., & Kent, D. L. (1992). What can the history and physical examination tell us about low back pain? *Journal of the American Medical Association, 268*(6), 760–765.

Dickinson, E. (1872). Dickinson/Higginson correspondence: Late 1872. *Dickinson Electronic Archives.* Institute for Advanced Technology in the Humanities (IATH), University of Virginia. Retrieved July 21, 2004, from *http://jefferson.village.virginia.edy/cgi-bin/AT-Dickinsonsearch.cgi.*

Didonna, F. (Ed.). (2009). *Clinical handbook of mindfulness.* New York: Springer.

Dodson-Lavelle, B. (2011, July 21). *Cognitive-based compassion training (CBCT).* Paper presented at the Max-Planck Institute for Human and Cognitive Brain Sciences conference, "How to Train Compassion," Berlin, Germany.

Duckworth, A. (2007). Grit: Perseverance and passion for long-term goals. *Journal of Personality and Social Psychology, 92*(6), 1087–1101.

Duncan, B., Hubble, M., & Miller, S. (1997). *Psychotherapy with "impossible" cases: The efficient treatment of therapy veterans.* New York: Norton.

Duncan, B., & Miller, S. (2000). *The heroic client: Doing client-centered, outcome-informed therapy.* San Francisco, CA: Jossey-Bass.

Duncan, L. G., Coatsworth, J. D., & Greenberg, M. T. (2009). A model of mindful parenting: Implications for parent–child relationships and prevention research. *Clinical Child and Family Psychology Review, 12,* 255–270.

Duncan, L. G., Moskowitz, J., Neilands, T., Dilworth, S., Hecht, F., & Johnson, M. (2012). Mindfulness-based stress reduction for HIV treatment side effects: A randomized, wait-list controlled trial. *Journal of Pain and Symptom Management, 43*(2), 161–171.

Dunn, E.W., Aknin, L.B., & Norton, M.I. (2008). Spending money on others promotes happiness. *Science, 319,* 1687–1688.

Ehlers A. A. (1995). 1-year prospective study of panic attacks: Clinical course and factors associated with maintenance. *Journal of Abnormal Psychology, 104,* 164–172.

Eisenberger, N.I., & Lieberman, M. D. (2004). Why rejection hurts: A common neural alarm system for physical and social pain. *Trends in Cognitive Sciences, 8,* 294–300.

Ekman, P. (2010). Darwin's compassionate view of human nature. *Journal of the American Medical Association, 303*(6), 557–558.

Eliot, T. S. (1930). *Ash Wednesday, the waste land and other poems* (1934). New York: Harcourt.

Elliot, R., Bohart, A., Watson, J., & Greenberg, L. (2011). Empathy. *Psychotherapy, 48*(1), 43–49.

Ellis, A. (1962). *Reason and emotion in psychotherapy.* New York: Lyle Stuart.

Epstein, M. (1995). *Thoughts without a thinker.* New York: Basic Books.

Epstein, M. (2008). *Psychotherapy without the self: A Buddhist perspective.* New Haven, CT: Yale University Press

Erikson, E. H. (1950). *Childhood and society.* New York: Norton.

Etkin, A., & Wager, T. (2007). Reviews and overviews functional neuroimaging of anxiety: A meta-analysis of emotional processing in PTSD, social anxiety disorder, and specific phobia. *American Journal of Psychiatry, 164,* 1476–1488.

Evans, S., Ferrando, S., Findler, M., Stowell, C., Smart, C., & Haglin D. (2008). Mindfulness-based cognitive therapy for generalized anxiety disorder. *Journal of Anxiety Disorders, 22,* 716–721.

Excuriex, B., & Labbé, E. (2011). Health care providers' mindfulness and treatment outcomes: A critical review of the literature. *Mindfulness, 2*(3), 242–253.

Faber, A., & Mazlish, E. (1999). *How to talk so kids will listen and listen so kids will talk.* New York: Avon.

Fadiga, L., Fogassi, L., Pavesi, G., & Rizzolatti, G. (1995). Motor facilitation during action observation: A magnetic stimulation study. *Journal of Neurophysiology, 73,* 2608–2611.

Farb, N .A., Anderson, A. K., Mayberg, H., Bean, J., McKeon, D., & Segal, Z. V. (2010). Minding one's emotions: Mindfulness training alters the neural expression of sadness. *Emotion, 10*(1), 25–33.

Farb, N., Segal, Z., & Anderson, A. (in press). Mindfulness meditation training alters cortical representations of interoceptive attention. *Social Cognitive and Affective Neuroscience.*

Farb, N. A., Segal, Z. V., Mayberg, H., Bean, J., McKeon, D., Fatima, Z., et al. (2007). Attending to the present: Mindfulness meditation reveals distinct neural modes of self-reference. *Social Cognitive and Affective Neuroscience, 2*(4), 313–322.

Farber, B. A., & Doolin, E. M. (2011). Positive regard and affirmation. In J. C. Norcross (Ed.), *Psychotherapy relationships that work: Evidence-based responsiveness* (2nd ed.). New York: Oxford University Press.

Farchione, T., Fairholme, C., Ellard, K., Boisseau, C., Thompson-Hollands, J., Carl, J., et al. (2012). Unified protocol for transdiagnostic treatment of emotional disorders: A randomized controlled trial. *Behavior Therapy, 43*(3), 666–678.

Feldman, C. (2001). *The Buddhist path to simplicity: Spiritual practice for everyday life.* London, UK: HarperCollins.

Feldman, C., & Kornfield, J. (1991). *Stories of the spirit, stories of the heart.* New York: HarperCollins.

Feldman, C., & Kuyken, W. (2011). Compassion in the landscape of suffering. *Contemporary Buddhism, 12*(1), 143–155.

Fields, R. (1992). *How the swans came to the lake: The narrative history of Buddhism in America.* Boston: Shambhala.

Figley, C. (2002). Compassion fatigue: Psychotherapists' chronic lack of self-care. *Journal of Clinical Psychology, 58*, 1433–1441.

Fjorback, L., Arendt, M., Ornbol, E., Fink, P., & Walach, H. (2011). Mindfulness-based stress reduction and mindfulness-based cognitive therapy: A systematic review of randomized controlled trials. *Acta Psychiatrica Scandinavica, 123*(2), 102–119.

Flanagan, O. (2011, October 6). *Buddhist ethics naturalized: Contemporary perspectives on Buddhist ethics.* Presentation given at Columbia University conference, New York, NY.

Flor, H., Turk, D. C., & Birbaumer, N. (1985). Assessment of stress-related psychophysiological reactions in chronic back pain patients. *Journal of Consulting and Clinical Psychology, 53*(3), 354–364.

Foa, E. B., Franklin, M., & Kozak, M. (1998). Psychosocial treatments for obsessive–compulsive disorder: Literature review. In R. Swinson, M. Anthony, S. Rachman, & M. Richter (Eds.), *Obsessive–compulsive disorder: Theory, research, and treatment* (pp. 258–276). New York: Guilford Press.

Foa, E. B., Huppert, J. D., & Cahill, S. P. (2006). Emotional processing theory: An update. In B.O. Rothbaum (Ed.), *Pathological anxiety: Emotional processing in etiology and treatment* (pp. 3–24). New York: Guilford Press.

Follette, V. M., Palm, K. M., & Hall, M. L. R. (2004). Acceptance, mindfulness, and trauma. In S. C. Hayes, V. M. Follette, & M. M. Linehan (Eds.), *Mindfulness and acceptance: Expanding the cognitive-behavioral tradition* (pp. 192–208). New York: Guilford Press.

Follette, V.M., & Vijay, A. (2009). Mindfulness for trauma and posttraumatic stress disorder. In F. Didonna (Ed.), *Clinical handbook of mindfulness* (pp. 299–317). New York: Springer.

Fonagy, P., & Target, M. (1997). Attachment and reflective function: Their role in self-organization. *Development and Psychopathology, 9*(4), 679–700.

Forsyth, J., & Eifert, G. (2008). *The mindfulness and acceptance workbook for anxiety: A guide to breaking free from anxiety, phobias, and worry using acceptance and commitment therapy.* Oakland, CA: New Harbinger.

Fox, S. D., Flynn, E., & Allen, R. H. (2011). Mindfulness meditation for women with chronic pelvic pain: A pilot study. *Journal of Reproductive Medicine, 56*(3–4), 158–162.

Frank, J. (1961). *Persuasion and healing: A comparative study of psychotherapy.* London, UK: Oxford University Press.

Fraser, R. D., Sandhu, A., & Gogan, W. J. (1995) Magnetic resonance imaging findings 10 years after treatment for lumbar disc herniation. *Spine, 20*(6), 710–714.

Fredrickson, B. L. (2003). The value of positive emotions. *American Scientist, 91,* 330–335.

Fredrickson, B. L. (2009). *Positivity: Top-notch research reveals the 3 to 1 ratio that will change your life.* New York: Three Rivers Press.

Fredrickson, B. L. (2012). Building lives of compassion and wisdom. In. C. K. Germer & R. D. Siegel (Eds.), *Wisdom and compassion in psychotherapy: Deepening mindfulness in clinical practice* (pp. 48–58). New York: Guilford Press.

Fredrickson, B. L., & Branigan, C. (2005). Positive emotions broaden the scope of attention and thought–action repertoires. *Cognition and Emotion, 19*(3), 313–332.

Fredrickson, B. L., Cohn, M. A., Coffey, K. A., Pek, J., & Finkel, S. M. (2008). Open hearts build lives: Positive emotions, induced through loving-kindness meditation, build consequential personal resources. *Journal of Personality and Social Psychology, 95,* 1045–1062.

Freud, S. (1961a). Beyond the pleasure principle. In J. Strachey (Ed. & Trans.), *The standard edition of the complete psychological works of Sigmund Freud* (Vol. 18, pp. 1–64). London, UK: Hogarth Press. (Original work published 1920)

Freud, S. (1961b). Civilization and its discontents. In J. Strachey (Ed. & Trans.), *The standard edition of the complete psychological works of Sigmund Freud* (Vol. 21, pp. 57–145). London, UK: Hogarth Press. (Original work published 1930)

Freud, S. (1961c). Mourning and melancholia. In J. Strachey (Ed. & Trans.), *The standard edition of the complete psychological works of Sigmund Freud* (Vol. 14, pp. 237–260). London, UK: Hogarth Press. (Original work published 1917)

Freud, S. (1961d). Recommendations to physicians practicing psychoanalysis. In J. Strachey (Ed. & Trans.), *The standard edition of the complete psychological works of Sigmund Freud* (Vol. 21, pp. 111–120). London, UK: Hogarth Press. (Original work published 1912)

Freud, S., & Breuer, J. (1961). Studies on hysteria. In J. Strachey (Ed. & Trans.), *The standard edition of the complete psychological works of Sigmund Freud* (Vol. 2, pp. 19–305). London, UK: Hogarth Press. (Original work published 1895)

Fromm, E., Suzuki, D. T., & DeMartino, R. (1960). *Zen Buddhism and psychoanalysis.* New York: Harper & Row.

Galantino, M., Baime, M., Maguire, M., Szapary, P., & Farrer, J. (2005). Association of psychological and physiological measures of stress in health-care professionals during an 8-week mindfulness meditation program: Mindfulness in practice. *Stress and Health: Journal of the International Society for the Investigation of Stress, 21*(4), 255–261.

Gard, T., Hölzel, B. K., Sack, A. T., Hempel, H., Lazar, S. W., Vaitl, D., et al. (2012). Pain attenuation through mindfulness is associated with decreased cognitive control and increased sensory processing in the brain. *Cerebral Cortex, 22*(11), 2692–2702.

Gardner, H. (1983). *Frames of mind.* New York: Basic Books.

Garland, E. L., Fredrickson, B. L., Kring, A. M., Johnson, D. P., Meyer, P. S., & Penn, D. L. (2010). Upward spirals of positive emotions counter downward spirals of negativity: Insights from the broaden-and-build theory and affective neuroscience on the treatment of emotion dysfunction and deficits in psychopathology. *Clinical Psychology Review, 30*, 849–864.

Garland, E. L., Gaylord, S. A., & Fredrickson, B. L. (2011). Positive reappraisal mediates the stress-reductive effects of mindfulness: An upward spiral process. *Mindfulness, 2*, 59–67

Garland, E. L., Gaylord, S. A., Palsson, O., Faurot, K., Douglas Mann, J., & Whitehead, W. E. (2011). Therapeutic mechanisms of a mindfulness-based treatment for IBS: Effects on visceral sensitivity, catastrophizing, and affective processing of pain sensations. *Journal of Behavioral Medicine, 35*(6), 591–602.

Gaser, C., & Schlaug, G. (2003). Brain structures differ between musicians and non-musicians. *Journal of Neuroscience, 23*(27), 9240–9245.

Gatchel, R. J., & Blanchard, E. B. (Eds.). (1998). *Psychophysiological disorders: Research and clinical applications.* Washington, DC: American Psychological Association.

Gaylord, S. A., Paisson, O. S., Garland, E. L., Faurot, K. R., Coble, R. S., Mann, J. D., et al. (2011). Mindfulness training reduces the severity of irritable bowel syndrome in women: Results of a randomized controlled trial. *American Journal of Gastoenterology, 106*, 1678–1688.

Geller, S., & Greenberg, L. (2002). Therapeutic presence: Therapists' experience of presence in the psychotherapy encounter in psychotherapy. *Person Centered and Experiential Psychotherapies, 1*(1–2), 71–86.

Geller, S., & Greenberg, L. (2012). *Therapeutic presence: A mindful approach to effective therapy.* Washington, DC: American Psychological Association.

Gendlin, E. T. (1996). *Focusing-oriented psychotherapy: A manual of the experiential method.* New York: Guilford Press.

Germer, C. K. (2005a). Anxiety disorders: Befriending fear. In C. K. Germer, R. D. Siegel, & P. R. Fulton (Eds.). *Mindfulness and psychotherapy* (pp. 152–172). New York: Guilford Press.

Germer, C. K. (2005b). Teaching mindfulness in therapy. In C. K. Germer, R. D. Siegel, & P. R. Fulton (Eds.), *Mindfulness and psychotherapy* (pp. 113–129). New York: Guilford Press.

Germer, C. K. (2009). *The mindful path to self-compassion: Freeing yourself from destructive thoughts and emotions.* New York: Guilford Press.

Germer, C. K. & Siegel, R. D. (Eds.). (2012). *Wisdom and compassion in psychotherapy: Deepening mindfulness in clinical practice.* New York: Guilford Press.

Geschwind, N., Peeters, F., Drukker, M., van Os, J., & Wichers, M. (2011). Mindfulness training increases momentary positive emotions and reward experience in adults vulnerable to depression: A randomized controlled trial. *Journal of Consulting and Clinical Psychology, 79*(5), 618–628.

Gilbert, B. D., & Christopher, M. S. (2009). Mindfulness-based attention as a moderator of the relationship between depressive affect and negative cognitions. *Cognitive Therapy and Research, 34,* 514–521.

Gilbert, P. (Ed.). (2005). *Compassion: Conceptualisations, research and use in psychotherapy.* London, UK: Routledge.

Gilbert, P. (2009a). *The compassionate mind: A new approach to life's challenges.* Oakland, CA: New Harbinger Press.

Gilbert, P. (2009b). Introducing compassion focused therapy. *Advances in Psychiatric Treatment, 15,* 199–208.

Gilbert, P. (2010a). Compassion focused therapy. *International Journal of Cognitive Therapy, 3,* 95–210.

Gilbert, P. (2010b). *Compassion focused therapy: The CBT distinctive features series.* London, UK: Routledge.

Gilbert, P. (2010c). An introduction to compassion focused therapy in cognitive behavior therapy. *International Journal of Cognitive Therapy, 3*(2), 97–112.

Gilbert, P., McEwan, K., Matos, M., & Rivis, A. (in press). Fears of compassion: Development of three self-report measures. *Psychology and Psychotherapy.*

Gilbert, P., & Proctor, S. (2006). Compassionate mind training for people with high shame and self-criticism: Overview and pilot study of a group therapy approach. *Clinical Psychology and Psychotherapy, 13,* 353–379.

Gilligan, C. (1982). *In a different voice.* Cambridge, MA: Harvard University Press.

Godfrin, K. A., & van Heeringen, C. (2010). The effects of mindfulness-based cognitive therapy on recurrence of depressive episodes, mental health and quality of life: A randomized controlled study. *Behaviour Research and Therapy, 48,* 738–746.

Goffman, E. (1971). *Relations in public.* New York: Harper Colophon.

Gold, D. B., & Wegner, D. M. (1995). Origins of ruminative thought: Trauma, incompleteness, nondisclosure, and suppression. *Journal of Applied Social Psychology, 25,* 1245–1261.

Goldapple, K., Segal, Z., Garson, C., Lau, M., Bieling, P., Kennedy, S., et al. (2004). Modulation of cortical–limbic pathways in major depression. *Archives of General Psychiatry, 61,* 34–41.

Goldenberg, D. L., Kaplan, K. H., Nadeau, M. G., Brodeur, C., Smith, S., & Schmid, C. H. (1994). A controlled study of a stress-reduction, cognitive-behavioral treatment program in fibromyalgia. *Journal of Musculoskeletal Pain, 2,* 53–66.

Goldin, P., & Gross, J. (2010). Effects of mindfulness-based stress reduction (MBSR) on emotion regulation in social anxiety disorder. *Emotion, 10*(1), 83–91.

Goldstein, J. (2010, May 7). *The meditative journey: Meditation and psychotherapy—refining the art.* Presentation given at Harvard Medical School conference, Cambridge, MA.

Goodman, T., Greenland, S.K., & Siegel, D. J. (2012). Mindful parenting as a path to wisdom and compassion. In C. K. Germer & R. D. Siegel (Eds.), *Wisdom and compassion in psychotherapy* (pp. 295–310). New York: Guilford Press.

Goss, K., & Allen, S. (2010). Compassion focused therapy for eating disorders. *International Journal of Cognitive Therapy, 3*(2), 141–158.

Grant, J. A., Courtemanche, J., Duerden, E. G., Duncan, G. H., & Rainville, P. (2010). Cortical thickness and pain sensitivity in Zen meditators. *Emotion, 10*(1), 43–53.

Grant, J. A., Courtemanche, J., & Rainville, P. (2011). A non-elaborative mental stance and decoupling of executive and pain-related cortices predicts low pain sensitivity in Zen meditators. *Pain, 152*(1), 150–156.

Grant, J. A., & Rainville, P. (2009). Pain sensitivity and analgesic effects of mindful states in Zen meditators: A cross-sectional study. *Psychosomatic Medicine, 71*(1), 106–114.

Greason, P. B., & Cashwell, C. S. (2009). Mindfulness and counseling self-efficacy: The mediating role of attention and empathy. *Counselor Education and Supervision, 49*(1), 2–19.

Green, R. (2001). *The explosive child: A new approach for understanding and parenting easily frustrated, chronically inflexible children.* New York: HarperCollins.

Greenberg, L. S. (2010). *Emotion-focused therapy (theories of psychotherapy).* Washington, DC: American Psychological Association.

Greenberg, L. S., & Safran, J.D. (1987). *Emotions in psychotherapy.* New York: Guilford Press.

Greenland, S. K. (2010). *The mindful child: How to help your kid manage stress and become happier, kinder, and more compassionate.* New York: Free Press.

Greeson, J. (2009). Mindfulness research update: 2008. *Complementary Health Practice Review, 14*(1), 10–18.

Gregg, J., Callaghan, G., Hayes, S., & Glenn-Lawson, J. (2007). Improving diabetes self-management through acceptance, mindfulness, and values: A randomized controlled trial. *Journal of Consulting and Clinical Psychology, 75*(2), 336–343.

Grepmair, L., Mietterlehner, F., Loew, T., Bachler, E., Rother, W., & Nickel, N. (2007). Promoting mindfulness in psychotherapists in training influences the treatment results of their patients: A randomized, double-blind, controlled study. *Psychotherapy and Psychosomatics, 76*, 332–338.

Grienenberger, J., Slade, A., & Kelly, K. (2005). Maternal reflective functioning, mother–infant affective communication, and infant attachment: Exploring the link between mental states and observed caregiving behavior in the intergenerational transmission of attachment. *Attachment and Human Development, 7*(3), 299–311.

Gross, C. R., Kreitzer, M. J., Reilly-Spong, M., Wall, M., Winbush, N. Y., Patterson, R., et al. (2011). Mindfulness-based stress reduction versus pharmacotherapy for chronic primary insomnia: A randomized controlled clinical trial. *Explore: The Journal of Science and Healing, 7*(2), 76–87.

Gross, J. J. (2002). Emotion regulation: Affective, cognitive, and social consequences. *Psychophysiology, 39,* 281–291.

Grossman, P. (2011). Defining mindfulness by how poorly I think I pay attention during everyday awareness and other intractable problems for psychology's (re)invention of mindfulness: Comment on Brown et al. (2011). *Psychological Assessment, 23*(4), 1034–40; discussion 1041–1046.

Grossman, P., Niemann, L., Schmidt, S., & Walach, H. (2004). Mindfulness-based stress reduction and health benefits: A meta-analysis. *Journal of Psychosomatic Research, 57,* 35–43.

Grossman, P., Tiefenthaler-Gilmer, U., Raysz, A., & Kesper, U. (2007). Mindfulness training as an intervention for fibromyalgia: Evidence of postintervention and 3-year follow-up benefits in well-being. *Psychotherapy and Psychosomatics, 76*(4), 226–233.

Gumley, A., Braehler, C., Laithwaite, H., MacBeth, A. & Gilbert, P. (2010). A compassion focused model of recovery after psychosis. *International Journal of Cognitive Therapy, 3*(2), 186–201.

Gunaratana, B. (2002). *Mindfulness in plain English.* Somerville, MA: Wisdom.

Gurman, S., & Messer, A. (2011). *Essential psychotherapies: Theory and practice* (3rd ed.). New York: Guilford Press.

Gusnard, D., & Raichle, M. (2001). Searching for a baseline: Functional imaging and the resting human brain. *Nature Reviews: Neuroscience, 2,* 685–694.

Guzman, J., Esmail, R., Karjalainen, K., Malmivaara, A., Irvin, E., & Bombardier, C. (2001). Multidisciplinary rehabilitation for chronic low back pain: Systematic review. *British Medical Journal, 323,* 1186–1187.

Gyatso, T. (2005, November 12). Our faith in science. *New York Times,* Op-Ed. Retrieved February 23, 2012, from *www.nytimes.com/2005/11/12/opinion/12dalai.html?pagewanted=all.*

Halifax, J. (1993). The road is your footsteps. In T. N. Hanh (Ed.), *For a future to be possible: Commentaries on the five wonderful precepts* (pp. 143–147). Berkeley, CA: Parallax Press.

Hall, H., McIntosh, G., Wilson, L., & Melles, T. (1998). Spontaneous onset of back pain. *Clinical Journal of Pain, 14*(2), 129–133.

Hanh, T. N. (1976). *The miracle of mindfulness.* Boston: Beacon Press.

Hanh, T. N. (1992). *Peace is every step: The path of mindfulness in everyday life.* New York: Bantam Books.

Hanh, T. N. (1998). *The heart of the Buddha's teachings.* Berkeley, CA: Parallax Press.

Hanh, T. N. (2003). *Joyfully together: The art of building a harmonious community.* Berkeley, CA: Parallax Press.

Hanh, T. N. (2007). *For a future to be possible: Buddhist ethics for everyday life*. Berkeley, CA: Parallax Press.

Hanson, R., & Mendius, R. (2009). *Buddha's brain: The practical neuroscience of happiness, love, and wisdom*. Oakland, CA: New Harbinger.

Harris, R., & Hayes, S. (2009). *ACT made simple: An easy-to-read primer on acceptance and commitment therapy*. Oakland, CA: New Harbinger.

Harris, S. (2006, March). Killing the Buddha. *Shambala Sun*. Retrieved on February 23, 2012 from *www.shambhalasun.com/index.php?option=com_content&task=view&id=2903&Itemid=0*.

Hart, S. (2010). *The impact of attachment*. New York: Norton.

Hartranft, C. (2003). *The yoga-sutra of Pantajali*. Boston: Shambhala.

Hasenkamp, W., & Barsalou, L. W. (2012). Effects of meditation experience on functional connectivity of distributed brain networks. *Frontiers in Human Neuroscience, 6*, 38.

Hasenkamp, W., Wilson-Mendenhall, C. D., Duncan, E., & Barsalou, L. W. (2012). Mind wandering and attention during focused meditation: A fine-grained temporal analysis of fluctuating cognitive states. *NeuroImage, 59*(1), 750–760.

Hatcher, R. (2010). Alliance theory and measurement. In J. Muran & J. Barber (Eds.), *The therapeutic alliance: An evidence-based guide to practice* (pp. 7– 28). New York: Guilford Press.

Hayes, S. (2002a). Acceptance, mindfulness, and science. *Clinical Psychology: Science and Practice, 9*(1), 101–106.

Hayes, S. (2002b). Buddhism and acceptance and commitment therapy. *Cognitive and Behavioral Practice, 9*, 58–66.

Hayes, S. (2011). Open, aware, and active: Contextual approaches as an emerging trend in the behavioral and cognitive therapies. *Annual Review of Clinical Psychology, 7*(1), 141–168.

Hayes, S. C., Follette, V. M., & Linehan, M. (2011). *Mindfulness and acceptance: Expanding the cognitive-behavioral tradition*. New York: Guilford Press.

Hayes, S. C., Luoma, J. B., Bond, F. W., Masuda, A., & Lillis, J. (2006). Acceptance and commitment therapy: Model, processes and outcomes. *Behaviour Research and Therapy, 44*(1), 1–25.

Hayes, S. C., Strosahl, K .D., & Wilson, K. G. (1999). *Acceptance and commitment therapy: An experiential approach to behavior change*. New York: Guilford Press.

Hayes, S. C., Strosahl, K. D., & Wilson, K. G. (2011). *Acceptance and commitment therapy: The process and practice of mindful change* (2nd ed.). New York: Guilford Press.

Hayes, S. C., Wilson, K. G., Gifford, E. V., Follette, V. M., & Strosahl, K. (1996). Experimental avoidance and behavioral disorders: A functional dimensional approach to diagnosis and treatment. *Journal of Consulting and Clinical Psychology, 64*(6), 1152–1168.

Hayes, S., & Smith, S. (2005). *Get out of your mind and into your life: The new acceptance and commitment therapy*. Oakland, CA: New Harbinger.

Hayes, S., Strosahl, K., & Houts, A. (Eds.). (2005). *A practical guide to acceptance and commitment therapy*. New York: Springer.

Hayes-Skelton, S. A., Roemer, L., & Orsillo, S. M. (in press). A randomized clinical trial comparing an acceptance-based behavior therapy to applied relaxation for generalized anxiety disorder. *Journal of Consulting and Clinical Psychology.*

Hein, G., & Singer, T. (2008). I feel how you feel but not always: The empathic brain and its modulation. *Current Opinion in Neurobiology, 18*(2), 153–158.

Hembree, E. A., & Foa, E. B. (2003). Interventions for trauma-related emotional disturbances in adult victims of crime. *Journal of Traumatic Stress, 16,* 187–199.

Henley, A. (1994). When the iron bird flies: A commentary on Sydney Walter's "Does a systemic therapist have Buddha nature?" *Journal of Systemic Therapies, 13*(3), 50–51.

Hermans, D., Craske, M. G., Mineka, S., & Lovibond, P. F. (2006). Extinction in human fear conditioning. *Biological Psychiatry, 60,* 361–368.

Hick, S., & Bien, T. (Eds.). (2010). *Mindfulness and the therapeutic relationship.* New York: Guilford Press.

Hill, C., & Updegraff, J. (2012). Mindfulness and its relationship to emotion regulation. *Emotion, 12*(1), 81–90.

Hillman, J. (2003). Foreword. In Heraclitus, *Fragments* (pp. xi–xviii). New York: Penguin Classics.

Hoffman, C., Ersser, S., Hopkinson, J., Nicholis, P., Harrington, J., & Thomas, P. (2012). Effectiveness of mindfulness-based stress reduction in mood, breast- and endocrine-related quality of life, and well-being in stage 0–III breast cancer: A randomized, controlled trial. *Journal of Clinical Oncology, 12,* 1335–1342.

Hofmann, S., Grossman, P., & Hinton, D. (2011). Loving-kindness and compassion meditation: Potential for psychological interventions. *Clinical Psychology Review, 31,* 1126–1132.

Hofmann, S., Sawyer, A., Witt, A., & Oh, D. (2010). The effect of mindfulness-based therapy on anxiety and depression: A meta-analytic review. *Journal of Clinical and Consulting Psychology, 78*(2), 169–183.

Hofmann, S. G., & Smits, J. J. (2008). Cognitive-behavioral therapy for adult anxiety disorders: A meta-analysis of randomized placebo-controlled trials. *Journal of Clinical Psychiatry, 69,* 621–632.

Hollis-Walker, L., & Colosimo, K. (2011). Mindfulness, self-compassion, and happiness in non-meditators: A theoretical and empirical examination. *Personality and Individual Differences, 50*(2), 222–227.

Hölzel, B. K., Carmody, J., Evans, K. C., Hoge, E. A., Dusek, J. A., Morgan, L., et al. (2010). Stress reduction correlates with structural changes in the amygdala. *Social Cognitive and Affective Neuroscience, 5,* 11–17.

Hölzel, B. K., Carmody, J., Vangel, M., Congleton, C., Yerramsetti, S. M., Gard, T., et al. (2011). Mindfulness practice leads to increases in regional brain gray matter density. *Psychiatry Research: Neuroimaging, 191,* 36–42.

Hölzel, B.K., Hoge, E.A., Greve, D.N., Gard, T., Creswell, J.D., Brown, K.W., et al. (2013). *Neural mechanisms of symptom improvements in generalized anxiety disorder following mindfulness meditation training.* Manuscript accepted for publication.

Hölzel, B. K., Lazar, S. W., Gard, T., Schuman-Olivier, Z., Vago, D. R., & Ott, U. (2011). How does mindfulness meditation work?: Proposing mechanisms of action from a conceptual and neural perspective. *Perspectives on Psychological Science, 6*(6), 537–559.

Hölzel, B. K., Ott, U., Gard, T., Hempel, H., Weygandt, M., Morgen, K., et al. (2008). Investigation of mindfulness meditation practitioners with voxel-based morphometry. *Social Cognitive and Affective Neuroscience, 3,* 55–61.

Hölzel, B. K., Ott, U., Hempel, H., Hackl, A., Wolf, K., Stark, R., et al. (2007). Differential engagement of anterior cingulate and adjacent medial frontal cortex in adept meditators and non-meditators. *Neuroscience Letters, 421*(1), 16–21.

Horney, K. (1945). *Our inner conflicts: A constructive theory of neurosis.* New York: Norton.

Horowitz, M. J. (1978). *Stress response syndromes.* New York: Jason Aronson.

Horvath, A., Del Re, A., Flückiger, C., & Symonds, D. (2011). Alliance in individual psychotherapy. In J. C. Norcross (Ed.), *Psychotherapy relationships that work: Therapist contributions and responsiveness to patients* (2nd ed.). New York: Oxford University Press.

Huppert, J., Bufka, L., Barlow, D., Gorman, J., & Shear, M. (2001). Therapists, therapist variables, and cognitive-behavioral therapy outcome in a multicenter trial for panic disorder. *Journal of Consulting and Clinical Psychology, 65,* 747–755.

Iacoboni, M. (2008). *Mirroring people.* New York: Farrar, Giroux & Strauss.

Immordino-Yang, M., McColl, A., Damasio, H., & Damasio, A. (2009). Neural correlates of admiration and compassion. *Proceedings of the National Academy of Sciences of the United States of America, 106*(19), 8021–8026.

Irving, J., Dobkin, P., & Park, J. (2009). Cultivating mindfulness in health care professionals: A review of empirical studies of mindfulness-based stress reduction (MBSR). *Complementary Therapies in Clinical Practice, 15,* 61–66.

Iyengar, B. K. S. (1966). *Light on yoga.* New York: Schocken Books.

James, H., & Chymis, A. (2004). *Are happy people ethical people?: Evidence from North America and Europe* (Working paper No. AEWP, 2004). Columbia, MO: University of Missouri, Department of Agricultural Economics.

James, W. (2007). *The principles of psychology* (Vol. 1). New York: Cosimo. (Original work published 1890)

Jang, J. H., Jung, W. H., Kanga, D. H., Byuna, M. S., Kwonc, S. J., Choid, C. H., et al. (2011). Increased default mode network connectivity associated with meditation. *Neuroscience Letters, 487,* 358–362.

Jensen, M. C., BrantZawadzki, M. D., Obucowski, N., Modic, M. T.,

Malkasian, D., & Ross, J. S. (1994). Magnetic resonance imaging of the lumbar spine in people without back pain. *New England Journal of Medicine, 331*(2), 69–73.

Jha, A., Krompinger, J., & Baime, M. (2007). Mindfulness training modifies subsystems of attention. *Cognitive, Affective, & Behavioral Neuroscience, 7*(2), 109–119.

Jimenez, S. S., Niles, B. L., & Park, C. L. (2010). A mindfulness model of affect regulation and depressive symptoms: Positive emotions, mood regulation expectancies, and self-acceptance as regulatory mechanisms. *Personality and Individual Differences, 49*, 645–650.

Jinpa, T., Rosenberg, E., McGonigal, K., Cullen, M., Goldin, P., & Ramel, W. (2009). *Compassion cultivation training (CCT): An eight-week course on cultivating compassionate heart and mind.* Unpublished manuscript. The Center for Compassion and Altruism Research and Education, Stanford University, Stanford, CA.

Johnson, J., Germer, C., Efran, J., & Overton, W. (1988). Personality as a basis for theoretical predilections. *Journal of Personality and Social Psychology, 55*(5), 824–835.

Jordan, J. V. (1991). Empathy and self boundaries. In J. V. Jordon, A. G. Kaplan, J. B. Miller, I. P. Stiver, & J.L. Surrey (Eds.), *Women's growth in connection: Writings form the Stone Center* (pp. 67–80). New York: Guilford Press.

Jordan, J. V., Kaplan, A. G., Miller, J. B., Stiver, I. P., & Surrey, J. L. (1991). *Women's growth in connection: Writings from the Stone Center.* New York: Guilford Press.

Joseph, S., Dalgleish, D., Williams, R., Yule, W., Thrasher, S., & Hodgkinson, P. (1997). Attitudes towards emotional expression and post-traumatic stress in survivors of the Herald of Free Enterprise disaster. *British Journal of Psychology, 36*, 133–138.

Jung, C. (2000). Psychological commentary. In W. Y. Evans-Wentz, *The Tibetan book of the dead* (pp. xxxv–lii). London: Oxford University Press. (Original work published 1927)

Junger, S. (2010). *War.* New York: Twelve.

Kabat-Zinn, J. (1982). An outpatient program in behavioral medicine for chronic pain patients based on the practice of mindfulness meditation: Theoretical considerations and preliminary results. *General Hospital Psychiatry, 4*, 33–47.

Kabat-Zinn, J. (1990). *Full catastrophe living: Using the wisdom of your body and mind to face stress, pain, and illness.* New York: Dell.

Kabat-Zinn, J. (1994). *Wherever you go, there you are.* New York: Hyperion.

Kabat-Zinn, J. (2002, Winter). At home in our bodies. *Tricycle: The Buddhist Review.*

Kabat-Zinn, J. (2003). Mindfulness-based interventions in context: Past, present, and future. *Clinical Psychology: Science and Practice, 10*(2), 144–156.

Kabat-Zinn, J. (2005). *Coming to our senses: Healing ourselves and the world through mindfulness.* New York: Hyperion.

Kabat-Zinn, J. (2011). *Mindfulness for beginners: Reclaiming the present moment—and your life.* Louisville, CO: Sounds True.

Kabat-Zinn, M., & Kabat-Zinn, J. (1998). *Everyday blessings: The inner work of mindful parenting.* New York: Hyperion.

Kabat-Zinn, J., Lipworth, L., & Burney, R. (1985). The clinical use of mindfulness meditation for the self-regulation of chronic pain. *Journal of Behavioral Medicine, 8*(2), 163–190.

Kabat-Zinn, J., Wheeler, E., Light, T., Skillings, Z., Scharf, M. J., Cropley, T. G., et al. (1998). Influence of a mindfulness meditation-based stress reduction intervention on rates of skin clearing in patients with moderate to severe psoriasis undergoing phototherapy (UVB) and photochemotherapy (PUVA). *Psychosomatic Medicine, 50,* 625–632.

Kahneman, D. (2011). *Thinking fast and slow.* New York: Farrar, Straus & Giroux.

Kaiser Greenland, S. (2010). *The mindful child: How to help your kid manage stress and become happier, kinder, and more compassionate.* New York: Free Press.

Kang, D., Jo, H. J., Jung, W. H., Kim, S. H., Jung, Y., & Choi, C. (in press). The effect of meditation on brain structure: Cortical thickness mapping and diffusion tensor imaging. *Social Cognitive and Affective Neuroscience.*

Kaplan, K. H., Goldenberg, D. L., & Galvin-Nadeau, M. (1993). The impact of a meditation-based stress reduction program on fibromyalgia. *General Hospital Psychiatry, 15*(5), 284–289.

Kar, N. (2011). Cognitive behavioral therapy for the treatment of post-traumatic stress disorder: A review. *Neuropsychiatric Disease and Treatment, 7,* 167–181.

Karlson, H. (2011). How psychotherapy changes the brain. *Psychotherapy Update, 28*(8). Retrieved September 23, 2012, from *www.psychiatrictimes.com/display/article/10168/1926705.*

Kazantzis, N., & Dattilio, F. M. (2010). Definitions of homework, types of homework, and ratings of the importance of homework among psychologists with cognitive behavior therapy and psychoanalytic theoretical orientations. *Journal of Clinical Psychology, 66*(7), 758–773.

Kearney, D. J., McDermott, K., Martinez, M., & Simpson, T. L. (2011). Association of participation in a mindfulness programme with bowel symptoms, gastrointestinal symptom-specific anxiety and quality of life. *Alimentary Pharmacology and Therapeutics, 34*(3), 363–373.

Kearney, M., Weininger, R., Vachon, M., Harrison, R., & Mount, B. (2009). Self-care of physicians caring for patients at the end of life: Being connected . . . "a key to my survival." *Journal of the American Medical Association, 301*(11), 1155–1165.

Keltner, D. (2009). *Born to be good: The science of a meaningful life.* New York: Norton.

Keltner, D., Marsh, J., & Smith, J. (2010). *The compassionate instinct.* New York: Norton.

Keng, S., Smoski, M., & Robins, C. J. (2011). Effects of mindfulness on psychological health: A review of empirical studies. *Clinical Psychology Review, 31,* 1041–1056.

Kerr, C. F., Josyula, K., & Littenberg, R. (2011). Developing an observing attitude: An analysis of meditation diaries in an MBSR clinical trial. *Clinical Psychology and Psychotherapy, 18,* 80–93.

Kesebir, P., & Diener, E. (2008). In defense of happiness: Why policymakers should care about subjective well-being. In L. Bruni, F. Comin, & M. Pugno (Eds.), *Capabilities and happiness* (pp. 60–80). New York: Oxford University Press.

Keysers, C. (2011). *The empathic brain.* Amsterdam, Netherlands: Social Brain Press.

Khazan, I. (2013). *The clinical handbook of biofeeback: A guide for training and practice with mindfulness.* New York: Wiley.

Killingsworth, M. A., & Gilbert, D. T. (2010). A wandering mind is an unhappy mind. *Science, 330,* 932.

Kilpatrick, L. A., Suyenobu, B. Y., Smith, S. R., Bueller, J. A., Goodman, T., Creswell, J. D., et al. (2011). Impact of mindfulness-based stress reduction training on intrinsic brain connectivity. *NeuroImage, 56,* 290–298.

Kim, D., Wampold, B., & Bolt, D. (2006). Therapist effects in psychotherapy: A random effects modeling of the NIMH TDCRP data. *Psychotherapy Research, 16,* 161–172.

Kim, J., Kim, S., Kim, J., Joeng, B., Park, C., Son, A., et al. (2011). Compassionate attitude towards others' suffering activates the mesolimbic neural system. *Neuropsychologia, 47,* 2073–2081.

Kimbrough, E., Magyari, T., Langenberg, P., Chesney, M. A., & Berman, B. (2010). Mindfulness intervention for child abuse survivors. *Journal of Clinical Psychology, 66,* 17–33.

Kingston, J., Chadwick, P., Meron, D., & Skinner, T. C. (2007). A pilot randomized control trial investigating the effect of mindfulness practice on pain tolerance, psychological well-being, and physiological activity. *Journal of Psychosomatic Research, 62*(3), 297–300.

Kleinman, A., Kunstadter, P., Alexander, E., Russell, G., & James, L. (Eds.). (1978). *Culture and healing in Asian societies: Anthropological, psychiatric and public health studies.* Cambridge, MA: Schenkman.

Klimecki, O., Leiberg, S., Lamm, C., & Singer, T. (in press). Functional neural plasticity and associated changes in positive affect. *Cerebral Cortex.*

Klimecki, O., & Singer, T. (2011). Empathic distress fatigue rather than compassion fatigue?: Integrating findings from empathy research in psychology and social neuroscience. In B. Oakley, A. Knafo, G. Madhavan, & D. S. Wilson (Eds.), *Pathological altruism* (pp. 368–384). New York: Oxford University Press.

Kocovski, N. L., Laurier, W., & Rector, N. A. (2009). Mindfulness and acceptance-based group therapy for social anxiety disorder: An open trial. *Cognitive and Behavioral Practice, 16,* 276–289.

Koerner, K., & Linehan, M. (2011). *Doing dialectical behavior therapy: A practical guide.* New York: Guilford Press.

Kohut, H. (1977). *The restoration of the self.* New York: International University Press.

Kolden, G. G., Klein, M. H., Wang, C. C., & Austin, S. B. (2011). Congruence/genuineness. *Psychotherapy, 48*(1), 65–71.

Kolts, R. (2011). *The compassionate mind approach to managing your anger.* London, UK: Constable & Robinson.

Kori, S.H., Miller, R.P., & Todd, D.D. (1990). Kinesiophobia: A new view of chronic pain behavior. *Pain Management, 3,* 35–43.

Koszycki, D., Benger, M., Shlik, J., & Bradwejn, J. (2007). Randomized trial of a meditation-based stress reduction program and cognitive behavior therapy in generalized social anxiety disorder. *Behaviour Research and Therapy, 45,* 2518–2526.

Kramer, G. (2007). *Insight dialogue: The interpersonal path to freedom.* Boston: Shambhala.

Kramer, G., Meleo-Meyer, F., & Turner, M. L. (2008). Cultivating mindfulness in relation: Insight dialogue and the interpersonal mindfulness program. In S. Hick & T. Bien (Eds.), *Mindfulness and the therapeutic relationship* (pp. 195–214). New York: Guilford Press.

Kramer, J. (2004). *Buddha mom.* New York: Penguin.

Krasner, M., Epstein, R., Beckman, H., Suchman, A., Chapman, A., Mooney, C., et al. (2009). Association of an educational program in mindful communication with burnout, empathy, and attitudes among primary care physicians. *Journal of the American Medical Association, 302,* 1284–1293.

Kristeller, J. L., & Wolever, R. (2011). Mindfulness-based eating awareness training for treating binge eating disorder: The conceptual foundation. *Eating Disorders, 19*(1), 49–61.

Krüger, E. (2010). *Effects of a meditation-based programme of stress reduction on levels of self-compassion.* Unpublished master's thesis, School of Psychology, Bangor University, Wales, UK.

Kurtz, R. (1990). *Body-centered psychotherapy: The Hakomi method.* Mendecino, CA: LifeRhythm.

Kuyken, W., Byford, S., Taylor, R. S., Watkins, E., Holden, E., White, K., et al. (2008). Mindfulness-based cognitive therapy to prevent relapse in recurrent depression. *Journal of Consulting and Clinical Psychology, 76*(6), 966–978.

Kuyken, W., Watkins, E., Holden, E., White, K., Taylor, R. S., Byford, S., et al. (2010). How does mindfulness-based cognitive therapy work? *Behavior Research and Therapy, 48,* 1105–1112.

Lambert, M. J., & Barley, D. E. (2001). Research summary on the therapeutic relationship and psychotherapy outcome. *Psychotherapy, 38,* 357–361.

Lambert, M. J., & Ogles, B. (2004). The efficacy and effectiveness of psychotherapy. In M. Lambert (Ed.), *Bergin and Garfield's handbook of psychotherapy and behavior change* (5th ed., pp. 139–193). New York: Wiley.

Lambert, M. J., & Okishi, J. C. (1997). The effects of the individual psychotherapist and implications for future research. *Clinical Psychology: Science and Practice, 4*, 66–75.

Lambert, N. M., Fincham, F. D., Stillman, T. F., & Dean, L. R. (2009). More gratitude, less materialism: The mediating role of life satisfaction. *Journal of Positive Psychology, 4*(1), 32–42.

Lamott, A. (1993). *Operating instructions: A journal of my son's first year.* New York: Pantheon.

Landis, S. K., Sherman, M. F., Piedmont, R. L., Kirkhart, M. W., Rapp, E. M., & Bike, D. H. (2009). The relation between elevation and self-reported prosocial behavior: Incremental validity over the five-factor model of personality. *Journal of Positive Psychology, 4*(1), 71–84.

Landreth, G. (2002). Play therapy: The art of the relationship. New York: Brunner-Routledge.

Langer, A., Cangas, A., Salcedo, E., & Fuentes, F. (2012). Applying mindfulness therapy in a group of psychotic individuals: A controlled study. *Behavioural and Cognitive Psychotherapy, 40*(1), 105–109.

Law, N. (2008, March 31). Scientists probe meditation secrets. *BBC News Online.* Retrieved from *http://news.bbc.co.uk/2/hi/health/7319043.stm*.

Lazar, S. W., Kerr, C. E., Wasserman, R. H., Gray, J. R., Greve, D. N., Treadway, M. T., et al. (2005). Meditation experience is associated with increased cortical thickness. *NeuroReport, 16*(17), 1893–1897.

Lazarus, A. (1993). Tailoring the therapeutic relationship, or being an authentic chameleon. *Psychotherapy, 30*, 404–407.

Lee, D. (1959). *Freedom and culture.* Englewood Cliffs, NJ: Prentice-Hall.

Lee, R., & Martin, J. (1991). *Psychotherapy after Kohut: A textbook of self-psychology.* Hillsdale, NJ: Analytic Press.

Lee, T., Leung, M., Hou, W., Tang, J., Yin, J., So, K., et al. (2012). Distinct neural activity associated with focused-attention meditation and loving-kindness meditation. *PLoS One, 7*(8), e40054.

Leeuw, M., Goossens, M. E., Linton, S. J., Crombez, G., Boersma, K., & Vlaeyen, J. W. (2007). The fear-avoidance model of musculoskeletal pain: Current state of scientific evidence. *Journal of Behavioral Medicine, 30*(1), 77–94.

Leiblich, A., McAdams, D., & Josselson, R. (2004). *Healing plots: The narrative basis of psychotherapy.* Washington, DC: American Psychological Association.

Leichsenring, F. (2001). Comparative effects of short-term psychodynamic psychotherapy and cognitive behavioural therapy in depression: A meta-analytic approach. *Clinical Psychology Review, 21*, 401–419.

Leung, M. K., Chan C. C., Yin J., Lee C. F., So K. F., & Lee T. M. (2012). Increased gray matter volume in the right angular and posterior parahippocampal gyri in loving-kindness meditators. *Social Cognitive and Affective Neuroscience, 8*(1), 34–39.

Levine, S., & Levine, O. (1995). *Embracing the beloved: Relationship as a path of awakening.* New York: Doubleday.

Levitt, J. T., Brown, T. A., Orsillo, S. M., & Barlow, D. H. (2004). The effects of acceptance versus suppression of emotion on subjective and psychophysiological response to carbon dioxide challenge in patients with panic disorder. *Behavior Therapy, 35,* 747–766.

Lewis, T., Amini, F., & Lannon, R. (2001). *A general theory of love.* New York: Random House.

Linehan, M. M. (1993a). *Cognitive-behavioral treatment of borderline personality disorder.* New York: Guilford Press.

Linehan, M. M. (1993b). *Skills training manual for treating borderline personality disorder.* New York: Guilford Press.

Linehan, M. M. (2009, May 2). *Radical compassion: Translating Zen into psychotherapy.* Presentation given at the Harvard Medical School conference Meditation and Psychotherapy: Cultivating Compassion and Wisdom, Cambridge, MA.

Linton, S. J. (1997). A population-based study of the relationship between sexual abuse and back pain: Establishing a link. *Pain, 73*(1), 47–53.

Litt, M. D., Shafer, D., & Napolitano, C. (2004). Momentary mood and coping processes in TMD pain. *American Psychological Association, 23*(4), 354–362.

Liu, X., Wang, S., Chang, S., Chen, W., & Si, M. (in press). Effect of brief mindfulness intervention on tolerance and distress of pain induced by cold-pressor task. *Stress Health.*

Lovibond, P., Mitchell, C., Minard, E., Brady, A., & Menzies, R. (2009). Safety behaviours preserve threat beliefs: Protection from extinction of human fear conditioning by an avoidance response. *Behaviour Research and Therapy, 47,* 716–720.

Lowens, I. (2010). Compassion focused therapy for people with bipolar disorder. *International Journal of Cognitive Therapy, 3*(2), 172–185.

Luborsky, L., Crits-Christoph, P., McLellan, T., Woody, G., Piper, W., & Imber, S. (1986). Do therapists vary much in their success?: Findings from four outcome studies. *American Journal of Orthopsychiatry, 51,* 501–512.

Luborsky, L., Rosenthal, R., Diguer, L., Andrusyna, T., Berman, J., Levitt, J., et al. (2002). The dodo bird is alive and well—mostly. *Clinical Psychology: Science and Practice, 9*(1), 2–12.

Lucas, R. E., Clark, A. E., Georgellis, Y., & Diener, E. (2003). Reexamining adaptation and the set point model of happiness: Reactions to changes in marital status. *Journal of Personality and Social Psychology, 84*(3), 527–539.

Luders, E., Clark, K., Narr, K. L., & Toga, A.W. (2011). Enhanced brain connectivity in long-term meditation practitioners. *NeuroImage, 57,* 1308–1316.

Luders, E., Thompson, P. M., Kurth, F., Hong, J.-Y., Phillips, O.R., Wang, Y. (in press). Global and regional alterations of hippocampal anatomy in long-term meditation practitioners. *Human Brain Mapping.*

Luders, E., Toga, A. W., Lepore, N., & Gaser, C. (2009). The underlying anatomical correlates of long-term meditation: Larger hippocampal and frontal volumes of gray matter. *NeuroImage, 45*(3), 672–678.

Lutz, A., Brefczynski-Lewis, J., Johnstone, T., & Davidson, R. (2008). Regulation of the neural circuitry of emotion by compassion meditation: Effects of meditative expertise. *PLoS ONE, 3*(3), e1897.

Lutz, A., Greischar, L. L., Perlman, D. M., & Davidson, R. J. (2009). BOLD signal in insula is differentially related to cardiac function during compassion meditation in experts vs. novices. *NeuroImage, 47*(3), 1038–1046.

Lutz, A., Greischar, L., Rawlings, N., Ricard, M., & Davidson, R. (2004). Long-term meditators self-induce high-amplitude synchrony during mental practice. *Proceedings of the National Academy of Sciences of the United States of America, 101,* 16369–16373.

Lutz, A., McFarlin, D. R., Perlman, D. M., Salomons, T. V., & Davidson, R. J. (2013). Altered anterior insula activation during anticipation and experience of painful stimuli in expert meditators. *NeuroImage, 64,* 538–546.

Lutz, A., Slagter, H. A., Dunne, J. D., & Davidson, R. J. (2008). Attention regulation and monitoring in meditation. *Trends in Cognitive Sciences, 12*(4), 163–169.

Lutz, A., Slagter, H. A., Rawlings, N., Francis, A., Greischar, L., & Davidson, R. (2009). Mental training enhances attentional stability: Neural and behavioral evidence. *Journal of Neuroscience, 29,* 13418–13427.

Lynch, T. R., Trost, W. T., Salsman, N., & Linehan, M. M. (2007). Dialectical behavior therapy for borderline personality disorder. *Annual Review of Clinical Psychology, 3,* 181–205.

Lyubomirsky, S. (2007). *The how of happiness: A scientific approach to getting the life you want.* New York: Penguin Press.

Ma, S. H., & Teasdale, J. D. (2004). Mindfulness-based cognitive therapy for depression: Replication and exploration of differential relapse prevention effects. *Journal of Consulting and Clinical Psychology, 72,* 31–30.

Magid, B. (2002). *Ordinary mind: Exploring the common ground of Zen and psychotherapy.* Somerville, MA: Wisdom.

Maharaj, N. (1997). *I am that: Talks with Sri Nisargadatta* (M. Frydman, Trans.). New York: Aperture.

Maharishi Mahesh Yogi. (2001). *Science of being and art of living: Transcendental meditation.* New York: Plume. (Original work published 1968)

Mahasi Sayadaw. (1971). *Practical insight meditation: Basic and progressive stages.* Kandy, Sri Lanka: Forest Hermitage.

Marlatt, G. A., & Donovan, D. M. (2007). *Relapse prevention: Maintenance strategies in the treatment of addictive disorders* (2nd ed.). New York: Guilford Press.

Marlatt, G. A., & Gordon, J. R. (1985). *Relapse prevention: Maintenance strategies in the treatment of addictive behaviors.* New York: Guilford Press.

Martin, D. J., Garske, J. P., & Davis, M. K. (2000). Relation of the therapeutic alliance with outcome and other variables: A meta-analytic review. *Journal of Consulting and Clinical Psychology, 68,* 438–450.

Martin-Asuero, A., & Garcia-Banda, G. (2010). The mindfulness-based stress reduction program (MBSR) reduces stress-related psychological distress in healthcare professionals. *Spanish Journal of Psychology, 13*(2), 897–905.

Mascaro., J., Rilling, J., Negi, L., & Raison, C. (2013). Pre-existing brain function predicts subsequent practice of mindfulness and compassion meditation. *Neuroimage, 60,* 35–42.

Maslow, A. H. (1954). *Motivation and personality.* New York: Harper.

Maslow, A. H. (1966). *The psychology of science: A reconnaissance.* New York: Harper & Row.

Mason, M., Norton, M., Van Horn, J., Wegner, D., Grafton, S., & Macrae, C. (2007). Wandering minds: The default netowrk and stimulus-independent thought. *Science, 315*(5810), 393–395.

Masters, W. H. (1970). *Human sexual inadequacy.* New York: Little, Brown.

Masters, W. H., & Johnson, V. E. (1966). *Human sexual response.* Philadelphia, PA: Lippincott, Williams & Wilkins.

May, C., Burgard, M., Mena, M., Abbasi, I., Bernhardt, N., Clemens, S., et al. (2011). Short-term training in loving-kindness meditation produces a state, but not a trait, alteration of attention. *Mindfulness, 2*(3), 143–153.

May, R. (1967). *The art of counseling.* New York: Abingdon Press.

Mayer, T. G., Gatchel, R. J., Mayer, H., Kishino, N. D., Keeley, J., & Mooney, V. (1987). A prospective two-year study of functional restoration in industrial low back injury: An objective assessment procedure. *Journal of the American Medical Association, 258*(13), 1763–1767.

McCarthy, K. (2012). *Self gratitude and personal success.* Retrieved November 3, 2012, from *http://ezinearticles.com/?Self-Gratitude-and-Personal-Success&id=800893.*

McCollum, E., & Gehart, D. (2010). Using mindfulness meditation to teach beginning therapists therapeutic presence: A qualitative study. *Journal of Marital and Family Therapy, 36*(3), 347–360.

McCown, D., Reibel, D., & Micozzi, M. (2011). *Teaching mindfulness. A practical guide for clinicians and educators.* New York: Springer.

McGrath, P. A. (1994). Psychological aspects of pain perception. *Archives of Oral Biology, 39*(Suppl.), 55S–62S.

McKay, K., Imel, Z., & Wampold, B. (2006). Psychiatrist effects in the psychopharmacological treatment of depression. *Journal of Affective Disorders, 92,* 287–290.

McKim, R. D. (2008). Rumination as a mediator of the effects of mindfulness: Mindfulness-based stress reduction with a heterogenous community sample experiencing anxiety, depression, and/or chronic pain. *Dissertation Abstracts International: Section B: Sciences and Engineering, 68,* 7673.

McWilliams, N. (2011). *Psychoanalytic psychotherapy: A practitioner's guide.* New York: Guilford Press.

Mechelli, A., Crinion, J. T., Noppeney, U., O'Doherty, J., Ashburner, J., Frackowiak, R. S., et al. (2004). Neurolinguistics: Structural plasticity in the bilingual brain. *Nature, 431,* 757.

Mehling, W. E., Hamel, K. A., Acree, M., Byl, N., & Hecht, F. M. (2005). Randomized, controlled trial of breath therapy for patients with chronic low-back pain. *Alternative Therapies in Health and Medicine, 11*(4), 44–52.

Melzack, R., & Wall, P. D. (1965). Pain mechanisms: A new theory. *Science, 150*(699), 971–979.

Mennin, D. S., & Fresco, D. M. (2010). Emotion regulation as an integrative framework for understanding and treating psychopathology. In A. M. Kring & D. M. Sloan (Eds.), *Emotion regulation and psychopathology: A transdiagnostic approach to etiology and treatment* (pp. 356–379). New York: Guilford Press.

Meyer, B., Pilkonis, P., Krupnick, J., Egan, M., Simmens, S., & Sotsky, S. (2002). Treatment expectancies, patient alliance, and outcome: Further analyses from the National Institute of Mental Health Treatment of Depression Collaborative Research Program. *Journal of Consulting and Clinical Psychology, 70*(4), 1051–1055.

Michalak, J., Burg, J., & Heidenreich, T. (2012). Don't forget your body: Mindfulness, embodiment, and the treatment of depression. *Mindfulness, 3*(3), 190–199.

Michelson, S. E., Lee, J. K., Orsillo, S. M., & Roemer, L. (2011). The role of values-consistent behavior in generalized anxiety disorder. *Depression and Anxiety, 28*, 358–366.

Miller, J. B., & Stiver, I.P. (1997). *The healing connection: How women form relationships in therapy and in life.* Boston: Beacon Press.

Miller, K. (2006). *Momma Zen: Walking the crooked path of motherhood.* Boston: Shambhala.

Miller, S., Duncan, B., & Hubble, M. (1997). *Escape from Babel: Toward a unifying language for psychotherapy practice.* New York: Norton.

Mitra, R., Jadhav, S., McEwen, B. S., Vyas, A., & Chattarji, S. (2005). Stress duration modulates the spatiotemporal patterns of spine formation in the basolateral amygdala. *Proceedings of the National Academy of Sciences of the United States of America, 102*(26), 9371–9376.

Molino, A. (Ed.). (1998). *The couch and the tree.* New York: North Point Press.

Mongrain, M., Chin, J., & Shapira, L. (2010). Practicing compassion increases happiness and self-esteem. *Journal of Happiness Studies, 12*, 963–981.

Monteiro, L., Nuttal, S., & Musten, F. (2010). Five skillful habits: An ethics-based mindfulness intervention. *Counseling and Spirituality, 29*(1), 91–104.

Moore, A., & Malinowski, P. (2009). Meditation, mindfulness, and cognitive flexibility. *Consciousness and Cognition, 18*, 176–186.

Moore, P. (2008). Introducing mindfulness to clinical psychologists in training: An experiential course of brief exercises. *Journal of Clinical Psychology in Medical Settings, 15*(4), 331–337.

Morgan, S. P. (2005). Depression: Turning toward life. In C.K. Germer, R. D. Siegel, & P. R. Fulton (Eds.), *Mindfulness and psychotherapy* (pp. 130–151). New York: Guilford Press.

Morina, N. (2007). The role of experiential avoidance in psychological functioning after war-related stress in Kosovar civilians. *Journal of Nervous and Mental Disease, 195*, 697–700.

Morita, S. (1998). *Morita therapy and the true nature of anxiety-based disorders: Shinkeishitsu.* Albany, NY: State University of New York Press. (Original work published 1928)

Morone, N. E., Rollman, B. L., Moore, C. G., Li, Q., & Weiner, D. K. (2009). A mind–body program for older adults with chronic low back pain: Results of a pilot study. *Pain Medicine, 10*(8), 1395–1407.

Morrison, I., Lloyd, D., DiPellegrino, G., & Roberts, N. (2008). Vicarious responses to pain in anterior cingulate cortex: Is empathy a multisensory issue? *Cognitive, Affective, and Behavioral Neuroscience, 4*(2), 270–278.

Murphy, S. (2002). *One bird, one stone.* New York: Renaissance Books.

Murray, C., & Lopez, A. (1998). *The global burden of disease: A comprehensive assessment of mortality and disability from disease, injuries and risk factors in 1990 and projected to 2020.* Boston: Harvard University Press.

Nader, K. (2006). Childhood trauma: The deeper wound. In J. P. Wilson (Ed.), *The posttraumatic self: Restoring meaning and wholeness to personality* (pp. 117–156). London, UK: Routledge.

Najmi, S., & Wegner, D. M. (2008). Thought suppression and psychopathology. In A. J. Elliot (Ed.), *Handbook of approach and avoidance motivation* (pp. 447–459). New York: Psychology Press.

Nalanda Translation Committee. (2004). Morning liturgy for Mahayana students. In *Bodhisattva vow and practice* (pp. 6–7). Halifax, NS, Canada: Nalanda Translation Committee.

Nanamoli, B. (Trans.) & Bodhi, B. (Ed.). (1995). Bhayabherava Sutta: Fear and dread. In *The middle length discourses of the Buddha* (pp. 102–107). Boston: Wisdom.

Napoli, M., Krech, P., & Holley, L. (2005). Mindfulness training for elementary school students: The Attention Academy. *Journal of Applied School Psychology, 21*(1), 99–125.

Napthali, S. (2003). *Buddhism for mothers: A calm approach to caring for yourself and your children.* Crows Nest, NSW, Australia: Allen & Unwin.

Nargeot, R., & Simmers, J. (2011). Neural mechanisms of operant conditioning and learning-induced behavioral plasticity in *Aplysia. Cellular and Molecular Life Sciences, 68*(5), 803–816.

National Center for Complementary and Alternative Medicine. (2007). Mind–body medicine: An overview. Retrieved November 7, 2012 from: *http://nccam.nih.gov/health/meditation/overview.htm.*

National Center for PTSD, U.S. Department of Veteran Affairs. (2011). Mindfulness practice in the treatment of traumatic stress. Retrieved from *www.ptsd.va.gov/public/pages/mindful-ptsd.asp.*

Neff, K. (2003). The development and validation of a scale to measure self-compassion. *Self and Identity, 2*(3), 223–250.

Neff, K. (2011). *Self-compassion: Stop beating yourself up and leave insecurity behind.* New York: Morrow.

Neff, K. D. (2012). The science of self-compassion. In C. K. Germer & R. D. Siegel (Eds.). *Wisdom and compassion in psychotherapy: Deepening mindfulness in clinical practice* (pp. 79–92). New York: Guilford Press.

Neff, K. D., & Germer, C. K. (2013). A pilot study and randomized controlled trial of the mindful self-compassion program. *Journal of Clinical Psychology, 69*(1), 28–44.

Neff, K., & Germer, C. (in press). Being kind to yourself: The science of self-compassion. In T. Singer & M. Bolz (Eds.), *Compassion: Bridging theory and practice*. Leipzig, Germany: Max-Planck Institut.

Neff, K., Kirkpatrick, K., & Rude, S. S. (2007). Self-compassion and its link to adaptive psychological functioning. *Journal of Research in Personality, 41*, 139–154.

Neumann, M., Bensing, J., Mercer, S., Ernstmann, N., Ommen, O., & Pfaff, H. (2011). Analyzing the "nature" and "specific effectiveness" of clinical empathy: A theoretical overview and contribution towards a theory-based research agenda. *Patient Education and Counseling, 74*, 339–346.

Nhat Hanh, Thich. (2011). *Planting seeds: Practicing mindfulness with children*. Berkeley, CA: Parallax Press.

Norcross, J. C. (Ed.). (2001). Empirically supported therapy relationships: Summary report of the Division 29 Task Force. *Psychotherapy, 38*(4).

Norcross, J. C. (Ed.). (2011). *Psychotherapy relationships that work* (2nd ed.). New York: Oxford University Press.

Norcross, J. C., & Beutler, L. (1997). Determining the therapeutic relationship of choice in brief therapy. In J. Butcher (Ed.), *Personality assessment in managed health care: A practitioner's guide* (pp. 42–60). New York: Oxford University Press.

Norcross, J. C., & Lambert, M. (2011). Evidence-based therapy relationships. In J. C. Norcross (Ed.), *Psychotherapy relationships that work* (2nd ed.). New York: Oxford University Press.

Norcross, J. C., & Wampold, B. (2011). Evidence-based therapy relationships: Research Conclusions and Clinical Practices. *Psychotherapy, 48*(1) 98–102.

Nyanaponika, T. (1965). *The heart of Buddhist meditation*. York Beach, ME: Red Wheel/Weiser.

Nyanaponika, T. (1972). *The power of mindfulness*. San Fransisco, CA: Unity Press.

Nyanaponika, T. (1998). *Abhidhamma studies*. Boston: Wisdom. (Original work published 1949)

Nye, N. (1995). Kindness. In *Words under the words* (pp. 42–43). Portland, OR: Eighth Mountain Press.

Ochsner, K. N., Bunge, S. A., Gross, J. J., & Gabrieli, J. D. (2002). Rethinking feelings: An fMRI study of the cognitive regulation of emotion. *Journal of Cognitive Neuroscience, 14*(8), 1215–1229.

Ogden, P., Minton, K., & Pain, C. (2006). *Trauma and the body: A sesnorimotor approach to psychotherapy*. New York: Norton.

Olendzki, A. (Trans.). (1998). Maha Niddesa 1.42. In *Upon the Tip of a Needle. Insight Journal*. Barre, MA: Barre Center for Buddhist Studies.

Olendzki, A. (2010). *Unlimiting mind: The radically experiential psychology of Buddhism*. Somerville, MA: Wisdom.

Olendzki, A. (2011). The construction of mindfulness. *Contemporary Buddhism, 12*(1), 55–70.

Olendzki, A. (2012, May 12). *Lovingkindness and compassion: What the*

Buddha discovered. Presentation given at Harvard Medical School Meditation and Psychotherapy: Practicing Compassion for Self and Others conference, Cambridge, MA.

Ong, J. C., Shapiro, S. L., & Manber, R. (2009). Mindfulness meditation and cognitive behavioral therapy for insomnia: A naturalistic 12-month follow-up. *Explore, 5*(1), 30–36.

O'Regan, B. (1985). Placebo: The hidden asset in healing. *Investigations: A Research Bulletin, 2*(1), 1–3.

Orlinsky, D., Ronnestad, M., & Willutzki, U. (2004). Fifty years of psychotherapy process–outcome research: Continuity and change. In M. Lambert (Ed.), *Handbook of psychotherapy and behavior change* (5th ed., pp. 307–390). New York: Wiley.

Orsillo, S. M., & Batten, S. (2005). Acceptance and commitment therapy in the treatment of posttraumatic stress disorder. *Behavior Modification, 29*, 95–129.

Orsillo, S. M., & Roemer, L. (2011). *The mindful way through anxiety: Break free from worry and reclaim your life.* New York: Guilford Press.

Pace, T., Negi, L., Adams, D., Cole, S., Sivilli, T., Brown, T., et al. (2009). Effect of compassion meditation on neuroendocrine, innate immune, and behavioral responses to psychosocial stress. *Psychoneuroendocrinology, 34*(1), 87–98.

Padilla, A. (2011). Mindfulness in therapeutic presence: How mindfulness of therapist impacts treatment outcome. *Dissertation Abstracts International: Section B: The Sciences and Engineering, 71*(9-B), 5801.

Pagnoni, G., & Cekic, M. (2007). Age effects on gray matter volume and attentional performance in Zen meditation. *Neurobiology of Aging, 28*(10), 1623–1627.

Pagnoni, G., Cekic, M., & Guo, Y. (2008). "Thinking about not-thinking": Neural correlates of conceptual processing during Zen Meditation. *PLoS ONE 3*(9), e3083.

Paracelsus. (2012). Unsourced quote retrieved November 23, 2012, from *https://en.wikiquote.org/wiki/Paracelsus.*

Patsiopoulos, A., & Buchanan, M. (2011). The practice of self-compassion in counseling: A narrative inquiry. *Professional Psychology: Research and Practice, 42*(4), 301–307.

Patterson, G. (1977). *Living with children: New methods for parents and teachers.* Champaign, IL: Research Press.

Pauley, G., & McPherson, S. (2010). The experience and meaning of compassion and self-compassion for individuals with depression or anxiety. *Psychology and Psychotherapy: Theory, Research, and Practice, 83*, 129–143.

Pearlman, L. A., & Courtois, C. A. (2005). Clinical applications of the attachment framework: Relational treatment of complex trauma. *Journal of Traumatic Stress, 18*, 449–459.

Pecukonis, E. V. (1996) Childhood sex abuse in women with chronic intractable back pain. *Social Work in Health Care, 23*(3), 1–16.

Pennebaker, J. W., Keicolt-Glaser, J. K., & Glaser, R. (1988). Disclosure of traumas and immune function: Health implications for psychotherapy. *Journal of Consulting and Clinical Psychology, 56*(2), 239–245.

Pepper, S. (1942). *World hypotheses.* Berkeley, CA: University of California Press.

Perlman, D. M., Salomons, T. V., Davidson, R. J., & Lutz, A. (2010). Differential effects on pain intensity and unpleasantness of two meditation practices. *Emotion, 10*(1), 65–71.

Perls, F. (2012). *Fritz Perls: The founder of Gestalt therapy.* Retrieved on September 23, 2012, from *www.fritzperls.com/autobiography.*

Peterson, C. (2007). Teleclass teaching: *North of neutral 2: Applications in action.* Bethesda, MD: MentorCoach.

Peterson, C. (2008). Teleclass teaching: *Positive psychology immersion master class: North of neutral.* Bethesda, MD: MentorCoach.

Peterson, C., & Park, N. (2007). Attachment security and its benefits in context. *Psychological Inquiry, 18*(3), 172–176.

Peterson, C., & Seligman, M. E. P. (2004). *Character strengths and virtues: A handbook and classification.* American Psychological Association: Washington, DC.

Phillips, M. L., Drevets, W. C., Rauch, S. L., & Lane, R. (2003). Neurobiology of emotion perception. I: The neural basis of normal emotion perception. *Biological Psychiatry, 54*(5), 504–514.

Picavet, H. S., Vlaeyen, J. W., & Schouten, J. S. (2002). Pain catastrophizing and kinesiophobia: Predictors of chronic low back pain. *American Journal of Epidemiology, 156*, 1028–1034.

Piet, J., & Hougaard, E. (2011). The effect of mindfulness-based cognitive therapy for prevention of relapse in recurrent major depressive disorder: A systematic review and meta-analysis. *Clinical Psychology Review, 31*(6), 1032–1040.

Piet, J., Hougaard, E., Hecksher, M. S., & Rosenberg, N. K. (2010). A randomized pilot study of mindfulness-based cognitive therapy and group cognitive-behavioral therapy for young adults with social phobia. *Scandinavian Journal of Psychology, 51*, 403–410.

Pietrzak, R. H., Goldstein, R. B., Southwick, S. M., & Grant, B. F. (2011). Personality disorders associated with full and partial posttraumatic stress disorder in the U.S. population: Results from Wave 2 of the National Epidemiologic Survey on Alcohol and Related Conditions. *Journal of Psychiatric Research, 45*, 678–686.

Pinker, S. (2008, January 13). The moral instinct. *New York Times Magazine,* pp. 32–58.

Placone, P. (2011). *Mindful parent, happy child: A guide to raising joyful and resilient children.* Palo Alto, CA: Alaya Press.

Pollak, S. M., Pedulla, T., & Siegel, R. D. (in press). *Sitting together: Essential skills for mindfulness-based psychotherapy.* New York: Guilford Press.

Pope, K., & Vasquez, M. (2011). *Ethics in psychotherapy and counseling: A practical guide.* New Jersey: Wiley.

Porges, S. W. (2011a). *The polyvagal theory: Neurophysiological foundations of emotions, attachment, communication, and self-regulation.* New York: Norton.

Porges, S. W. (2011b, June). *The polyvagal theory for treating trauma* [Video podcast]. [With R. Buczynski]. [Transcript]. Mansfield Center, CT: National Institute for the Clinical Application of Behavioral Medicine. Available at *www.stephenporges.com.*

Pradhan, E. K., Baumgarten, M., Langenberg, P., Handwerger, B., Gilpin, A. K., Magyari, T., et al. (2007). Effect of mindfulness-based stress reduction in rheumatoid arthritis patients. *Arthritis and Rheumatism, 57*(7), 1134–1142.

Proust, M. (2003). *In search of lost time.* New York: Modern Library. (Original work published 1925)

Raes, F. (2010). Rumination and worry as mediators of the relationship between self-compassion and depression and anxiety. *Journal of Personality and Individual Differences, 48,* 757–761.

Raes, F. (2011). The effect of self-compassion on the development of depression symptoms in a nonclinical sample. *Mindfulness, 2*(1), 33–36.

Rainville, J., Sobel, J., Hartigan, C., Monlux, G., & Bean, J. (1997). Decreasing disability in chronic back pain through aggressive spine rehabilitation. *Journal of Rehabilitation Research and Development, 34*(4), 383–393.

Ramel, W., Goldin, P. R., Carmona, P. E., & McQuaid, J. R. (2004). The effects of mindfulness meditation on cognitive processes and affect in patients with past depression. *Cognitive Therapy and Research, 28,* 433–455.

Raque-Bogdan, R., Ericson, S., Jackson, J., Martin, H., & Bryan, N. (2011). Attachment and mental and physical health: Self-compassion and mattering as mediators. *Journal of Consulting Psychology, 58*(2), 272–278.

Reik, T. (1949). *Listening with the third ear.* New York: Farrar, Stauss.

Reis, D. (2007). Mindfulness meditation, emotion, and cognitive control: Experienced meditators show distinct brain and behaviour responses to emotional provocations. *Dissertation Abstracts International: Section B, 69*(6-B), 3869.

Reynolds, D. (2003). Mindful parenting: A group approach to enhancing reflective capacity in parents and infants. *Journal of Child Psychotherapy, 29*(3), 357–374.

Ricard, M. (2010). The difference between empathy and compassion. *HuffPost Living.* Retrieved October 15, 2010, from *www.huffingtonpost.com/matthieu-ricard/could-compassion-meditati_b_751566.html.*

Richards, K., Campenni, C., & Muse-Burke, J. (2010). Self-care and well-being in mental health professionals: The mediating effects of self-awareness and mindfulness. *Journal of Mental Health Counseling, 32*(3), 247–264.

Rimes, K., & Winigrove, J. (in press). Mindfulness-based cognitive therapy for people with chronic fatigue syndrome still experiencing excessive fatigue after cognitive behavior therapy: A pilot randomized study. *Clinical Psychology and Psychotherapy.*

Robinson, M. E., & Riley, J. L. (1999). The role of emotion in pain. In R. J.

Gatchel & D. C. Turk (Eds.), *Psychosocial factors in pain: Critical perspectives* (pp. 74–88). New York: Guilford Press.

Roemer, L., & Orsillo, S. M. (2007). An open trial of an acceptance-based behavior therapy for generalized anxiety disorder. *Behavior Therapy, 38*, 72–85.

Roemer, L., & Orsillo, S. M. (2009). *Mindfulness- and acceptance-based behavioral therapies in practice.* New York: Guilford Press.

Roemer, L., Orsillo, S. M., & Salters-Pedneault, K. (2008). Efficacy of an acceptance-based behavior therapy for generalized anxiety disorder: Evaluation in a randomized controlled trial. *Journal of Consulting and Clinical Psychology, 76*(6), 1083–1089.

Rogers, C. R. (1957). The necessary and sufficient conditions of therapeutic personality change. *Journal of Consulting Psychology, 21*, 95–103.

Rogers, C. R. (1961). *On becoming a person: A therapist's view of psychotherapy.* New York: Houghton Mifflin.

Rogers, C. R. (1980). *A way of being.* Boston: Houghton Mifflin.

Rogers, C. R., Gendlin, E., Kiesler, D., & Truax, C. (Eds.). (1967). *The therapeutic relationship and its impact.* Madison, WI: University of Wisconsin Press.

Rogers, S. (2005). *Mindful parenting: Meditations, verses, and visualizations for a more joyful life.* Miami Beach, FL: Mindful Living Press.

Rosenberg, L. (1998). *Breath by breath: The liberating practice of insight meditation.* Boston: Shambhala.

Rosenthal, J. Z., Grosswald, S., Ross, R., & Rosenthal, N. (2011). Effects of transcendental meditation in veterans of Operation Enduring Freedom and Operation Iraqi Freedom with posttraumatic stress disorder: A pilot study. *Military Medicine, 176*, 626–630.

Rosenthal, N. (2012). *Transcendence: Healing and transformation through Transcendental Meditation.* New York: Tarcher.

Rosenzweig, S. (1936). Some implicit common factors in diverse methods of psychotherapy. *American Journal of Orthopsychiatry, 6*, 412–415.

Rosenzweig, S., Greeson, J. M., Reibel, D. K., Green, J. S., Jasser, S. A., & Beasley, D. (2010). Mindfulness-based stress reduction for chronic pain conditions: Variation in treatment outcomes and role of home meditation practice. *Journal of Psychosomatic Research, 68*(1), 29–36.

Rosenzweig, S., Reibel, D., Greeson, J., Brainard, G., & Hojat, M. (2003). Mindfulness-based stress reduction lowers psychological distress in medical students. *Teaching and Learning in Medicine, 15*, 88–92.

Rothbaum, B. O., & Davis, M. (2003). Applying learning principles to the treatment of post-trauma reactions. *Annals of the New York Academy of Sciences, 1008*, 112–121.

Roy, D. (2007). *Momfulness; Mothering with mindfulness, compassion, and grace.* San Francisco, CA: Jossey Bass.

Rubia, K. (2009). The neurobiology of meditation and its clinical effectiveness in psychiatric disorders. *Biological Psychiatry, 82*, 1–11.

Rude, S. S., Maestas, K. L., & Neff, K. (2007). Paying attention to distress: What's wrong with rumination. *Cognition and Emotion, 21*(4), 843–864.

Rumi, J. (1995). Childhood friends. In *The essential Rumi* (C. Barks, Trans.). San Francisco, CA: HarperCollins.

Ryan, A., Safran, J., Doran, J., & Moran, C. (2012). Therapist mindfulness, alliance, and treatment outcome. *Psychotherapy Research, 23*(3), 289–297.

Ryan, R. M., & Deci, E. L. (2001). On happiness and human potentials: A review of research on hedonic and eudaimonic well-being. *Annual Review Psychology, 52*, 141–166.

Ryan, T. (2102). *A mindful nation: How a simple practice can help us reduce stress, improve performance, and recapture the American spirit.* Carlsbad, CA: Hay House.

Safran, J. D. (Ed.). (2003). *Psychoanalysis and Buddhism: An unfolding dialogue.* Somerville, MA: Wisdom.

Safran, J. D., Muran, J. C., & Eubacks-Carter, C. (2011). Repairing alliance ruptures. In J. C. Norcross (Eds.), *Psychotherapy relationships that work* (2nd ed.). New York: Oxford University Press.

Sakyong, J. T. D. (2012). *Enlightened society treatise.* Halifax, NS, Canada: Shambhala Media.

Sakyong, M. J. M. (2003). *Turning the mind into an ally.* New York: Riverhead Books.

Salam, A. (1990). *Unification of fundamental forces.* Cambridge, UK: Cambridge University Press. Retrieved November 23, 2012, from *https:// en.wikiquote.org/wiki/Albert_Einstein#On_the_Generalized_Theory_ of_Gravitation_.281950.29.*

Salzberg, S. (1995). *Lovingkindness: The revolutionary art of happiness.* Boston: Shambhala.

Salzberg, S. (2002). *Lovingkindness: The revolutionary art of happiness* (2nd ed.). Boston: Shambhala.

Salzberg, S. (2011). *Real happiness: The power of meditation.* New York: Workman.

Sapolsky R. M. (2004). *Why zebras don't get ulcers* (3rd ed.). New York: Henry Holt.

Sauer, S., & Baer, R. A. (2010). Mindfulness and decentering as mechanisms of change in mindfulness- and acceptance-based interventions. In R. Baer (Ed.), *Assessing mindfulness and acceptance processes in clients* (pp. 25–50). Oakland, CA: Context Press.

Schacht, T. (1991). Can psychotherapy education advance psychotherapy integration?: A view from the cognitive psychology of expertise. *Journal of Psychotherapy Integration, 1*, 305–320.

Schanche, E., Stiles, T., McCollough, L., Swartberg, M., & Nielsen, G. (2011). The relationship between activating affects, inhibitory affects, and self-compassion in patients with Cluster C personality disorders. *Psychotherapy: Theory, Research, Practice, Training, 48*(3), 293–303.

Scheel, M. J., Hanson, W. E., & Razzhavaikina, T. I. (2004). *The process of recommending homework in psychotherapy: A review of therapist delivery methods, client acceptability, and factors that affect compliance* (Faculty Publications, Paper 372). Lincoln: Department of Psychology, University of Nebraska.

Schneider, K., & Leitner, L. (2002). Humanistic psychotherapy. In M. Hersen & W. H. Sledge (Eds.), *Encyclopedia of psychotherapy* (Vol. 1, pp. 949–957). New York: Elsevier Science/Academic Press.

Schofferman, J., Anderson, D., Hines, R., Smith, G., & Keane, G. (1993). Childhood psychological trauma and chronic refractory low-back pain. *Clinical Journal of Pain, 9*(4), 260–265.

Schonstein, E., Kenny, D. T., Keating, J., & Koes, B. W. (2003). Work conditioning, work hardening, and functional restoration for workers with back and neck pain. *Cochrane Database Systematic Review, 1,* CD001822.

Schore, A. N. (1994). *Affect regulation and the origin of the self: The neurobiology of emotional development.* Hillsdale, NJ: Erlbaum.

Schottenbauer, M. A., Glass, C. R., Arnkoff, D. B., Tendick, V., & Gray, S. H. (2008). Nonresponse and dropout rates in outcome studies on PTSD: Review and methodological considerations. *Psychiatry, 71,* 134–168.

Schur, E. A., Afari, N., Furberg, H., Olarte, M., Goldberg, J., Sullivan, P. F., et al. (2007). Feeling bad in more ways than one: Comorbidity patterns of medically unexplained and psychiatric conditions. *Journal of General Internal Medicine, 22*(6), 818–821.

Schutze, R., Rees, C., Preece, M., & Schutze, M. (2010). Low mindfulness predicts pain catastrophizing in a fear-avoidance model of chronic pain. *Pain, 148*(1), 120–127.

Schwartz, B., & Sharpe, K. (2010). *Practical wisdom: The right way to do the right thing.* New York: Riverhead Books.

Schwartz, G. E. (1990). Psychobiology of repression and health: A systems approach. In J. L Singer, (Ed.), *Repression and dissociation: Defense mechanisms and personality styles—current theory and research* (pp. 405–434). Chicago, IL: University of Chicago Press.

Segal, Z. V., Bieling, P., Young, T., MacQueen, G., Cooke, R., Martin, L., et al. (2010). Antidepressant monotherapy vs. sequential pharmacotherapy and mindfulness-based cognitive therapy, or placebo, for relapse prophylaxis in recurrent depression. *Archives of General Psychiatry, 67*(12), 1256–1264.

Segal, Z. V., Williams, J. M. G., & Teasdale, J. D. (2002). *Mindfulness-based cognitive therapy for depression: A new approach to preventing relapse.* New York: Guilford Press.

Segal, Z. V., Williams, J. M. G., & Teasdale, J. D. (2012). *Mindfulness-based cognitive therapy for depression* (2nd ed.). New York: Guilford Press.

Segall, S. R. (2003). Psychotherapy practice as Buddhist practice. In S. R. Segall (Ed.), *Encountering Buddhism: Western psychology and Buddhist teachings* (pp. 165–178). Albany, NY: State University of New York Press.

Seligman, M. E. P. (1995). The effectiveness of psychotherapy: The Consumer Reports Study. *American Psychologist, 50*(12), 965–974.

Seligman, M. E. P. (2002). *Authentic happiness: Using the new positive psychology to realize your potential for lasting fulfillment.* New York: Free Press.

Seligman, M. E. P. (2003). Teleclass teaching: *Vanguard authentic happiness teleclass*. Bethesda, MD: MentorCoach.

Seligman, M. E. P. (2004). VIA signature strengths survey. Retrieved October 29, 2012, from *www.authentichappiness.sas.upenn.edu/default.aspx*.

Seligman, M. E. P. (2011). *Flourish: A visionary new understanding of happiness and well-being*. New York: Free Press.

Seligman, M. E. P., & Csikszentmihalyi, M. (2000). Positive psychology. An introduction. *American Psychologist, 55*(1), 5–14.

Seligman, M. E. P., Steen, T. A., Park, N., & Peterson, C. (2005). Positive psychology progress: Empirical validation of interventions. *American Psychologist, 60*, 410–421.

Selye, H. (1956). *The stress of life*. New York: McGraw-Hill.

Semple, R. J. (2010). Does mindfulness meditation enhance attention?: A randomized controlled trial. *Mindfulness, 1*(2), 121–130.

Semple, R. J., Lee, J., Rosa, D., & Miller, L. F. (2010). A randomized trial of mindfulness-based cognitive therapy for children: Promoting mindful attention to enhance social–emotional resiliency in children. *Journal of Child and Family Studies, 19*(2), 218–229.

Sephton, S. E. (2007). Mindfulness meditation alleviates depressive symptoms in women with fibromyalgia: Results of a randomized clinical trial. *Arthritis and Rheumatism, 57*(1), 77–85.

Shahrokh, N., & Hales, R. (Eds.). (2003). *American psychiatric glossary* (8th ed.). Washington, DC: American Psychiatric Publishing.

Shankland, W. E. (2011). Factors that affect pain behavior. *Cranio: Journal of Craniomandibular Practice, 29*(2), 144–154.

Shantideva. (1979). *Bodhicaryavatara: A guide to the bodhisattva's way of life* (S. Bachelor, Trans.). Dharamshala, India: Library of Tibetan Works & Archives.

Shapira, L., & Mongrain, L. (2010). The benefits of self-compassion and optimism exercises for individuals vulnerable to depression. *Journal of Positive Psychology, 5*(5), 377–389.

Shapiro, D. H. (1992). Adverse effects of meditation: A preliminary investigation of long-term meditators. *International Journal of Psychosomatics, 39*, 62–66.

Shapiro, D. H., & Shapiro, D. (1982). Meta-analysis of comparative therapy outcome studies: A replication and refinement. *Psychological Bulletin, 92*, 581–604.

Shapiro, S. L. (2009). The integration of mindfulness and psychology. *Journal of Clinical Psychology, 65*(6), 555–560.

Shapiro, S. L., Astin, J. A., Bishop, S. R., & Cordova, M. (2005). Mindfulness-based stress reduction for health care professionals: Results from a randomized trial. *International Journal of Stress Management, 12*, 164–176.

Shapiro, S. L., Brown, K. W., & Biegel, G. M. (2007). Teaching self-care to caregivers: Effects of mindfulness-based stress reduction on the mental health of therapists in training. *Training and Education in Professional Psychology, 1*(2), 105–115.

Shapiro, S. L., & Carlson, L. E. (2009). *The art and science of mindfulness: Integrating mindfulness into psychology and the helping professions.* Washington, DC: American Psychological Association.

Shapiro, S. L., Carlson, L. E., Astin, J., & Freedman, B. (2006). Mechanisms of mindfulness. *Journal of Clinical Psychology, 62*(3), 373–386.

Shapiro, S. L., & Izett, S. (2008). Meditation: A universal tool for cultivating empathy. In S. Hick & T. Bien (Eds.), *Mindfulness and the therapeutic relationship* (pp. 161–175). New York: Guilford Press.

Shapiro, S. L., Schwartz, G., & Bonner, G. (1998). Effects of mindfulness-based stress reduction on medical and premedical students. *Journal of Behavioral Medicine, 21,* 581–599.

Shay, J. (1995). *Achilles in Vietnam: Combat trauma and the undoing of character.* New York: Touchstone.

Shoham-Salomon, V., & Rosenthal, R. (1987). Paradoxical interventions: A meta-analysis. *Journal of Consulting and Clinical Psychology, 55,* 22–28.

Siegel, D. (1999). *The developing mind: How relationships and the brain interact to shape who we are.* New York: Guilford Press.

Siegel, D. (2007). *The mindful brain: Reflection and attunement in the cultivation of well-being.* New York: Norton.

Siegel, D. (2009a). Emotion as integration: A possible answer to the question, What is emotion? In D. Fosha & D. Siegel (Eds.), *The healing power of emotion: Affective neuroscience, development, and clinical practice* (pp. 145–171). New York: Norton.

Siegel, D. (2009b). Mindful awareness, mindsight, and neural integration. *The Humanistic Psychologist, 37,* 137–158.

Siegel, D. (2010a). *The mindful therapist: A clinician's guide to mindsight and neural integration.* New York: Norton.

Siegel, D. (2010c). *Mindsight: The new science of personal transformation.* New York: Bantam.

Siegel, R. D. (2010b). *The mindfulness solution: Everyday practices for everyday problems.* New York: Guilford Press.

Siegel, R. D. (2011, September/October). East meets west. *Psychotherapy Networker, 36*(5), 26.

Siegel, R. D. (in press). Mindfulness in the treatment of trauma-related chronic pain. In V. Follette, D. Rozelle, J. Hopper, D. Rome, & J. Briere (Eds.), *Contemplative methods in trauma treatment: Integrating mindfulness and other approaches.* New York: Guilford Press.

Siegel, R. D., & Germer, C. K. (2012). Wisdom and compassion: Two wings of a bird. In C. K. Germer & R. D. Siegel (Eds.), *Wisdom and compassion in psychotherapy: Deepening mindfulness in clinical practice* (pp. 7–34). New York: Guilford Press.

Siegel, R. D., Urdang, M. H., & Johnson, D. R. (2001). *Back sense: A revolutionary approach to halting the cycle of back pain.* New York: Broadway Books.

Siev, J., Huppert, J., & Chambless, D. (2009). The dodo bird, treatment technique, and disseminating empirically supported treatments. *The Behavior Therapist, 32*, 69–75.

Silverstein, R. G., Brown, A. C., Roth, H. D., & Britton, W. B. (2011). Effects of mindfulness training on body awareness to sexual stimuli: Implications for female sexual dysfunction. *Psychosomatic Medicine, 73*(9), 817–825.

Singer, T., & Decety, J. (2011). Social neuroscience of empathy. In J. Decety & J. T. Cacioppo (Eds.), *The Oxford handbook of social neuroscience* (pp. 551–564). New York: Oxford University Press.

Singer, T., & Lamm, C. (2009). The social neuroscience of empathy. *Annals of the New York Academy of Sciences, 1156*, 81–96.

Singer, W. (2005, November). *Synchronization of brain rhythms as a possible mechanism for the unification of distributed mental processes.* Paper presented at the Mind and Life Institute conference, The Science and Clinical Applications of Meditation, Washington, DC.

Singer-Kaplan, H. (1974). *New sex therapy: Active treatment of sexual dysfunctions.* New York: Crown.

Singh, N. N., Singh, A. N., Lancioni, G. E., Singh, J., Winton, A. S. W., & Adkins, A. D. (2010). Mindfulness training for parents and their children with ADHD increases children's compliance. *Journal of Child and Family Studies, 19*, 157–166.

Singh, N. N., Wahler, R., Adkins, A. D., & Myers, R. (2003). Soles of the feet: A mindfulness-based self-control intervention for aggression by an individual with mild mental retardation and mental illness. *Research in Developmental Disabilities, 24*(3), 158–169.

Skinner, B. F. (1974). *About behaviorism.* New York: Knopf.

Slagter, H., Lutz, A., Greischar, L., Francis, A., Nieuwenhuis, S., Davis, J., et al. (2007). Mental training affects distribution of limited brain resources. *PLoS Biology, 5*, e138.

Smith, J. C. (1975). Meditation as psychotherapy: A review of the literature. *Psychological Bulletin, 82*(4), 558–564.

Smith, J. C. (2004). Alterations in brain and immune function produced by mindfulness meditation: Three caveats. *Psychosomatic Medicine, 66*, 148–152.

Smith, M. T., & Neubauer, D. N. (2003). Cognitive behavior therapy for chronic insomnia. *Clinical Cornerstone, 5*(3), 28–40.

Snyder, C. R., Lopez, S. J., & Pedrotti, J. T. (2011). *Positive psychology: The scientific and practical explorations of human strengths* (2nd ed.). Thousand Oaks, CA: Sage.

Sprang, G., & Clark, J. (2007). Compassion fatigue, compassion satisfaction, and burnout: Factors impacting a professional's quality of life. *Journal of Loss and Trauma, 12*, 259–280.

Springer, K. W., Sheridan, J., Kuo, D., & Carnes, M. (2007). Long-term physical and mental health consequences of childhood physical abuse: Results from a large population-based sample of men and women. *Child Abuse and Neglect, 31*(5), 517–530.

Stahl, B., & Goldstein, E. (2010). *A mindfulness-based stress reduction workbook*. Oakland, CA: New Harbinger.

Stanley, S., Reitzel, L. R., Wingate, L. R., Cukrowicz, K. C., Lima, E. N., & Joiner, T. E. (2006). Mindfulness: A primrose path for therapists using manualized treatments? *Journal of Cognitive Psychotherapy, 20*, 327–335.

Steger, M. F., Kashdan, T. B., & Oishi, S. (2008). Being good by doing good: Daily eudaimonic activity and well-being. *Journal of Research in Personality, 42*, 22–42.

Steil, R., Dyer, A., Priebe, K., Kleindienst, N., & Bohus, M. (2011). Dialectical behavior therapy for posttraumatic stress disorder related to childhood sexual abuse: A pilot study of an intensive residential treatment program. *Journal of Traumatic Stress, 24*, 102–106.

Stein, G. (1993). Sacred Emily. In G. Stein, *Geography and plays*. Madison, WI: University of Wisconsin Press. (Original work published 1922)

Stern, D. (2003). The present moment. *Psychology Networker, 27*(6), 52–57.

Stern, D. (2004). *The present moment in psychotherapy and everyday life*. New York: Norton.

Stiles, W. (2009). Responsiveness as an obstacle for psychotherapy outcome research: It's worse than you think. *Clinical Psychology: Science and Practice, 16*, 86–91.

Stratton, P. (2006). Therapist mindfulness as a predictor of client outcomes. *Dissertation Abstracts International: Section B: Science and Engineering, 66*, 6296.

Strosahl, K. D., & Robinson, P. (2008). *The mindfulness and acceptance workbook for depression*. Oakland, CA: New Harbinger.

Surrey, J., & Jordan, J. V. (2012). The wisdom of connection. In C. K. Germer & R. D. Siegel (Eds.), *Wisdom and compassion in psychotherapy* (pp. 163–175). New York: Guilford Press.

Sussman, R., & Cloninger, C. (Eds.). (2011). *Origins of altruism and cooperation*. New York: Springer.

Suzuki, S. (1973). *Zen mind, beginner's mind*. New York: John Weatherhill.

Sweet, M., & Johnson, C. (1990). Enhancing empathy: The interpersonal implications of a Buddhist meditation technique. *Psychotherapy: Theory, Research, Practice, Training, 27*(1), 19–29.

Szasz, T. (2004). *Words to the wise*. New Brunswick, NJ: Transaction.

Tacon, A. M., McComb, J., Caldera, Y., & Randolph, P. (2003). Mindfulness meditation, anxiety reduction, and heart disease: A pilot study. *Family and Community Health, 26*(1), 25–33.

Tang, Y. Y., Lu, Q., Fan, M., Yang, Y., & Posner, M. I. (2012). Mechanisms of white matter changes induced by meditation. *Proceedings of the National Academy of Sciences of the United States of America, 109*, 10570–10574.

Tang, Y. Y., Lu, Q., Geng, X., Stein, E. A., Yang, Y., & Posner, M. I. (2010). Short-term meditation induces white matter changes in the anterior cingulate. *Proceedings of the National Academy of Sciences of the United States of America, 107*, 15649–15652.

Tang, Y. Y., Ma, Y., Fan, Y., Feng, H., Wang, J., Feng, S., et al. (2009). Central and autonomic nervous system interaction is altered by short-term meditation. *Proceedings of the National Academy of Sciences of the United States of America, 106,* 8865–8870.

Tang, Y. Y., Ma, Y., Wang, J., Fan, Y., Feng, S., Lu, Q., et al. (2007). Short-term meditation training improves attention and self-regulation. *Proceedings of the National Academy of Sciences, 104,* 17152–17156.

Tang, Y. Y., & Posner, M. I. (2010). Attention training and attention state training. *Trends in Cognitive Sciences, 13*(5), 222–227.

Taylor, D. J., & Roane, B. M. (2010). Treatment of insomnia in adults and children: A practice-friendly review of research. *Journal of Clinical Psychology, 66*(11), 1137–1147.

Taylor, V.A., Daneault, V., Grant, J., Scavone, G., Breton, E., Roffe-Vidal, S., et al. (2013). Impact of meditation training on the default mode network during a restful state. *Social Cognitive and Affective Neuroscience, 8*(1), 1–3.

Taylor, V. A., Grant, J., Daneault, V., Scavone, G., Breton, E., Roffe-Vidal, S., et al. (2011). Impact of mindfulness on the neural responses to emotional pictures in experienced and beginner meditators. *NeuroImage, 57*(4), 1524–1533.

Teasdale, J. D., Segal, Z. V., & Williams, J. M. G. (2003). Mindfulness and problem formulation. *Clinical Psychology: Science and Practice, 10,* 157–160.

Teasdale, J. D., Segal, Z. V., Williams, J. M. G., Ridgeway, V. A., Soulsby, J. M., & Lau, M. A. (2000). Prevention of relapse/recurrence in major depression by mindfulness-based cognitive therapy. *Journal of Consulting and Clinical Psychology, 68,* 615–623.

Thomas, L. (1995). *The lives of a cell: Notes of a biology watcher.* New York: Penguin.

Thompson, B. L., & Waltz, J. (2007). Everyday mindfulness and mindfulness meditation: Overlapping constructs or not? *Personality and Individual Differences, 43,* 1875–1885.

Thompson, M., & McCracken, L. M. (2011). Acceptance and related processes in adjustment to chronic pain. *Current Pain and Headache Reports, 15*(2), 144–151.

Thompson, N., & Walsh, M. (2010). The existential basis of trauma. *Journal of Social Work Practice: Psychotherapeutic Approaches in Health, Welfare and the Community, 24,* 377–389.

Thomson, R. (2000). Zazen and psychotherapeutic presence. *American Journal of Psychotherapy, 54*(4), 531–548.

Thoreau, H. (2012). *Walden, or life in the woods.* CreateSpace.com: CreateSpace Independent Publishing Platform. (Original work published 1854)

Tirch, D. (2011). *The compassionate mind guide to overcoming anxiety.* London, UK: Constable.

Tonelli, M. E., & Wachholtz, A. B. (2012). Meditation-based treatement yielding immediate relief of meditation-naïve migraineurs. *Pain Management Nursing, 49*(9), 1155–1164.

Treanor, M. (2011). The potential impact of mindfulness on exposure and extinction learning in anxiety disorders. *Clinical Psychology Review, 31,* 617–625.

Treat, T. A., Kruschke, J. K., Viken, R. J., & McFall, R. M. (2011). Application of associative learning paradigms to clinically relevant individual differences in cognitive processing. In T. R. Schachtman & S. Reilly (Eds.), *Associative learning and conditioning theory: Human and non-human applications* (pp. 376–398). New York: Oxford University Press

Tremlow, S. (2001). Training psychotherapists in attributes of mind from Zen and psychoanalytic perspectives, Part II: Attention, here and now, nonattachment, and compassion. *American Journal of Psychotherapy, 55*(1), 22–39.

Tronick, E. (1989). Emotions and emotional communication in infants. *American Psychologist, 44*(2), 112–119.

Tronick, E. (2007). *The neurobehavioral and social–emotional development of infants and children.* New York: Norton.

Trungpa, C. (1984). *Shambhala: The sacred path of the warrior.* Boston: Shambhala.

Tryon, G. S., & Winograd, G. (2011). Goal consensus and collaboration. In J. C. Norcross (Ed.), *Psychotherapy relationships that work* (2nd ed.). New York: Oxford University Press.

Tugrade, M. M., & Frederickson, B.L. (2012). Resilient individuals use positive emotions to bounce back from negative emotional experiences. *Journal of Personality and Social Psychology, 86*(2), 320–333.

Tullberg, T., Grane, P., & Isacson, J. (1994). Gadolinium-enhanced magnetic resonance imaging of 36 patients one year after lumbar disc resection. *Spine, 19*(2), 176–182.

Twohig, M. P., Hayes, S. C., Plumb, J. C., Pruitt, L. D., Collins, A. B., Hazlett-Stevens, H., et al. (2010). A randomized clinical trial of acceptance and commitment therapy versus progressive relaxation training for obsessive–compulsive disorder. *Journal of Consulting and Clinical Psychology, 78*, 705–716.

Unno, M. (2006). *Buddhism and psychotherapy across cultures: Essays on theories and practices.* Somerville, MA: Wisdom.

Valentine, E., & Sweet, P. (1999) Meditation and attention: A comparison of the effects of concentrative and mindfulness meditation on sustained attention. *Mental Health, Religion, and Culture, 2*(1), 59–70.

Van Dam, T., Sheppard, S., Forsyth, J., & Earleywine, M. (2011). Self-compassion is a better predictor than mindfulness of symptom severity and quality of life in mixed anxiety and depression. *Journal of Anxiety Disorders, 25*, 123–130.

van den Hurk, P., Giommi, F., Gielen, S., Speckens, A., & Barendregt, H. (2010). Greater efficiency in attentional processing related to mindfulness meditation. *Quarterly Journal of Experimental Psychology B (Colchester), 63*, 1168–1180.

van der Kolk, B. A., Pelcovitz, D., Roth, S., Mandel, F. S., McFarlane, A., & Herman, J. L. (1996). Dissociation, somatization, and affect dysregulation: The complexity of adaptation of trauma. *American Journal of Psychiatry, 153*(Suppl.), 83–93.

van der Oord, S., Bögels, S., & Pejnenburg, D. (2012). The effectiveness of mindfulness training for children with ADHD and mindful parenting for their parents. *Journal of Child and Families Studies, 21*(1), 139–147.

Veehof, M. M., Oskam, M. J., Schreurs, K. M., & Bohlmeijer, E. T. (2011). Acceptance-based interventions for the treatment of chronic pain: A systematic review and meta-analysis. *Pain, 152*(3), 533–542.

Vestergaard-Poulsen, P., van Beek, M., Skewes, J., Bjarkam, C. R., Stubberup, M., Bertelsen, J., et al. (2009). Long-term meditation is associated with increased gray matter density in the brain stem. *NeuroReport, 20*(2), 170–174.

Vianello, M., Galliani, E. M., & Haidt, J. (2010). Elevation at work: The effects of leaders' moral excellence. *Journal of Positive Psychology, 5*(5), 390–441.

Vinca, M., & Hayes, J. (2007, June). *Therapist mindfulness as predictive of empathy, presence, and session depth.* Paper presented at the annual meeting of the Society for Psychotherapy Research, Madison, WI.

Vlaeyen, J. W., & Linton, S. J. (2000). Fear-avoidance and its consequences in chronic musculoskeletal pain: A state of the art. *Pain, 85*(3), 317–332.

Volinn, E. (1997). The epidemiology of low back pain in the rest of the world. A review of surveys in low middle income countries. *Spine, 22*, 1747–1754.

Vøllestad, J., Nielsen, M., & Nielsen, G. (2011). Mindfulness- and acceptance-based interventions for anxiety disorders: A systematic review and meta-analysis. *British Journal of Clinical Psychology, 51*(3), 239–260.

Vujanovic, A. A., Niles, B. L., Pietrefesa, A., Schmertz, S. K., & Potter, C. M. (2011). Mindfulness in the treatment of posttraumatic stress disorder among military veterans. *Professional Psychology, 42*, 24–31.

Waddell, G., Newton, M., Henderson, I., & Somerville, D. (1993) A fearavoidance beliefs questionnaire (FABQ) and the role of fearavoidance beliefs in chronic low back pain and disability. *Pain, 52*(2), 157–168.

Waddington, L. (2002). The therapy relationship in cognitive therapy: A review. *Behavioural and Cognitive Psychotherapy, 30*, 179–191.

Wagner, A. W., & Linehan, M. M. (2006). Applications of dialectical behavior therapy to posttraumatic stress disorder and related problems. In V. M. Follette & J. I. Ruzek (Eds.), *Cognitive-behavioral therapies for trauma* (2nd ed., pp. 117–145). New York: Guilford Press.

Wallace, B. A. (2007). *Contemplative science.* New York: Columbia University Press.

Wallace, B. A. (2012, Fall). Popping pills for depression: A Buddhist view. *Inquiring Mind, 29.* Retrieved from *www.inquiringmind.com/Articles/PoppingPills.html.*

Wallin, D. (2007). *Attachment in psychotherapy.* New York: Guilford Press.

Walser, R., & Westrup, D. (2007). *Acceptance and commitment therapy for the treatment of post-traumatic stress disorder and trauma-related problems: A practitioner's guide to using mindfulness and acceptance strategies.* Oakland, CA: New Harbinger.

Walsh, R., & Shapiro, S. (2006). The meeting of meditative disciplines and Western psychology: A mutually enriching dialogue. *American Psychologist, 61*(3), 227–239.

Wampold, B. (2001). *The great psychotherapy debate: Models, methods, and findings.* Hillsdale, NJ: Erlbaum.

Wampold, B. (2012). *The basics of psychotherapy: An introduction to theory and practice.* Washington, DC: American Psychological Association.

Wampold, B., Imel, Z., & Miller, S. (2009). Barriers to the dissemination of empirically supported treatments: Matching messages to the evidence. *The Behavioral Therapist, 32,* 144–155.

Wang, P., & Gao, F. (2010). Mindful communication to address burnout, empathy, and attitudes. *Journal of the American Medical Association, 303*(4), 330–331.

Warkentin, J. (1972). The paradox of being alive and intimate. In A. Burton (Ed.), *Twelve therapists.* San Francisco: Jossey-Bass.

Warnecke, E., Quinn, S., Ogden, K., Towle, N., & Nelson, M. (2011). A randomised controlled trial of the effects of mindfulness practice on medical student stress levels. *Medical Education, 45*(4), 381–388.

Wells, A. (1999). A metacognitive model and therapy for generalized anxiety disorder. *Clinical Psychology and Psychotherapy, 6,* 86–95.

Welwood, J. (2000). *Toward a psychology of awakening.* Boston: Shambhala.

West, W. (2002). Some ethical dilemmas in counseling and counseling research. *British Journal of Guidance and Counseling, 30,* 261–268.

Westen, D. (1999). *Psychology: Mind, brain and culture* (2nd ed.). New York: Wiley.

Wilkinson, M. (2010). *Changing minds in therapy: Emotion, attachment, trauma, and neurobiology.* New York: Norton.

Willard, C. (2010). *Child's mind: Mindfulness practices to help our children be more focused, calm, and relaxed.* Berleley, CA: Parallax Press.

Williams, J. M. G., & Kabat-Zinn, J. (2011). Mindfulness: Diverse perspectives on its meaning, origins, and multiple applications at the intersection of science and dharma. *Contemporary Buddhism, 12*(1), 1–18.

Williams, J. M. G., & Swales, M. (2004). The use of mindfulness-based approaches for suicidal patients. *Archives of Suicide Research, 8,* 315–329.

Williams, M., Teasdale, J., Segal, Z., & Kabat-Zinn, J. (2007). *The mindful way through depression: Freeing yourself from chronic unhappiness.* New York: Guilford Press.

Wilson, K. G., & Dufrene, T. (2011). *Mindfulness for two: An acceptance and commitment therapy approach to mindfulness in psychotherapy.* Oakland, CA: New Harbinger.

Wilson, K. G., & Murrell, A. R. (2004). Values work in acceptance and commitment therapy. In S. C. Hayes, V. M . Follette, & M. M. Linehan (Eds.), *Mindfulness and acceptance: Expanding the cognitive-behavioral tradition* (pp. 120–151). New York: Guilford Press.

Winnicott, D. W. (1965). *The maturational processes and the facilitating environment: Studies in the theory of emotional development.* London, UK: Hogarth Press.

Winnicott, D. W. (1971). *Playing and reality.* New York: Basic Books.

Witkiewitz, K., & Bowen, S. (2010). Depression, craving, and substance use following a randomized trial of mindfulness-based relapse prevention. *Journal of Consulting and Clinical Psychology, 78*(3), 362–374.

Witkiewitz, K., Bowen, S., Douglas, H., & Hsu, S. (2013). Mindfulness-based relapse prevention for substance craving. *Addictive Behaviors, 38*(2), 1563–1571.

Wolever, R., Bobinet, K., McCabe, K., Mackenzie, E., Fekete, E., Kusnick, C., et al. (2012). Effective and viable mind–body stress reduction in the workplace: A randomized, controlled trial. *Journal of Occupational Health Psychology, 17*(2), 246–258.

Wong, S. Y., Chan, F. W., Wong, R. L., Chu, M. C., Kitty Lam, Y. Y., Mercer, S. W., et al. (2011). Comparing the effectiveness of mindfulness-based stress reduction and multidisciplinary intervention programs for chronic pain: A randomized comparative trial. *Clinical Journal of Pain, 27*(8), 724–734.

Wright, I., Rabe-Hesketh, S., Woodruff, P., David, A., Murray, R., & Bullmore, E. (2000). Meta-analysis of regional brain volumes in schizophrenia. *American Journal of Psychiatry, 157*(1), 16–25.

Yaari, A., Eisenberg, E., Adler, R., & Birkhan, J. (1999). Chronic pain in Holocaust survivors. *Journal of Pain and Symptom Management, 17*(3), 181–187.

Yehuda, R. (Ed.). (1998). *Psychological trauma.* Washington, DC: American Psychiatric Publishing.

Yoga for anxiety and depression. (2009). *Harvard Health Publications.* Retrieved May 9, 2011, from *www.health.harvard.edu/newsletters/Harvard_Mental_Health_Letter/2009/April/Yoga-for-anxiety-and-depression.*

Yontef, G. (1993). *Awareness, dialogue, and process: Essays on Gestalt therapy.* Highland, NY: Gestalt Journal Press.

Yook, K., Lee, S. H., Ryu, M., Kim, K. H., Choi, T. K., Suh, S. Y., et al. (2008). Usefulness of mindfulness-based cognitive therapy for treating insomnia in patients with anxiety disorders: A pilot study. *Journal of Nervous and Mental Disease, 196*(6), 501–503.

Zangi, H. A., Mowinckel, P., Finset, A., Eriksson, L. R., Hoystad, T. O., Lunde, A. K., et al. (2012). A mindfulness-based group intervention to reduce psychological distress and fatigue in patients with inflammatory rheumatic joint diseases: A randomised controlled trial. *Annals of the Rheumatic Diseases, 71*(6) 911–917.

Zeidan, F., Gordon, N. S., Merchant, J., & Goolkasian, P. (2010). The effects of brief mindfulness meditation training on experimentally induced pain. *Journal of Pain, 11*(3), 199–209.

Zernicke, K., Campbell, T., Blustein, P., Fung, T., Johnson, J., Bacon, S., et al. (in press). Mindfulness-based stress reduction for the treatment of irritable bowel syndrome symptoms: A randomized wait-list controlled trial. *International Journal of Behavioral Medicine.*

Zetzel, E. (1970). *The capacity for emotional growth.* New York: International Universities Press.

Index

Page numbers followed by *f* indicate figure, *t* indicate table.